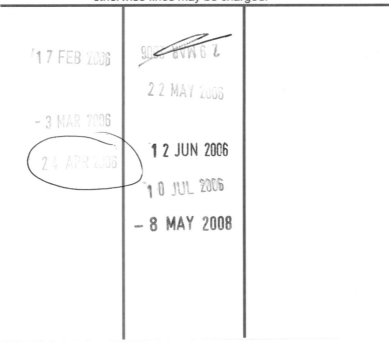

Clinical Oral Physiology

Clinical Oral Physiology

EDITED BY:

Timothy S. Miles
Birgitte Nauntofte
Peter Svensson

Quintessence Publishing Co. Ltd

Copenhagen, London, Berlin, Chicago, Paris, Milan, Barcelona,
Istanbul, São Paulo, Tokyo, New Dehli, Moscow, Prague, Warsaw

British Library Cataloguing in Publication Data
Clinical oral physiology
1. Mouth – Physiology 2. Mouth – Pathophysiology 3. Dentistry
I. Miles, Timothy S. II. Nauntofte, Birgitte III. Svensson, Peter

ISBN 1-85097-091-2

Cover design by Maria Elskær

Printed in Denmark by P. J. Schmidt Grafisk A/S

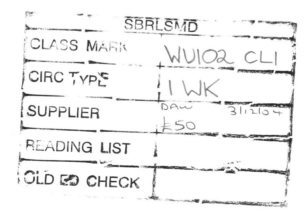

CONTRIBUTORS

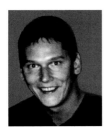

Allan Bardow
Assistant Professor, DDS, PhD
Faculty of Health Sciences
University of Copenhagen
Nørre Alle 20
DK-2200 Copenhagen N
Denmark
ab@odont.ku.dk

Graduated as a dentist from the University of Copenhagen in 1994, Obtained PhD degree in 2001. Assistant Professor at the Department of Oral Medicine, Clinical Oral Physiology, Oral Pathology and Anatomy, University of Copenhagen since 2001.

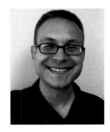

Tim Bressmann
Assistant Professor, PhD
Graduate Department of
Speech-Language Pathology
University of Toronto
500 University Avenue
Toronto ON M5G 1V7
tim.bressmann@utoronto.ca

Dr. Tim Bressmann studied Linguistics at the universities of Freiburg, Dublin and Bielefeld. He obtained his PhD from the University of Munich and is currently Assistant Professor in the Graduate Department of Speech-Language Pathology at the University of Toronto. His main research interests concern the structurally related speech disorders in craniofacial syndromes as well as head and neck cancer.

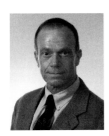

Greg Essick
Professor, DDS, PhD
Department of Prosthodontics
School of Dentistry
University of North Carolina
Chapel Hill
NC 27599 7450
USA
greg_essick@dentistry.unc.edu

Dr. Greg Essick is Professor, Department of Prosthodontics and Curriculum in Neurobiology at the University of North Carolina at Chapel Hill, USA. He received a BS degree in mathematics, a DDS degree, and a PhD degree in physiology at the university, and completed postdoctoral training at the Salk Institute, La Jolla, CA, USA, Dr. Essick teaches neuro- and orofacial physiology and supervises dental students in the clinic. He researches mechanisms underlying tactile perception and pain in healthy individuals and patients with sensory disorders.

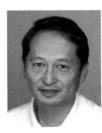

James W. Hu
Professor, PhD
Faculty of Dentistry
University of Toronto
124 Edward Street
Toronto, Ontario M5G 1G6
Canada
james.hu@utoronto.ca

James W. Hu is a professor of Dentistry at the University of Toronto. Trained in the National Institute of Dental Research as a neurophysiologist, specialized in pain research in late 70s and joined the University of Toronto since 1977. Published more than 95 papers or chapters related to craniofacial pain.

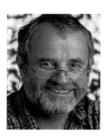

Timothy S. Miles
Professor, BDS, PhD, DSc,
FRACDS
Discipline of Physiology
School of Molecular and
Biomedical Science
University of Adelaide
Adelaide SA 5005
Australia
timothy-miles@adelaide.edu.au

Timothy Miles graduated in Dentistry at the University of Adelaide, Australia in 1969. After a short period of clinical practice, he completed a PhD in Physiology at the University of Western Ontario in Canada, writing his dissertation on the subject of trigeminal inputs to the cerebellum. He has subsequently held academic appointments at the University of Zürich, the University of Adelaide, the University of Montreal, Fribourg University, the University of British Columbia, Oxford University, the Institute for Neurology, London, and the University of Aalborg, Denmark. He currently holds the first personal Chair in Physiology at the University of Adelaide. He is the author of more than 120 peer-reviewed scientific papers in international journals. These widely-cited papers have established the mechanisms underlying the reflex and cortical control of the human masticatory system.

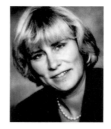

Birgitte Nauntofte
Professor, DDS, PhD, dr.odont
Faculty of Health Sciences
University of Copenhagen
Nørre Alle 20
DK-2200 Copenhagen N
Denmark
bn@odont.ku.dk

Graduated as dentist from the Royal Dental College in Copenhagen in 1982. Obtained PhD degree in 1985 and dr. odont degree in 1993. Professor in Clinical Oral Physiology at the Department of Oral Medicine, Clinical Oral Physiology, Oral Pathology and Anatomy, University of Copenhagen since 2000.

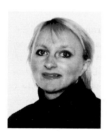

Anne Marie Lynge Pedersen
Associate Professor, DDS, PhD
Faculty of Health Sciences
University of Copenhagen
Nørre Alle 20
DK-2200 Copenhagen
Denmark
amp@odont.ku.dk

Graduated as a dentist from the Royal Dental College in Copenhagen in 1992, Obtained PhD degree in 1997. Associate Professor at the Department of Oral Medicine, Clinical Oral Physiology, Oral Pathology and Anatomy, University of Copenhagen since 2003.

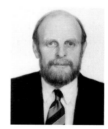

Dr. Barry J. Sessle
FRSC Professor, and Canada
Research Chair, BDS, MDS,
BSc, PhD, DSc (hc)
Faculty of Dentistry University
of Toronto
124 Edward Street Toronto
Ontario M5G 1G6
Canada
barry.sessle@utoronto.ca

Dr. Barry J. Sessle is Professor and Canada Research Chair, Faculty of Dentistry, University of Toronto. He is a Fellow of the Royal Society of Canada, Editor-in-Chief of the Journal of Orofacial Pain, and Past-President of the International Association for Dental Research, and the International Association for the Study of Pain. He has co-authored 9 books and published 300 articles.

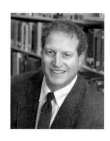

Jonathan A. Ship
Professor, Director, Bluestone Center for
Clinical Research, DMD
Department of Oral
Medicine, DMD
New York University College
of Dentistry
421 First Avenue, 2nd Floor
New York, NY 10010-4086
USA
jonathan.ship@nyu.edu

Dr. Jonathan A. Ship, is a Professor of Oral Medicine and Director of the Bluestone Center for Clinical Research at the New York University College of Dentistry, New York, NY. He is a Diplomate of the American Board of Oral Medicine, a Fellow of the Gerontological Society of America, and a Fellow of the Royal College of Surgeons (Edinburgh).

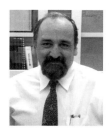

Andrew I. Spielman
Professor, Associate Dean for
Academic Affairs DMD, PhD
New York University College of
Dentistry
345E 24th Street
USA
andrew.spielman@nyu.edu

Andrew I. Spielman, is a Professor of Basic Science at NYU College of Dentistry in New York City. Dr. Spielman holds a dental degree, a certificate in Maxillo-facial Surgery, MS and PhD degrees in Oral Biology/Biochemistry. Dr. Spielman has published 60 peer-reviewed articles, chapters, and co-edited a textbook on taste and smell.

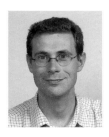

Peter Svensson
Professor, DDS, PhD, dr.odont
Dental School
University of Aarhus
Vennelyst Boulevard
DK-8000 Aarhus C
Denmark
psvensson@odont.au.dk

Date of Birth: May 21, 1963. Graduated from the Dental School, University of Aarhus 1987 (DDS). Earned his PhD degree in 1993 and Doctor of Odontology in 2000. In 2001 promoted to full professor and chairman of Department of Clinical Oral Physiology. Appointed clinical consultant at Department of Oral Maxillofacial Surgery, Aarhus University Hospital in 2002.

The research has focused on orofacial pain and temporomandibular disorders with more than 145 contributions to peer-reviewed journals and book chapters. Presented more than 80 lectures, talks and courses on orofacial pain mechanisms and TMD problems around the world. Awarded the Codan Young Investigator Research Prize in 1995, the Strathmann Research Award in 1998 and the Zendium-Hoogendoorn Award in 2000. Reviewer and editorial board member of several international dental and neuroscience journals. Editor-in-Chief of Journal of Oral Rehabilitation.

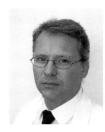

Mats Trulsson
Associate Professor, DDS, PhD
Department of Prosthetic
Dentistry
Institute of Odontology
Karolinska Institute
S-141 04 Huddinge, Sweden
mats.trulsson@ofa.ki.se

Dr. Mats Trulsson is an Associate Professor at the Department of Prosthetic Dentistry, Karolinska Institute, Stockholm, Sweden. He received his basic training in dentistry (DDS) and physiology (PhD) at Umeå University. After his relocation to the Karolinska Institute (2000) he holds a position as a Senior Research Fellow at the Swedish Medical Research Council and also continues to practise part-time as a prosthodontist. Dr Trulsson and his colleagues are particularly renowned for their work in characterising the properties of mechanoreceptors in the orofacial area, including the periodontal mechanoreceptors.

TABLE OF CONTENTS

CHAPTER 6

CHAPTER 7

CHAPTER 10

CHAPTER 11

CHAPTER 12

INDEX

Introduction

Timothy S. Miles
Birgitte Nauntofte
Peter Svensson

Dentistry is an area of biomedical science that is changing constantly and rapidly in both the biological and the technological domains. The emphasis in dental practice has expanded dramatically from its traditional primary focus on the care of the teeth to include the care of the soft and hard tissues that support the dentition, and the many other systems that are important for the care of oral environment in health and disease. These advances in Dentistry have arisen from an ever-expanding body of research in the relevant basic and applied sciences. The challenge for dentists today is to remain abreast of these changes and to incorporate them into their professional practice. This can happen only when they have a clear understanding of the underlying biosciences.

The development of prosthetic implants to replace missing teeth is an excellent example of how an understanding of physiology underpins dental research and modern clinical practice. This technology has now entered the mainstream of dentistry, and is giving hitherto unattainable levels of comfort and function to large numbers of patients. The scientific development of oral implants arose from a profound understanding of bone physiology. A sound physiological knowledge is equally important to practitioners who are involved with the provision of implants. It is interesting to note that in many ways, dentistry led medicine in this field, with many of the advances in this field subsequently being adopted in orthopaedic surgery for bony implants in the limbs.

Another area in which dental scientists have made major contributions is in the understanding of pain. A quick scan of any major scientific journal devoted to the study of pain will reveal the disproportionately large number of contributions that relate to orofacial pain.

Conventional physiology textbooks are helpful in describing general physiological issues, but many have a strong emphasis on the needs of medical, nursing or science students. Such books provide a good basis for an understanding of the major physiological systems that is required for Dentistry students. However, the special needs of Dentistry students for specialised information on how various physiological mechanisms are relevant to the orofacial area, or to the practice of Dentistry, are largely unacknowledged.

The present volume aims to address this gap both by emphasising the general physiological mechanisms that are important in Dentistry, and by summarising the current understanding of specific orofacial mechanisms that represent vital knowledge to the practising dentist. We envisage that this

15

book will be read to supplement the information that is available in more general physiological textbooks.

The book is focused on the topic "Clinical Oral Physiology" which is the part of Dentistry linking physiological and pathophysiological knowledge to a variety of frequently encountered problems in dental practice. As always, an understanding of disturbances affecting functions such as saliva formation, taste, chewing, swallowing, and speech and sensation (including pain) is gained only through understanding how these systems function normally.

One of the major developments in dental education is the move towards problem-based and/or cased-based curricula. If anything, this has increased the importance of having relevant basic science resources for Dentistry students to access when considering their problems and cases, to ensure that these vital concepts necessary to understanding clinical issues are presented in an integrated and clinically-relevant fashion.

As Editors of this volume, we are delighted that leading research workers across the whole scope spectrum of fields relevant to Dentistry agreed to write chapters in this book. These chapters present the current understanding in these fields in an easy-to-read format. Because this book is aimed particularly at the understanding of clinical oral physiological mechanisms, we have, where possible, steered away from the related fields of Anatomy and Biochemistry, except when some discussion of these areas was necessary. Thus, this textbook provides a comprehensive overview of the underlying basic physiological mechanisms and their clinical implications. The book targets dental undergraduate and postgraduate students as well as practising clinicians who want to remain abreast of the latest scientific thinking on these topics.

In addition to the authors, a number of other people made valuable contributions to this book. We wish in particular to acknowledge the invaluable assistance of expert colleagues who gave freely of their time to comment on drafts of various chapters of this book. These include, in alphabetical order:

Dr Allan Bardow, University of Copenhagen
Dr Mark Bartold, The University of Adelaide
Dr Mina Borromeo, The University of Melbourne
Professor Alan Bretag, University of South Australia
Dr Svend Kirkeby, University of Copenhagen
Professor Michael Nordstrom, The University of Adelaide
Dr Guiseppe Posterino, The University of Adelaide
Dr Peter O'Loughlin, The Hanson Centre, Adelaide
Dr Catriona Steele, University of Toronto

We also greatly acknowledge the designer of the cover, Mrs. Maria Elskær, Copenhagen.

Finally, we acknowledge the assistance of our ever-patient publisher, Dr. Lone Schou and Jens Wejsmark, who has brought this whole enterprise together into its final published form.

Timothy S. Miles, BDS, PhD, DSc, FRACDS.
Birgitte Nauntofte, DDS, PhD, dr.odont.
Peter Svensson, DDS, PhD, dr.odont.

CHAPTER 1

Saliva

Allan Bardow, Anne Marie Lynge Pedersen and Birgitte Nauntofte

---

Goals:
- To describe the functions of saliva and relate these functions to its specific constituents.
- To describe the mechanisms underlying the formation of saliva and the factors that influence saliva flow rate and composition under normal and pathophysiological conditions.
- To describe the role of saliva for oral clearance and pH regulation.
- To describe the role of saliva in pellicle formation and tooth solubility.
- To discuss the identification of patients with salivary dysfunction, the measurement of saliva production and oral dryness, and the management of dry mouth.

Key words:
Salivary glands; salivary reflexes; saliva formation; saliva electrolytes and proteins; buffer capacity; oral clearance; hyposalivation and oral sequelae; xerostomia; management of dry mouth.

▦ Introduction

Impaired saliva secretion and changes in the saliva composition whether temporary or permanent are common conditions. On a population basis it is assumed that at least 10% of the adults suffer from dryness of the mouth. However, the prevalence of oral dryness increases with age due to a higher frequency of systemic diseases and intake of medicines amongst the elderly. Thus, about 30% of the population aged 65 years and above suffers from oral dryness. Impaired saliva secretion (hyposalivation) increases the risk of oral diseases like dental caries and oral candidal infection. In addition, the sensation of oral dryness (xerostomia) may compromise the patient's health-related quality of life. Assessment of saliva flow and its composition as well as dry mouth symptoms combined with a thorough medical and oral history taking provide valuable clues for the dentist in the process of differential diagnosis. Nevertheless, understanding the pathology behind salivary gland dysfunctions and the abnormal saliva composition requires detailed insight into both the normal physiology and the pathophysiology of the salivary glands.

▦ Functions of saliva

Saliva protects the teeth and the oro-oesophageal mucosa through a number of mechanisms. Besides maintenance of the integrity of these tissues, saliva also has multiple functions in relation to digestion in the upper

17

gastrointestinal tract. It facilitates food intake by dissolving food taste-substances, it clears and dilutes food detritus and bacterial matter, rinses the mouth, lubricates oral soft tissues, and facilitates mastication, swallowing and speech. As shown in Table 1 and Figure 10, some of these important functions relates to the fluid characteristics and others to specific components of the saliva. Clearly, therefore, changes that compromise salivary gland function are likely to affect oral function and health.

The salivary glands

The mixed fluid in the mouth is called whole saliva. It is derived predominantly from three pairs of major salivary glands (Figure 1) that account for about 90% of the total fluid secretion, and from the minor salivary glands in the oral mucosa that contribute somewhat less than 10% of the total volume. In addition, whole saliva also contains gingival crevicular fluid (depending upon the periodontal status of the patient), microorganisms from dental plaque, and food debris. Saliva is a hypotonic fluid relative to plasma and it is composed of more than 99% water and less than 1% of dry matter such as proteins and salts. The normal daily production of saliva ranges between 0.5–1.5 litre.

In the resting state, about two-thirds of the volume of whole saliva is produced by the submandibular glands. However, when salivary glands are stimulated, the parotids can account for at least half of the whole saliva volume in the mouth. Only a small percentage of unstimulated or stimulated whole saliva comes from the sublingual glands. Although the minor glands, which are distributed in groups throughout the oral mucosa,

Table 1. Principal functions of saliva related to fluid characteristics and specific components.

Functions	Salivary fluid characteristics and specific components
Protection	
Mechanical cleansing of the mouth	Water
Clearance of food/microorganisms	Water
Lubrication of oral surfaces	Water, mucins, proline-rich glycoproteins
Mucosal intergrity and coating	Water, mucins, electrolytes, epidermal growth factor, nerve growth factor
Tooth mineralisation	Cystatins, histatins, proline-rich proteins, statherins Ca^{2+}, and phosphate
Buffering	Bicarbonate, phosphate and protein
Antimicrobial activity	Anti-bacterial: amylases, cystatins, histatins, mucins, lactoperoxidase, lysozyme, lactoferrin, calprotectin, immunoglobulins, chromogranin A, von Ebner glands protein, secretory leukocyte proteinase inhibitor Anti-fungal: histatins, immunoglobulins, chromogranin A Anti-viral: cystatins, mucins, immunoglobulins, secretory leukocyte proteinase inhibitor
Digestion and speech	
Formation of bolus	Water, mucins
Mastication and swallowing	Water, mucins
Initial digestion	Water, mucins, amylases, lipases, ribonucleases, proteases
Taste	Water, gustin, Zn^{2+}
Speech	Water, mucins

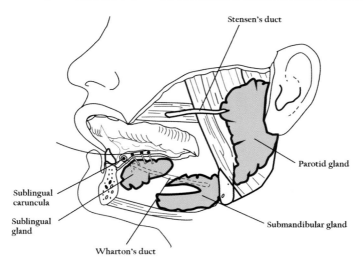

● **Figure 1.** *The salivary glands.*
Human major salivary glands: the parotid, the submandibular, and the sublingual gland. The parotid duct (Stensen's duct) is about 5 cm long and opens into the mouth in the buccal mucosa opposite the second maxillary molar. The saliva from the submandibular and sublingual glands enters the mouth mostly through the around 5 cm long submandibular duct (Wharton's duct), which ends on the sublingual caruncula behind the mandibulary incisors. But the sublingual gland also secretes through several small ducts along the sublingual fold in the floor of the mouth lateral to the side of the tongue.

make only a small contribution to the total saliva volume, they play an important role in the lubrication of the mucosa since they secrete a large fraction of the salivary proteins.

Some of the salivary glands are purely serous (like the parotids), others are mucous (like the minor palatine glands), and others are mixed gland types (submandibular, sub-

Table 2. Morphological and biochemical characteristics of the salivary glands.

Salivary gland	Acinar cell type	Fluid characteristics	Innervation*
The major salivary glands			
Parotid gland	Serous	watery, amylase-rich	IX
Submandibular gland	Mixed, mainly mucous	viscous, mucin-rich	VII
Sublingual gland	Mixed, mainly mucous	viscous, mucin-rich	VII
The minor salivary glands			
Palatinal	Mucous	mucin rich	VII
Buccal	Seromucous	mucin rich	VII
Labial	Seromucous	mucin rich	VII
Lingual (von Ebner's glands)	Serous	watery, lipase-rich fluid	IX
Retromolar	Mainly mucous	mucin rich	VII/IX

*Parasympathetic nerve supply. The sympathetic nerve supply is derived from the superior cervical ganglion.

lingual and minor buccal glands). Table 2 summarizes the acinar characteristics of the salivary gland types, their innervation and their fluid characteristics.

In general, the acinar cells ("secretory end-pieces") comprise about 80% of the gland mass. Primary saliva is formed in this region of the gland. The saliva then moves into the

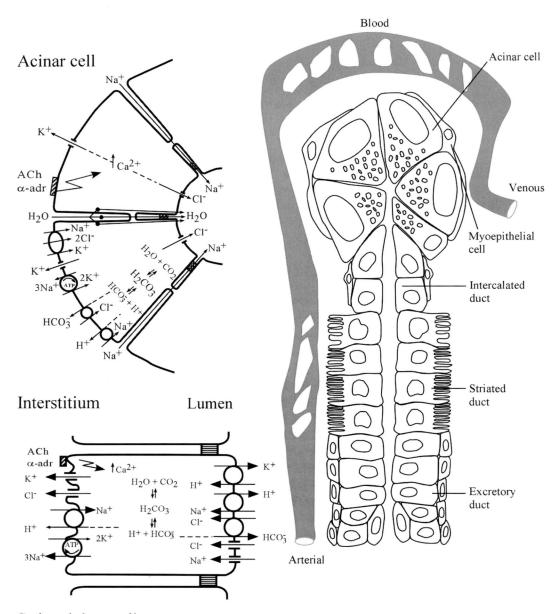

duct system where it continuously undergoes modification until it is secreted into the mouth.

The length and the diameter of the ducts vary depending on the gland type. The duct system of the human parotid and submandibular glands is branched and contains intercalated, striated and excretory duct segments with the striated ducts making up the bulk of the duct system (Figure 2). In the parotid and submandibular glands, each segment of the duct system is well developed.

Figure 2. *Intracellular ion and water transport in different gland segments.*
Salivary glands consist of many thousands of secretory units comprising acini (arrangement of acinar cells) and an intercalated and a striated duct segment. A large number of such secretory units converge into a main excretory duct that drains the saliva into the mouth. **To the right:** Although the duct system is branched thereby serving several secretory units, this illustration is a simplified schematic drawing of a major gland and its blood supply. The blood flows in opposite direction to the saliva flow. To increase salivary secretion upon autonomic stimulation, vasodilatation and increased blood flow takes place. **To the left:** Main membrane transport mechanisms of the acinar and striated duct cells. In both cell types, the specific neurotransmitters bind to their specific receptor complexes and, via a number of intracellular biochemical events, the outcome is activation of plasma membrane ion transporters leading to the formation of saliva. For simplistic reasons two acinar cells illustrate in combination the transporters that are activated in a single acinar cells. The upper acinar cell illustrates the Ca^{2+}-activated loss of K^+ and Cl^- that occurs initially on stimulation/receptor activation whereas the lower acinar cell illustrates the transporters involved in the re-establishment of the prestimulatory ion gradients across the plasma membrane. Note that the cells have two transport mechanisms, the parallel operating exchange systems for Na^+/H^+ and Cl^-/HCO_3^- as well as the $Na^+/K^+/2Cl^-$ cotransporter, that both result in cellular uptake of Na^+ and Cl^-. It should also be noted that the important mechanism involved the intracellular pH regulation is the conversion of CO_2 (arising from the metabolic turn over) and H_2O into equal amount of HCO_3^- and H^+ catalyzed by the presence of cytosolic carbonic-anhydrase.

These ducts are quite long and have relatively large diameters. Conversely, the sublingual glands as well as a number of minor glands have only sparsely distributed intercalated and striated duct segments, which may even be absent in short, small diameter ducts. Myoepithelial cells envelop the secretory end-pieces and intercalated ducts. When they contract, these cells are believed to promote the flow of primary saliva into the ducts (Figure 2).

The secretory end-piece consists of polarized acinar cells, which surround a central lumen that is connected to the intercalated ducts ("intercalated" means "placed between", and refers to the location of the ducts, which lie between the acinus and the striated duct). The nucleus and a major part of the endoplasmic reticulum (ER) are located in the basal part of each acinar cell, whereas the protein-containing granules are placed at the luminal pole. Gap junctions connect the cytoplasm of the acinar cells and allow for electrical coupling within the acini. However, there are also tight junction structures that connect the acinar cells with each other. These are selectively leaky to cations and water and serve to separate the luminal (primary saliva) and interstitial fluids. Furthermore, the acinar cell membranes are highly permeable to water.

The intercalated duct cells are believed to be the stem cells for the acinar and ductal cell types, and they also are believed to aid in primary saliva secretion. The striated ducts consist of columnar cell types with deep membrane infolding and many mitochondria in the basal surface facing the interstitium. These duct cells modify the primary saliva formed in the acinus. In contrast to the acinar cells, the membranes of duct cells have a low permeability to water, and the tight junctions connecting the duct cells have a very low permeability to both ions

and water. Nevertheless, some water reabsorption may occur in the duct cells at very
low flow rates, especially in the intralobular
ducts due to the osmotic gradient or as a
result of the influence of circulating antidi-
uretic hormone (ADH).

Finally, the intralobular ducts drain into
an extralobular excretory duct system that
carries the saliva to the main excretory duct
which is lined with stratified columnar epithelium.

Blood supply to the salivary glands

The rich blood supply of the major salivary
glands is important for saliva production
since the fluid in saliva originates from the
capillaries and the interstitial fluid. This
blood supply is organised as a portal system
with two capillary networks in series, a
dense one around the duct system and another around the secretory end-piece (Figure
2). The secretory activity of the salivary
glands is entirely under autonomic control.
The blood vessels of the salivary glands are
controlled by the sympathetic nervous system, which makes them constrict. However,
parasympathetic stimulation of the glands
can overcome this sympathetic vasoconstrictor tone and lead to vasodilatation and increased blood flow to the secreting gland.
Parasympathetic stimulation induces the
production of a number of substances which
participate in the regulation of local blood
flow and hence the secretory activity of the
gland. These substances include mediators
such as vasoactive intestinal polypeptide
(VIP) and nitric oxide (NO) that are synthesised and released by the salivary glands
and their surrounding tissues comprising
nerves, endothelium, and blood vessels. In
addition, the striated ducts release a serine
protease, kallikrein, which acts on circulating plasma proteins to induce the formation of the vasodilator bradykinin: this in

turn participates in the regulation of local
blood flow to the gland.

■ Nervous control of salivary secretion

The secretion of saliva is regulated by reflexes involving the autonomic nervous system. The reflex pathways are unilateral, since
stimulation of one side of the mouth induces
only ipsilateral salivation. The act of chewing
and the sensation of taste initiate action potentials in various sensory receptors (Figure
3). The *masticatory-salivary reflex* involves
sensory inputs mainly from mechanical receptors in the mouth. These arise predominantly from mechanoreceptors in the periodontal ligament, but other proprioceptors
in the trigeminal innervation including
muscle spindles in the masticatory muscles
and oral nociceptive stimuli may contribute.
The *gustatory-salivary reflex*, however, util-
ises sensory signals from taste-activated
chemoreceptors in the taste buds within the
lingual papillae and in the tonsillar region,
the epiglottis, the pharyngeal wall and
oesophagus: these are conducted along the
facial (VII), glossopharyngeal (IX), and
vagus (X) nerves to the salivatory nuclei in
the medulla oblongata of the brain. Here,
the signals are integrated and activate the secretomotor pathways of the reflex that consist of parasympathetic and sympathetic
autonomic nerve bundles that travel along
separate pathways to the salivary glands. The
submandibular and sublingual glands are
controlled by the superior salivatory nucleus, whereas the parotid is controlled by
the inferior salivatory nucleus.

Selective parasympathetic or sympathetic
stimulation of the salivary glands elicits secretion. But the parasympathetic fibres carried in the VII and IX nerves and the sym-

● **Figure 3.** *Regulation of secretion.*
The reflexes involved in salivary secretion. Afferents nerves carry impulses to salivary nuclei, the center of salivary secretion placed in the medulla. From here signals are directed to the efferent part of the reflex, which stands under autonomic regulation by parasympathetic and sympathetic nerves. Besides the afferents shown in this figure, other afferents arising from olfaction and stretch of the stomach can initiate salivation. Concerning the efferents, the sympathetic nerves run from the sympathetic trunk, follow the blood vessels supplying the glands, and then separately innervate the glands. The parotid gland receives parasympathetic signals from the glossopharyngeal nerve that synapses in the otic ganglion placed relatively close to the gland. The submandibular and sublingual glands receive parasympathetic signals from the facial nerve that synapse in the submandibular ganglion. Release of neurotransmitters from the postganglionic neurons of both branches of the nervous system elicits secretion of saliva.

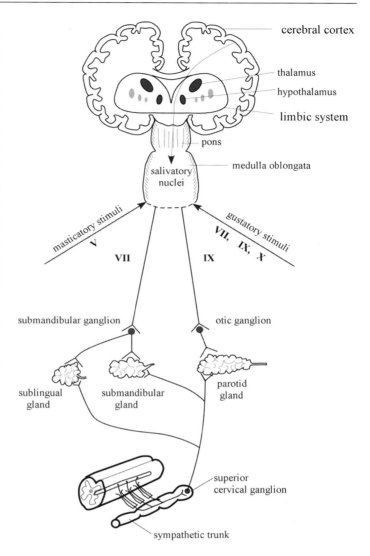

pathetic fibres following the blood vessels supplying the glands normally act in concert to produce saliva. The release of neurotransmitters from autonomic nerve endings activates specific cell surface membrane receptors on the salivary gland tissue thereby determining the flow rate and composition of saliva.

The classical neurotransmitters released from the peripheral postganglionic parasym-

pathetic and sympathetic nerve endings are acetylcholine (ACh) and noradrenaline (NA) respectively. However, other substances that are co-released such as adenosine triphosphate (ATP), substance P, VIP, neuropeptide Y also have important modulatory effects on the formation of saliva.

The saliva flow rate depends not only on the nature of the stimulus but also on its duration and intensity. Thus stimuli like strongly acidic taste, high chewing frequency and/or high bite force result in elevated saliva flow rates. Generally, the parasympathetic branch provides the main stimulus for salivation giving rise to a high flow rate of watery saliva, compared with sympathetic stimulation which leads to a lower flow rate of saliva that is much more viscous because of its high content of mucins.

The reflexes mentioned above are known as "unconditioned" reflexes. However, salivary secretion can also be initiated by "conditioned" reflexes that are programmed in higher centres in the brain (Figure 3). Thus, positive experiences with foods in the past may lead to the secretion of saliva induced by the sight or thought of food (Pavlov's classical dog experiments). Emotional state also influences the saliva flow rate. Dental students will be familiar with the experience that fear or anxiety can lead to a dry mouth due to central inhibition of the reflex pathway. Salivation may also be diminished in untreated depression. Furthermore, during sleep, saliva secretion from the major glands is normally very low.

In summary, therefore, many signals from a variety of peripheral receptors and from higher centres are being constantly integrated in the salivatory nuclei, the result of which may be either facilitation or inhibition of salivation.

Formation of saliva

According to the secretion model for formation of saliva proposed by Thaysen and colleagues more than 50 years ago, saliva is formed basically in two steps. The secretory end-piece produces primary saliva which is isotonic, having an ionic composition similar to that of plasma. This fluid is then modified in the duct system by selective re-absorption of Na^+ and Cl^- (but not water) and by a certain secretion of K^+ and HCO_3^- to yield the final saliva which is secreted into the mouth. Thus the secretion rate and thereby the volume of final saliva is determined directly by the formation rate of primary saliva by the acinar cells.

Figure 4 shows that the ionic composition of primary saliva resembles that of plasma or interstial fluid. However, the formation of primary saliva is not the result of pressure filtration of blood. Rather, it is the result of active transport of solutes by the gland tissue that arises from a dramatic, stimulation-induced increase in metabolic activity.

Stimulus-secretion coupling

The secretion of electrolytes, water and the exocytotic release of proteins from the acinar cells upon stimulation involve a multitude of biochemical signalling processes: a few important ones are illustrated in Figure 5. The key event is the rise in the free Ca^{2+} concentration ($[Ca^{2+}]$) in the acinus that is initiated by specific activation of receptors in the plasma membrane by neurotransmitters. However, the mechanism by which the various activated receptor systems induce a rise in Ca^{2+} involves different signalling routes.

ACh binds to muscarinic cholinergic receptors and the NA to α_1-adrenergic receptors in the salivary gland cell membranes: both are G protein-coupled receptors of the so-called Gq/11 type. Binding induces phospholipase C-mediated hydrolysis of the plasma membrane component phosphatidylinositol 4,5 bisphosphate (PIP_2) that forms the second messengers inositol 1,4,5 trisphosphate (IP_3) and diacylglycerol (DAG).

The water-soluble IP_3 binds to specific IP_3- receptors on the endoplasmic reticulum (ER) that induces Ca^{2+} release from this store within the cell, giving rise to an in-

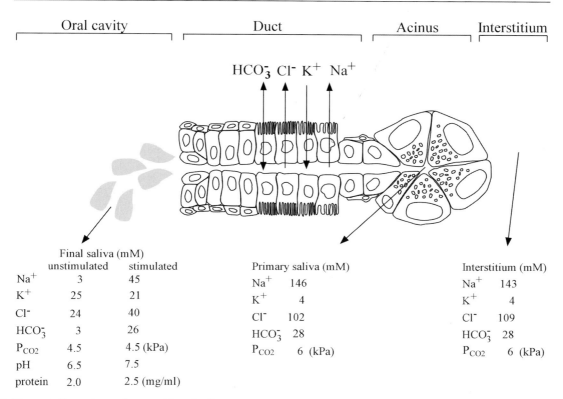

| Oral cavity | | Duct | | Acinus | Interstitium |

HCO_3^- Cl⁻ K⁺ Na⁺

	Final saliva (mM)			Primary saliva (mM)		Interstitium (mM)
	unstimulated	stimulated				
Na⁺	3	45		Na⁺	146	Na⁺	143
K⁺	25	21		K⁺	4	K⁺	4
Cl⁻	24	40		Cl⁻	102	Cl⁻	109
HCO_3^-	3	26		HCO_3^-	28	HCO_3^-	28
P_{CO2}	4.5	4.5 (kPa)		P_{CO2}	6 (kPa)	P_{CO2}	6 (kPa)
pH	6.5	7.5					
protein	2.0	2.5 (mg/ml)					

Figure 4. *Formation and composition of saliva.*
The formation of saliva occurs in two steps. Step 1: The secretory end pieces produce a primary saliva resembling plasma in ionic composition. Step 2: This fluid undergoes major changes and become hypotonic as it passes down the duct system, primarily by reaborption of Na⁺ and Cl⁻ without water. However, the ductal modification strongly depends on the secretion rate. The figure also shows typical electrolyte concentrations for unstimulated as well as stimulated whole saliva.

crease in the free intracellular $[Ca^{2+}]$ in the range from 10^{-7} M to 10^{-6} M. This pathway is particularly important for initiating electrolyte transport.

Another receptor-coupled signalling pathway that leads to an increase in the intracellular free $[Ca^{2+}]$ is the β-adrenergic activation (by NA) of a G_s-protein and adenylate cyclase, which elicits the synthesis of cyclic adenosine monophosphate (cAMP). This cAMP then activates protein kinase A, which in turn causes intracellular $[Ca^{2+}]$ to increase. The cAMP pathway has been impli-

cated in protein synthesis in the rough ER, and in exocytosis of protein-containing secretory granules across the cell membranes involving a number of small GTP binding proteins. In addition, protein synthesis also occurs as a consequence of DAG formation: this activates protein kinase C, another mediator of cellular protein synthesis and secretion. Protein secretion from the salivary gland tissues comprises a continuous so-called "constitutive exocytosis" of protein-containing vesicles that contribute to the protein secretion and is ongoing at all times.

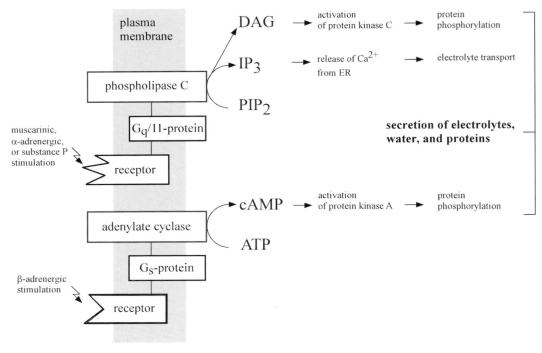

Figure 5. *Membrane receptors and cell signaling pathways.*
Binding of a variety of neurotransmitters to specific cell surface receptors in the acinar plasma membrane initiates a number of biochemical cascade reactions within the cell membranes and cytoplasm that leads to secretion of primary saliva from the secretory end piece. This schematic drawing illustrates some receptor-coupled processes generating increased cytosolic concentration of the second messengers: calcium and cyclic adenosine monophosphate (cAMP). Generally, activation of muscarinic cholinergic, α_1-adrenergic or substance P receptors leads to an increased intracellular calcium concentration resulting in electrolyte and water transport and protein synthesis and secretion whereas activation of the β-adrenergic receptor results in an increased cAMP concentration, which triggers protein synthesis and secretion. The basic signaling pathways shown in this figure are also involved in the ductal cell types where activation of transport mechanisms occur leading to modification of the primary saliva by the reaborption of some electrolytes and secretion of others as well as by protein synthesis and release.

The constitutive exocytosis can be accelerated to the regulatory exocytosis that occurs as a result of appropriate firing impulse frequency and specific receptor activation of the salivary glands. This regulated exocytotic protein secretion from the major salivary glands is controlled by the dual parasympathetic and sympathetic secretomotor innervation. However, the minor glands secrete a protein rich (mucin) secretion continuously.

Electrolyte transport by the acinar cells
The plasma membranes of the acinar cells are freely permeable to water and to lipid-soluble substances, but not to small, charged molecules such as ions. Thus electrolyte transport across the plasma membrane must occur through specific transport mechanisms such as ion channels, pumps, cotransporters and exchange systems (Figure 2). The general principle behind the formation of primary saliva is that the acinar cell re-

sponds to a receptor-activated increase in the intracellular free $[Ca^{2+}]$ by losing K^+ to the interstitium and Cl^- (and some HCO_3^-) to the lumen *via* activated Ca^{2+}-regulated K^+ and Cl^- channels in the basolateral and luminal surfaces of the cell membrane, respectively. Because of the simultaneous activation of these ion channels, the membrane potential of about -60 mV remains virtually unchanged upon secretion. The accumulation of Cl^- ions in the lumen creates a negative intracellular potential that drives interstitial Na^+ into the lumen *via* a paracellular transport route through cation-selective tight junctions to preserve electroneutrality. A transepithelial water flux, probably occurring by trans- and paracellular pathways, follows the net movement of salt into the lumen osmotically, resulting in acinar cell shrinkage (presumably by water loss *via* water channels "aquaporins") and formation of isotonic, plasma-like primary saliva.

As a result of this initial receptor-activated acinar cell loss of K^+ and Cl^- and water (cell shrinkage), the intracellular Na^+ concentration in the acinar cell increases mainly by downhill Na^+ influx *via* activation of the Na^+/H^+ exchanger and/or $Na^+/K^+/2Cl^-$ cotransporter. This elevated acinar Na^+ concentration in turn activates the central membrane element, the Na^+/K^+-pump (ATPase). This active pumping mechanism, utilizing energy in the form of ATP, then re-establishes the original, prestimulatory (unstimulated) ion gradients across the acinar plasma membrane by active uphill extrusion of Na^+ and influx of K^+. The prestimulatory acinar Cl^- concentration is re-established by uphill influx of the Cl^- ion against an electrochemical gradient *via* the Cl^-/HCO_3^- exchangers (that operate in parallel with the Na^+/H^+ exchangers) and/or *via* the $Na^+/K^+/2\ Cl^-$ cotransporter. Osmosis

causes water to follow the inward movements of ions and the cell swells back to its prestimulatory volume. Accordingly, when the stimulus is removed, the free intracellular $[Ca^{2+}]$, the cell volumes, the cytoplasmic pH and the activity of the transporters including the ion channels return to their original prestimulatory levels, and the acinus is again ready to produce substantial amounts of primary saliva in response to a new stimulatory challenge.

Ductal modification of electrolyte composition of primary saliva

As for the secretory end-pieces the parasympathetic and sympathetic nerve fibres control the activity of the saliva ducts. Furthermore, the membrane transporters and the cell-signalling mechanisms of the duct cells are similar to those of the acinar cells. However, the ductal epitheliums possess both absorptive and secretory functions. Most of the reabsorption of Na^+ and Cl^- occurs in the striated duct and, because of the low water permeability of the duct, the final saliva secreted into the mouth becomes hypotonic to plasma, i.e., with much lower concentrations of Na^+ and Cl^- than primary saliva.

The driving force for the Na^+ reabsorption from the primary saliva across the luminal membrane is generated from the activity of basolateral ATP-consuming Na^+/K^+-pumps in the infoldings of the membrane in the striated duct cells (Figure 2). This pump mechanism maintains extrusion of Na^+ from the duct cell to the interstitium (and ductal uptake of K^+). This creates an inwardly directed Na^+ gradient, allowing Na^+ to pass into the duct cell from the primary saliva. The ductal uptake of Na^+, which is activated by circulating adrenal mineralocorticoids (e.g. aldosterone), occurs *via* Na^+ channels and presumably also by Na^+/H^+ exchange mechanisms. The uptake of Na^+ into the duct is to a large extent balanced by parallel uptake of Cl^- *via* Cl^- channels and Cl^-/HCO_3^- exchange mechanisms. Besides the uptake of Cl^-, some secretion of K^+ into the saliva occurs to preserve electroneutrality. These transporters are the most important mechanisms for the modification of primary saliva by the ducts. Stimulation of receptors in the duct cells by neurotransmitters and peptides induces a rise in intracellular free $[Ca^{2+}]$ and cAMP in a manner similar to that in acinar cells, but the regulatory role of these messengers for the modification of saliva in the duct is still not clear.

From a clinical point of view, it is important to stress that medicines that inhibit the muscarinergic or adrenergic receptor systems (like some antidepressants, neuroleptics, antihistamines, and hypertensives) or that directly affect the membrane transporters in the salivary gland tissues (like some diuretics), have the potential to induce changes in the flow rate and composition of saliva.

Saliva and its inorganic composition

The final composition of the saliva arising from the major salivary glands depends strongly on the flow rate. However, the final product secreted to the mouth is always hypotonic. Depending on the flow rate, whole saliva contains 3–6 times less electrolytes than plasma. As the flow rate increases, the most dramatic increases occur in the Na^+, Cl^-, and HCO_3^- concentration (see Figures 4 and 6).

Because the ductal transport mechanisms involved in Na^+ (and Cl^-) reabsorption from the primary saliva have a maximal transport capacity, and because there is limited time within the duct system to modify the electrolyte composition at high stimulated flow rates, stimulated saliva is less hypotonic than unstimulated saliva (i.e., it has higher concentrations of Na^+ and Cl^-). The concentration of HCO_3^-, which is the principal buffer in saliva, also varies with the flow rate: unstimulated saliva contains very little HCO_3^- whereas stimulated saliva contains much higher concentrations. With very powerful stimulation (including pharmacological stimulation), the salivary HCO_3^- concentration certainly exceeds the plasma level and can even become the predominant anion in the stimulated saliva. The secreted HCO_3^- is derived from CO_2 from salivary gland metabolism. It is, however, not clear how much originates from the acinar and ductal gland segments. It is possible that the striated ducts

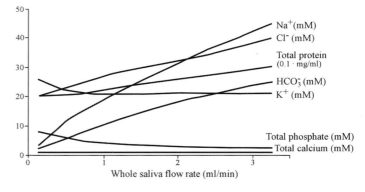

Figure 6. *Inorganic saliva composition.* The saliva inorganic and organic composition as a function of the saliva flow rate. As shown the salivary concentrations of Na^+, Cl^-, and HCO_3^- increases with increasing flow rates, whereas the saliva concentrations of total phosphate and to some extend K^+ decreases with increasing flow rates. The concentrations of total calcium and total protein also increase upon stimulation although not substantially.

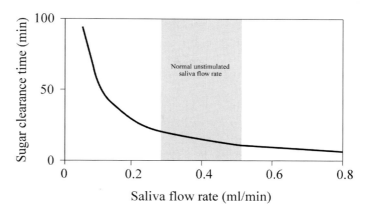

Figure 7. *Oral sugar clearance.* Oral sugar clearance (to a very low level of sugar) as a function of the unstimulated saliva flow rate calculated from a mathematical model (Dawes, 1983). In this model the volume of saliva just before swallowing as well as the volume of saliva swallowed are set to a constant level. As shown the oral sugar clearance is highly dependent on the unstimulated saliva flow rate increasing substantially when the unstimulated saliva flow rate is below 0.2 ml/min.

can both absorb HCO_3^- (at low flow rates) and secrete it (at high flow rates).

An essential aspect of the HCO_3^- buffer system is that it can diffuse freely across the epithelial boundaries in form of gaseous CO_2 driven by the CO_2 gradient within the different gland compartments. However, because the partial pressure of CO_2 (P_{CO_2}) in saliva remains almost constant at all flow rates and at various metabolic rates, its HCO_3^- concentration (and thereby pH) increases with flow rate (see Figure 4 and later for the equilibrium of the HCO_3^- buffer system).

The membrane transporters believed to govern the HCO_3^- concentration in saliva may comprise ductal Cl^-/HCO_3^- exchangers. In parotid saliva, for example, HCO_3^- concentration correlates positively to that of Cl^-. Accordingly, at low flow rates the Cl^- and HCO_3^- concentrations and pH are low, and *vice versa* at higher secretion rates.

Figure 6 shows that as flow rate increases, the whole saliva concentrations of Na^+, Cl^-, HCO_3^-, total calcium and total protein increase to varying extents, while the concentration of K^+ and total phosphate decreases. However, the saliva flow rate and composition also depend on the type of gland from which it is secreted, as well as on the nature and the duration of stimulation. Thus,

stimulated saliva collected during the first few minutes has a composition that is different from that of saliva collected following several minutes of sustained stimulation. Furthermore, many solutes show circadian variations that are independent of the variation in salivary flow rate.

Oral clearance

The time taken to clear the food that enters the mouth varies from one subject to another (Figure 7). This clearance is primarily due to swallowing and the flushing effect of saliva. The dilution of substances in the mouth and their removal is crucial for the protection of the oral tissues. If substances that are harmful to teeth such as sugars or acids accumulate in the mouth, destructive processes such as dental caries or erosion are accelerated. The normal procedure for measuring oral clearance is to introduce a certain substance (e.g., sugar) into the mouth in high concentration after an initial swallow. The substance is then diluted by the 0.8 ml or so of saliva that remains in the mouth after swallowing (the so-called residual volume). The *oral clearance rate* is the time taken either to clear the substance from the mouth or to reduce it to a very low concentration. This is strongly dependent on the saliva flow rate as well as on the volume of saliva in the mouth before and after swallowing.

When a substance is introduced to the mouth in a high concentration it will, depending on its taste, initially stimulate saliva production. The resulting increase in saliva flow rate will then increase the volume of saliva in the mouth. When this volume reaches the threshold for swallowing (about 1.1 ml), a swallow will occur, removing part of the ingested substance. The remainder will then be diluted with new saliva coming from the glands until the threshold is again reached and the next swallow occurs. Each time the subject swallows, some of the substance will be removed which will in turn reduce the stimulus to secretion. Accordingly, oral clearance occurs non-linearly with time especially during the first minutes after introduction of the substance to the mouth. When the substance in the mouth has reached a certain low level, it will no longer stimulate saliva flow and the production of saliva will return to the unstimulated level. Hence the unstimulated flow of saliva has the greatest overall impact on the oral clearance time (Figure 7) because it is present throughout the longest period of the clearance time. When this is less than 0.2 ml/min, the time taken to clear sugar from the oral cavity increases dramatically. Therefore individuals with impaired unstimulated saliva flow rates have a slow oral clearance time and are at higher risk of developing dental caries and erosion.

■ Saliva buffer capacity

One of the important roles of saliva is to maintain a non-harmful pH in the mouth during the time taken to clear acids that are ingested orally, such as carbonated drinks, fruit juices, and wines. The ability of the saliva to maintain the pH when exposed to acids is termed buffer capacity. This is determined in the laboratory by titration of the saliva within the pH range of interest. The saliva pH, which in healthy individuals varies between 6.0–7.5, depends strongly on the secretion rate with the most alkaline fluid being secreted during stimulated flow. A drop in saliva pH below 5.5–5.0 is potentially harmful to the oral tissues, particularly enamel/dentine. Thus from a dental point of view the most interesting pH range for determination of the buffer capacity is from the saliva's original pH in the mouth down to pH 5. Typical titration curves illustrating the saliva pH as a function of added acid (HCl) are shown in Figure 8. From such titration curves the saliva buffer capacity (β) can be determined in mmol H^+/(litre saliva · pH unit) in a certain pH interval:

$$\beta = \Delta C_A / \Delta pH$$

Where ΔC_A is the increase in saliva acid concentration and ΔpH is the change in saliva pH caused by the addition of acid.

If addition of large amounts of acid results in only a minor pH change, the buffer capacity of the saliva is high and *vice versa*. Note that, regardless of the concentration of buffers, the buffer capacity will gradually increase when the pH decreases because of the logarithmic nature of the pH scale ($-\log [H^+]$). Buffer capacity is not to be confused with the term "buffer effect" of saliva often used in dental literature. In the dental office, the buffer effect is often determined by adding a fixed amount of acid to a fixed amount of saliva and then reading off the final pH. Although this gives a handy clue about the buffering capacity of the saliva, it gives no information about the buffers present in the mouth or about variations in the saliva buffer capacity at different pH values.

The buffer capacity of human saliva increases with increasing flow rates and is maximal around pH 6. Figure 8 shows that the buffer capacity of both unstimulated and stimulated saliva at pH 6 is considerable higher than that of tap water. The buffer capacity of highly stimulated parotid saliva is even higher than that of a relatively viscous fluid, like milk. However, the buffer capacity of human saliva is never as high as that of blood, which is partly due to the high protein concentration of blood. The three im-

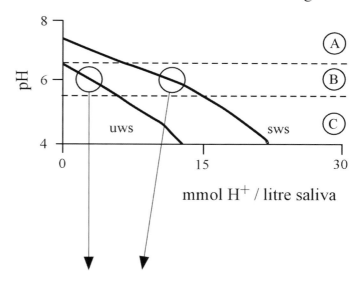

Titration of whole saliva with strong acid

Buffer capacity at pH 6

Figure 8. *Titration and buffer capacity of saliva.*
Titration curves of unstimulated and stimulated human whole saliva. As shown stimulated whole saliva (SWS) is better in maintaining its pH upon addition of acid compared to unstimulated saliva (UWS) indicating a higher buffer capacity. The buffer capacity in (A) originates mainly from the salivary contents of phosphate, in (B) from the salivary contents of bicarbonate, and in (C) from the salivary proteins. The area where both curves have the flattest slope, and therefore the highest buffer capacity, is around pH 6 indicated at the figure. Below is shown the buffer capacity at pH 6 of unstimulated and stimulated whole saliva as well as stimulated parotid saliva (SPS) in comparison to the buffer capacity of other fluids. It can be seen that the buffer capacity of saliva is higher than the buffer capacity of water at all times, that the buffer capacity of stimulated parotid saliva is higher than that of milk, and that the buffer capacity of saliva never becomes as high as it is in blood.

portant buffer systems in human saliva are the bicarbonate, the phosphate, and the protein buffer systems.

The bicarbonate buffer system and saliva pH regulation

The concentration of bicarbonate, the main buffer in human saliva, varies under physiological conditions from about 2–5 mM in unstimulated saliva up to plasma-like levels of about 28 mM in stimulated saliva. The equilibrium for the bicarbonate buffer system in a partly open compartment like the mouth is:

$$CO_2 + H_2O \overset{CA}{\leftrightarrow} H_2CO_3 \leftrightarrow HCO_3^- + H^+$$

Where CO_2 is the CO_2 in saliva and in the air surrounding the saliva in the mouth and CA is carbonic anhydrase that catalyses the hydration of CO_2 to carbonic acid.

The bicarbonate buffer system makes its highest contribution to the overall buffer capacity of saliva at the pK value for carbonic acid that is close to pH 6 in saliva (Figure 8). At pH 6, the contribution of the bicarbonate buffer system to the overall buffer capacity varies from 50% in unstimulated/resting saliva up to more than 90% in stimulated saliva produced at high flow rates. This difference is due to the flow-dependent variations in the saliva bicarbonate concentration.

Figure 4 shows that in the normal pH range of the parotid saliva (6.0–7.5) the partial pressure of CO_2 (P_{CO_2}) is 6.0 kPa, which is equal to that of blood. However, when saliva enters the mouth, some CO_2 is lost which results in a drop in its P_{CO_2} to around 4.5 kPa. Nevertheless, the P_{CO_2} of the whole saliva is still more than 1000 times higher than the P_{CO_2} in the atmosphere (4 Pa). Accordingly, any exposure of saliva to the atmosphere (during saliva collection or during sialochemical measurements) will result in major losses of saliva CO_2 that decrease the concentration

of the whole bicarbonate buffer system and increase the salivary pH shifting the equilibrium to the left. CO_2 is also lost from the saliva if it is mixed with acid because the equilibrium of the bicarbonate buffer system shifts to the left, which results in an increased salivary P_{CO_2}. Thus acidification to pH 4.0 of whole saliva containing 25 mM of bicarbonate results in a 25-fold increase in its P_{CO_2} level. Such acidification will give rise to a P_{CO_2} in saliva that is 25,000 times higher than the P_{CO_2} in the atmosphere. Accordingly, the driving force for CO_2 loss to the atmosphere from such acidified saliva is as high as for carbonated drink exposed to the atmosphere. The ability of the bicarbonate buffer system to go from one form to another during buffering is called phase buffering and this ability further increases the buffering of the system.

The saliva bicarbonate concentration is most commonly determined from the saliva P_{CO_2} and pH by the Henderson-Hasselbalch equation:

$$HCO_3^- = (0.225 \ P_{CO_2}) \ (10^{pH - pK})$$

Where P_{CO_2} is the saliva P_{CO_2} in kPa, and pK the pK value of carbonic acid in saliva.

To summarise: in order to determine the bicarbonate concentration and pH of saliva as well its buffer capacity accurately, it is essential to avoid the loss of CO_2. To achieve this, the saliva has to be collected and analysed in closed systems using techniques similar to those used for arterial blood samples.

The phosphate buffer system

Figure 6 shows that the total phosphate concentration in saliva also depends on the flow rate. However, while the salivary bicarbonate concentration increases with increasing flow rates, the saliva total phosphate concentration decreases with increasing flow rates. Thus resting/unstimulated saliva may contain up to 10 mM of total phosphate, whereas stimulated saliva secreted at high flow rates may contain well under 3 mM. The different ionic forms of phosphate are determined by their pK values and thus by the pH value of the saliva (Figure 9).

Within the normal pH range of the saliva (6.0–7.5), most phosphate will be present as dihydrogen phosphate (pK around 6.8 in saliva), and hydrogen phosphate. However, the two other forms of phosphate (i.e. H_3PO_4 and PO_4^{3-}) will also be present in the pH range from 6.0–7.0, although in very low concentrations. Accordingly, in saliva phosphate is most effective as a buffer at pH 6.8 (Figure 8).

The phosphate buffer system normally contributes about 50% of the buffer capacity in unstimulated/resting saliva. However, due to the flow-dependent decrease in saliva total phosphate concentration upon stimulation together with the huge increase in the bicarbonate concentration, phosphate normally makes only a minor contribution to the stimulated saliva buffer capacity.

The protein buffer system

Saliva contains a variety of different proteins with specific biological functions (Figure 10). Most of these can act as buffers when the pH is above or below their isoelectric point (pI). Below their pI they can accept protons and thereby act as buffers, and above they can release protons. Because the pI of most salivary proteins is around pH 7.0, their buffering effect becomes pronounced mostly at acidic and alkaline pH values. Thus, they contribute substantially to the saliva buffer capacity at pH values of less than pH 5 (Figure 8). In addition to their chemical buffering, some of the saliva proteins also increase the viscosity of the saliva when the pH becomes acidic and thereby cover and physically protect the teeth against the acid load.

■ Saliva and its saturation with respect to hydroxyapatite

Under physiological conditions, teeth do not dissolve in saliva because it is supersaturated with respect to hydroxyapatite $Ca_{10}(PO_4)_6(OH)_2$, the main inorganic component of teeth. The solubility product for hydroxyapatite (KSP_{HA}) is 10^{-117} M^{18} (where 18 refers to the 18 ions present in the hydroxyapatite unit cell). This value corresponds to the ion activity product for hydroxyapatite (IAP_{HA}) in a solution saturated with respect to hydroxyapatite.

For saliva the IAP_{HA} can be calculated from its actual salivary ion activities (the free ionic concentration corrected for electrostatic effects) of Ca^{2+}, PO_4^{3-}, and OH^- as shown below:

$$IAP_{HA} = (Ca^{2+})^{10} \, (PO_4^{3-})^6 \, (OH^-)^2$$

From this expression it can be seen that IAP_{HA} increases with increasing activities of these ions in saliva and *vice versa*. The greatest impact on IAP_{HA}, however, comes from the saliva pH. Thus when pH decreases, the activities of both PO_4^{3-} (see Figure 9 for the equilibrium of the phosphate buffer system) and OH^- will decrease dramatically.

When KSP_{HA} and IAP_{HA} are known the degree of saturation of saliva with respect to hydroxyapatite (DS_{HA}) can be calculated as:

$$DS_{HA} = (IAP_{HA}/KSP_{HA})^{(1/18)}$$

where $^{(1/18)}$ also refers to the 18 ions present in the hydroxyapatite (i.e. $Ca_{10}(PO_4)_6(OH)_2$) unit cell.

If IAP_{HA} in saliva is larger than KSP_{HA}, (i.e. $DS_{HA} > 1$), the saliva is supersaturated with respect to hydroxyapatite. However, if IAP_{HA} is smaller than KSP_{HA} ($DS_{HA} < 1$), the saliva is undersaturated and the enamel/den-

Figure 9. *The phosphate buffer system.* The equilibrium of the phosphate buffer system as a function of pH. In the normal pH range for saliva most phosphate will be present as $H_2PO_4^-$ and HPO_4^{2-}. However, the two other forms of phosphate (i.e. H_3PO_4 and PO_4^{3-}) will also be present although in very low concentrations.

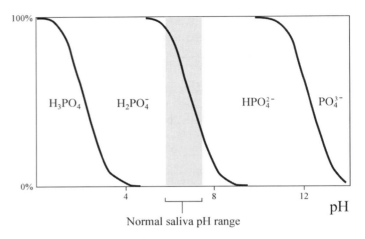

tine will dissolve, leading either to dental erosion or dental caries, depending on the origin of the acidic challenge.

Calculation "case" of DS_{HA} in saliva
A patient has an unstimulated saliva flow rate of 0.3 ml/min and a saliva pH of 6.0 (OH^- activity of 10^{-8} M). The saliva total calcium concentration is 1 mM corresponding to a Ca^{2+} activity of 0.4×10^{-3} M and the total phosphate concentration is 5 mM corresponding to a PO_4^{3-} activity of 1.7×10^{-10} M

IAP_{HA} of saliva$=(0.4 \times 10^{-3})^{10}$ $(1.7 \times 10^{-10})^6 (1 \times 10^{-8})^2 \approx 2.5 \times 10^{-109}$ M^{18}

Thus in this case IAP_{HA} is larger than the corresponding KSP_{HA} of 10^{-117} M^{18}

$DS_{HA}=(2.5 \times 10^{-109}/10^{-117})^{(1/18)}=2.9$

Thus in this case DS_{HA} becomes >1 and therefore the saliva is supersaturated with respect to hydroxyapatite

The value of pH in saliva at which IAP_{HA} equals KSP_{HA} (i.e. the condition where $DS_{HA}=1$) is often denoted the "critical" pH in the dental literature. The critical pH in human saliva is on average 5.5 under normal physiological conditions, but this is certainly not a fixed value since it depends on a number of ion activities that change dynamically as the saliva flow rates varies. Unstimulated saliva containing a high phosphate concentration, and therefore having a high phosphate activity, has generally a more acidic critical pH than stimulated saliva containing a low phosphate concentration. The critical pH in saliva normally varies from 5.3 to 5.5 depending on the flow rate: however, it may vary from 5.2 to 5.8 in extreme cases where the phosphate concentration is very high or very low, respectively.

Nucleation followed by precipitation of calcium-phosphate salts is likely to occur in a fluid that is supersaturated with these ions. Three-dimensional nucleation is the nucleation of the calcium-phosphate salt within a fluid followed by crystal growth of the salt (homogeneous and heterogeneous nucleation). Two-dimensional nucleation is surface- or seed-induced nucleation of the calcium-phosphate salt followed by crystal growth of the salt. Three-dimensional nucleation is not likely to occur in saliva because of the low calcium and phosphate concentrations as well as the many proteins that act as nucleation inhibitors. Two-dimensional nucleation, however, occurs quite often in the form of dental calculus where substances in the dental plaque and on the tooth surfaces serve as seeds for the process. Calculus formation normally occurs on teeth in the regions of the mouth where the salivary supersaturation of calcium-phosphate salts is highest, i.e. near the orifices of the submandibular, sublingual and parotid ducts. Here the pH is most alkaline due to the high bicarbonate concentration in the secreted saliva, as well as the CO_2 evaporation due to mouth breathing. Accordingly, calculus formation occurs most frequently around the mandibulary incisors and maxillary molars.

■ Organic saliva composition and its functions

Both the acinar and ductal cells secrete proteins into saliva (exocrine function) and the blood circulation (endocrine function); see also paragraph on stimulus-secretion coupling. These salivary proteins are the major organic components of saliva. There are more than 40 different proteins in human saliva whose molecular weights vary from a few kDa to more than one thousand kDa. The total protein concentration is on average 2.0 mg/ml saliva, which is nearly 40 times lower than in plasma. The protein concentration depends on both the duration of stimulation (long periods of stimulation results in high saliva total protein concentrations) and on the flow rate (high flow rates result in high total protein concentrations). However, the total protein concentration and composition is much less dependent on the flow rate than are the inorganic components. Instead, it is mainly influenced by individual genetic differences. Hence, the profile of saliva proteins in monozygous twins is similar.

Our understanding of the functions of the saliva proteins is based on *in vitro* experiments rather than clinical trials. So far therefore little is known about the impact of specific saliva proteins on oral health *in vivo*. Some studies have shown that differences in protein composition play a role in individuals' susceptibility to develop caries while other studies have not been able to demonstrate this.

Mixing dried saliva proteins with water gives a solution with a texture and viscosity that is similar to saliva. Not surprisingly, therefore, the distinct texture and viscosity of saliva is the result of its protein composition. Some saliva proteins protect the oral tissues against infections, others coat and lubricate the oral tissues, some play a role in maintaining high saliva concentrations of calcium, other are digestive enzymes, and some catalyse the hydration of CO_2 to carbonic acid. Although most have one major function, many have multifunctional roles. A few examples are discussed below in the context of their function and possible clinical impact.

Digestive enzymes
Human saliva contains α-amylase, an enzyme that hydrolyses the α-1,4 glycosidic linkages of starch molecules. Hence the breakdown of ingested starch to simple hexoses occurs in two phases starting in the oral cavity with salivary α-amylase and continuing in the intestine with pancreatic α-amylase. As shown in Figure 10, the salivary

Salivary proteins (size and function)

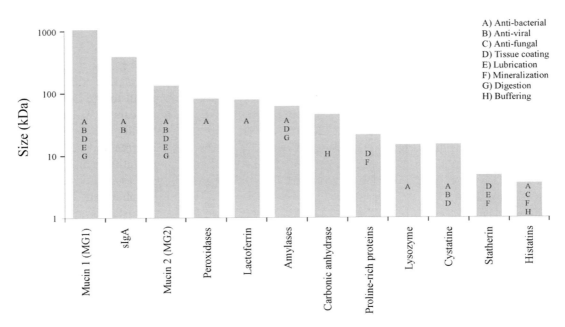

● **Figure 10.** *The major salivary proteins.*
Some of the major salivary proteins ranked according to their molecular weight (please note that the scale is logarithmic). For each protein its possible function in saliva is stated. Thus the high molecular weight mucin (MG1) is shown to have (A) anti-bacterial, (B) anti-viral, (D) tissue coating, (E) lubricating, and (G) digestive effects.

α-amylase family has molecular weights of around 55–60 kDa and they are therefore among the larger proteins found in saliva. The α-amylases are secreted particularly from the serous cells in the parotid and submandibular glands in response to parasympathetic stimulation and the α-amylases are secreted both to blood circulation and the saliva. The concentration of α-amylases in saliva is high and may constitute as much as 30–40% of the total protein in whole saliva. This is more than 1000 times higher than the total α-amylase concentration in human blood. Therefore injuries to the salivary glands due to irradiation, glandular obstruction, or surgery can result in elevated plasma α-amylase concentrations because it leaks from the salivary glands into the blood circulation. Salivary α-amylases are active above pH 6 and become inactivated by the low pH in the stomach. Since this limits the time available for salivary α-amylases to work, it is considered of minor importance in starch digestion. It may however be important for starch digestion in neonates with an insufficiently developed pancreas.

Human saliva also contains lipase, an enzyme able to break down dietary triglycerides. Salivary lipase is secreted from the serous cells in the parotid gland and from the von Ebner's glands on the tongue. Like salivary α-amylase, it is considered of minor importance in healthy individuals, but may play a role in neonates and patients with pancreatic dysfunction.

Proteins with lubricating functions

Human saliva contains mucins that are large glycoproteins, constituting more than 40% carbohydrate, which have lubricating functions on the oral tissues. Two specific types of mucins have been characterized in human saliva. MG1 is produced in the mucous acini in the submandibular and sublingual glands as well as in the palatal and labial glands. MG2 is produced in the serous cells in most glands except for the parotid. The MG1 mucin weighs more than 1000 kDa and is the largest protein present in saliva, whereas MG2 weighs 130 kDa (Figure 10). Due to the differences in weight, the two mucins are often referred to as high- and low- molecular weight mucins.

Mucins are hydrophilic and contain water: they work effectively to moisten and lubricate oral surfaces. They also form disulfide bridges with other mucin molecules and thereby create a network that covers and protects the oral tissues. The hydrophilic and network-forming abilities of salivary mucins give saliva its distinct texture and viscosity.

Calcium binding proteins

Human saliva under normal physiological conditions is always supersaturated with hydroxyapatite as well as with other calcium phosphate salts. However, these salts do not normally precipitate in saliva due to the presence of calcium-binding proteins. Statherin is an asymmetrical protein and one of the smallest proteins in human saliva (4–5 kDa), which is secreted from acinar cells. Statherin inhibits three-dimensional as well as two-dimensional nucleation and prevents the formation of calcified masses (sialoliths)

in the salivary ducts and glands, and reduces the formation of calculus. The acidic proline-rich proteins (PRPs) are also small molecules (10–30 kDa) that constitute around 30% of the proteins parotid and submandibular saliva. Like statherin, the PRPs are secreted from acinar cells. They inhibit two-dimensional nucleation by binding calcium and also bind tannins that are harmful to the oral tissues. Interestingly, there appears to be differences in the amount and quality of acidic proline-rich proteins in caries-free and caries-active individuals. Although statherin and the PRPs are the proteins mostly associated with inhibition of calcium-phosphate salt nucleation, other proteins like the histatins and cystatins also inhibit nucleation.

Carbon dioxide hydration

Carbonic anhydrase (CA) is an essential enzyme present in all cells. Carbonic anhydrase catalyse the reversible hydration of CO_2 to carbonic acid (see equilibrium for the bicarbonate buffer system). Several isoforms of CA have been characterized of which one (CA VI) that has a weight of around 42–45 kDa is present in saliva. In the parotid and submandibular glands the acinar cells secrete CA VI. In contrast to the well-known cytoplasmic forms of CA, CA VI is the only isoform of the enzyme that is known to occur in a secretory form. Some studies have suggested that CA VI isoforms play a protective role against dental caries.

Saliva proteins with antimicrobial functions

Most immunoglobulins in human saliva are in the form of secretory IgA (sIgA) that is a large hydrophilic protein (380 kDa). Salivary IgA is a product of plasma cells that is modified and secreted by acinar and duct cells in the salivary glands. This secretory immunoglobulin is a specific defence factor that is stimulated by the presence of bacteria. Because of its hydrophilic abilities, salivary IgA can mix and function in saliva where it aggregates bacteria. Salivary IgA also has affinity for other antimicrobial components in saliva like the mucins. This affinity may synergistically increase the antimicrobial aggregating effects of both proteins. Some studies have shown a protective effect of salivary IgA against dental caries. However, other studies have not been able to show such relationships.

In addition to specific antimicrobial defence mechanisms, human saliva contains a variety of unspecific or innate antimicrobial defence mechanisms that have attracted increasing interest in recent years. Mucins, in addition to their lubricating effect on the oral tissues, also give protection against microbes. Thus the coating and network-forming effects of the mucins function as a barrier protecting the underlying tissue. The mucins also agglutinate large numbers of bacteria in saliva and thereby increase their removal by swallowing.

Lysozyme and lactoferrin are examples of proteins secreted by duct cells. In contrast to acinar proteins, ductal proteins decrease in concentration upon increased saliva flow. Both these proteins belong to the innate antimicrobial defence mechanisms. Lysozyme (around 14 kDa) kills gram-positive bacteria by breaking down their cell walls. Because of its strong positive charge, lysozyme may also be able to activate bacterial autolysin. Lactoferrin is a relatively big protein (around 75–78 kDa) whose best-known function is to bind iron and thereby inhibit bacterial growth by reducing the concentration of this important co-factor for bacterial enzymes. Besides having an iron-binding effect, lactoferrin has hidden antimicrobial domains that are liberated from the protein after proteolytic activity. Thus lactoferrin is believed to have bacteriostatic, bacteriocidal, fungicidal, and antiviral properties. It has been reported that low levels of lactoferrin are related to high levels of potentially pathogenic oral bacteria. Human saliva also contains the enzyme peroxidase (75–78 kDa) another innate antimicrobial defence mechanisms that is secreted by the acini. This enzyme catalyses the oxygenation of thiocyanate (SCN^-) to hypothiocyanate ($OSCN^-$) and thereby reduces bacterial growth by blocking essential bacterial metabolic processes.

Histatins are small antimicrobial peptides of around 3–4 kDa that are known mainly for their potent lethal effect in vitro on oral fungi like *Candida albicans*. Histatins are present in high concentrations in parotid saliva. The killing effect of histatin 5 on *Candida albicans* depends on the ionic strength of saliva, and becomes higher with lower salt concentrations such as those in unstimulated saliva in which histatins bind to *Candida albicans*. Histatins have also been shown to kill bacteria such as *Streptococcus mutans*.

Growth factors in saliva

Since ancient times, saliva from various animals has been applied to wounds to accelerate the healing process. It is now known that the wound-healing effect of saliva arises from its intrinsic growth factors. These growth factors are secreted from ducts cells in the salivary glands. Some, like epidermal growth factor (EGF) have a local effect. EGF is a small protein found in the submandibular and parotid glands whose output is increased by mastication. When secreted in saliva, EGF enhances healing of ulcers and plays a protective role in oesophageal mucosal protection. Salivary EGF interacts with the innate salivary protein defence mechanisms to form a mucosal defence barrier. NGF that has stimulating effect on ganglionic function is also released from salivary glands.

Transforming growth factors (TGF-α and TGF-β) are other small proteins that have been found in saliva, and which can cause cell differentiation and growth. Finally, fibroblast growth factor (FGF), a potent regulator of wound healing, has also been found in saliva.

Formation and function of the pellicle

Under normal conditions in the mouth, i.e. with plenty of saliva, an organic film called the acquired pellicle covers the teeth. The term "acquired" refers to the fact that this film develops on the teeth after they have erupted and not, as assumed earlier, before eruption. While the exact composition of this film is not known, it is derived mainly from salivary proteins. Its protective effect is, however, well known from laboratory studies in which teeth with and without a pellicle have been exposed to acid. These studies have shown that teeth covered by the pellicle develop less demineralization than teeth without the pellicle. Studies in which pure hydroxyapatite crystals have been exposed to acid suggest that formation of a salivary protein pellicle on the crystal surfaces may decrease the rate of dissolution by more than 80%. The effect of differences in saliva protein composition on the protective effect of this pellicle is not yet fully understood. Nevertheless, the ability of the salivary proteins to form the acquired pellicle is certainly one of the major mechanisms by which saliva protects the teeth. Moreover, a recent study has shown an inverse relationship between the salivary pellicle thickness and the incidence of cervical erosive lesions, which suggests that dental erosion may also be depend on the pellicle-forming ability of saliva in a site-specific pattern.

When completely clean teeth are exposed to saliva, the pellicle begins to form in less than a minute and reaches equilibrium within 2 hours. However, a so-called maturation time of several days is necessary for it to reach its maximum protective capacity. Because the surface of enamel is negatively charged, the first layer that is formed (the hydration layer) has a positive charge arising mainly from calcium. This positively-charged hydration layer then attracts negatively-charged macromolecules. The proteins that are best known to be attracted to tooth surfaces and which are present in the pellicle are the acidic proline-rich proteins, sIgA, cystatin, MG1, lactoferrin, lysozyme, and amylase. The reason why some of the other salivary proteins have not been shown in the pellicle can be explained by their weaker ability to bind to hydroxyapatite. Apart from the purely chemical protection against acids, the acquired pellicle also seems to determine the initial attachment of bacteria onto the tooth surface. The acquired pellicle may thereby favour a non-harmful colonization pattern and hence further protect the teeth.

Other organic components in saliva

In addition to the proteins, there are numerous other organic components in saliva, including the circulating adrenal glucocorticoid cortisol. The concentration of cortisol in saliva reflects its concentration in plasma, although its concentration is 10–30 times lower in saliva (typically 10–20 nM). Under conditions of high stress, the salivary cortisol can increase above 30 nM. Since a collection of saliva is non-stressful compared with blood sampling, saliva has become widely used in measurements of cortisol for monitoring stress. Moreover, the cortisol found in saliva is unbound; that is, it is not combined with its carrier protein, so that its concentration is a good indicator of its bioavailability.

Saliva also contains many of the sex hormones present in blood. For example, the salivary concentration of estriol in pregnant women also correlates well with its plasma concentration and can therefore be used to monitor fetal well-being.

Under normal conditions, the glucose concentration in saliva follows that of plasma, although at much lower levels. Thus glucose is normally present in saliva only in very low concentrations less than 0.1 mM. However, patients with high plasma glucose from untreated diabetes have elevated salivary glucose concentrations that can reach nearly 1.0 mM. Since glucose serve as a bacterial substrate such patients are likely to develop dental caries at high rates.

Human saliva normally contains between 2 and 4 mM urea, which is a product of protein metabolism. Urea is not a buffer, but in the presence of bacterial urease it can alkalise pH by being broken down into CO_2 and ammonia (which picks up a proton). Patients who suffer from untreated renal failure have salivary urea concentrations as high as 85 mM. The resulting high pH of the saliva and plaque in these patients reduce the incidence of dental caries.

Finally saliva contains blood group substances from the ABO blood groups. Before genotyping by DNA testing, the presence of these substances in saliva was an important tool in forensic and palaeoserological science.

Saliva as a screening tool

Saliva is a convenient fluid to use for diagnostic purposes and has obvious benefits over plasma because it is easy to collect in a non-invasive and non-stressful manner in the field. The ability of some circulating drugs to enter the saliva by diffusion is of special interest in forensic and pharmaceutical science and in some legal situations. Only the free and biologically active fraction of a drug in plasma gets into saliva where the concentration of proteins is much lower compared to plasma. When a water-soluble drug enters saliva that has a lower pH than plasma, it ionises. Its concentration in saliva, and thus the ratio of the free drug concentration between plasma and saliva, is then determined by its pK_a, the pH of the saliva and the pH of plasma. The wide variation in the rate of salivary secretion and the resulting variation in pH limit its use as a diagnostic medium for some drugs (depending on their pK). Hence, some drugs are concentrated in saliva while others are present in much lower concentrations than in plasma.

However, for some illegal drugs, the issue is detection rather than quantification, and saliva provides a simple screening assay for this purpose. The salivary levels of "recreational" drugs like cocaine and marijuana as well as alcohol give a good reflection of their plasma levels. Tobacco products like nicotine and cotinine can also be measured in saliva, and correlate well with their plasma concentrations. This has made it possible for the life insurance industry to verify the smoking status of individuals by means of salivary tests. Pollutants like lead, cadmium and copper can also be detected in saliva and their concentrations show the extent of the individual's exposure to them.

In another domain, saliva can be used to determine the profile of infection of the oral cavity with pathogens such as Candida as well as giving *Lactobacillus* and *Streptococcus mutans* scores. Finally, saliva is also valuable for qualitative screening $(+/-)$ for much more serious systemic infections diseases like HIV.

Salivary gland dysfunction

Salivary gland dysfunction is defined as any quantitative and/or qualitative change in the output of saliva. Thus, salivary gland dysfunction includes either an increase in salivary output (hyperfunction) or a decrease (hypofunction). Genuine salivary hyperfunction, sialorrhoea, is relatively uncommon in adults. It may be caused by mucosal irritation or be idiopathic. Drooling often occurs as a result of an underlying neurological disorder, for example cerebral palsy, amyotrophic lateral sclerosis, and Parkinson's disease. Drooling may also be seen in mentally-handicapped individuals and as a side-effect of neuroleptic medication in adults. The problem is generally the result of decreased swallowing efficiency and frequency and is rarely related to genuine salivary hyperfunction. Drooling may, however, be a severe problem to the patient, since it can cause maceration of the skin at the angles of the mouth and on the chin followed by colonization of opportunistic microorganisms. Furthermore, constant drooling may have a negative impact on the patient's psychological well-being and social behaviour. Some patients complain of having too much saliva and develop an obsessive swallowing pattern, i.e. a need to swallow compulsively at frequent intervals, but objectively are found to have a normal production of saliva.

Salivary gland hypofunction, in contrast, is a common condition especially in people with other underlying diseases and in those who take certain types of medication. Salivary hypofunction may develop into hyposalivation, a term which is based on *objective* measures of the saliva production (see section on collection of saliva). Hyposalivation usually results in altered salivary composition and is often associated with *xerostomia* which is defined as the *subjective* feeling of dry mouth. Generally, this symptom occurs when the unstimulated salivary flow is reduced to approximately 50% of its normal value in any given individual, which means that more than one major salivary gland must be affected. Unstimulated whole salivary flow rates are more closely associated with the symptoms of xerostomia than stimulated rates. However, complaints of xerostomia can occur in the absence of hyposalivation and *vice versa.* In mouth-breathing, for example, xerostomia is related to mucosal dryness arising from increased evaporation of saliva. It should be emphasized that xerostomia is not solely related to decreased salivary flow rate, but also to changes in its composition.

Principal causes of salivary gland hypofunction and xerostomia

Several medical conditions and medications can affect the salivary glands and their secretions in a number of ways. The salivary reflex can be affected *via* effects on the central or peripheral neural regulation, or through the receptor systems in the salivary gland tissues, stimulus-secretion coupling, membrane transporters, protein synthesis and/or protein release mechanisms. The most common reasons for salivary gland hypofunction are listed in Table 3.

Age and hormonal changes
Salivary dysfunctions in children are rare and mostly temporary conditions. The adult levels of salivary flow rate are usually

Table 3. Common causes of hyposalivation and/or changes in saliva composition.

Iatrogenic	medications, e.g. antidepressants, diuretics, antihistamines, antihypertensives, antipsychotics and opiates, polypharmacy, chemotherapy; radiotherapy to the head and neck region, surgical trauma
Autoimmune diseases	rheumatoid arthritis, Sjögren's syndrome, sarcoidosis
Neurological disorders	mental depression, cerebral palsy, Bell's palsy, Holmes-Adie syndrome
Hormonal disorders	diabetes mellitus (labile), hyper- and hypothyroidism
Infections	HIV infection/AIDS, epidemic parotitis
Hereditary disorders	cystic fibrosis, ectodermal dysplasia
Metabolic disturbances	malnutrition, eating disturbances, bulimia, anorexia nervosa, dehydration, vitamin deficiency
Local salivary diseases	sialolithiasis, sialadenitis, carcinoma
Other conditions	menopause, impaired masticatory performance

reached by the age of 15 years. In healthy individuals, the stimulated whole saliva flow rate does not decline with age. However, an age-related decrease may occur in secretions from minor and submandibular glands, but not from the parotids. This functional decrease is consistent with age-related changes of the morphology of these glands in which the acinar volume may shrink by 40–50%. On the other hand, diverse morphological changes can occur in the various salivary glands with aging including increased adiposity, ductal proliferation and fibrosis. Complaints of oral dryness are common in older adults and may be explained by the age-related decrease in minor and submandibular gland secretions, even when chewing-stimulated whole saliva secretions are normal. It should be emphasised that, even though changes in the structure of the salivary gland might suggest hypofunction, there is no clinically significant reduction in the overall gland output with aging in healthy, non-medicated adults. Accordingly, the increased incidence of subjective symptoms and objective signs of salivary gland hypofunction in the elderly is more likely to be due to the increased incidence of systemic diseases and the increased likelihood of medication in this age group, than to age-related salivary gland hypofunction.

Menopause is often associated with salivary dysfunction, since the incidence of dry mouth and burning mouth symptoms is high among menopausal women. However, observations on the changes in flow rates and composition of saliva have given conflicting results. Generally, the salivary flow rates are not significantly decreased in healthy postmenopausal women compared with those of premenopausal women. Concentrations of phosphate in whole saliva are higher in postmenopausal women than in controls. Hormone replacement therapy increases salivary flow rates, as well as its buffer capacity and pH in postmenopausal women.

Iatrogenic-induced salivary hypofunction
Salivary gland hypofunction and xerostomia are side effects of many prescription drugs, including antidepressants, antihypertensives, diuretics, antihistamines, antipsychotics and opiates. Antidepressants and antihistamines act on muscarinic cholinergic receptors in salivary glands resulting in reduced saliva volume, whereas other drugs such as di-

uretics may induce changes in the composition of saliva through their action on mechanisms that control fluid and salt balance, and inhibitory effects on electrolyte transporters in the salivary gland cells.

There is also a relationship between the number of medications taken on a regular daily basis, with xerostomia and hyposalivation, irrespective of whether the medications specifically cause hyposalivation. Thus, patients taking more than four drugs (polypharmacy) have lower unstimulated and stimulated whole saliva flow rates than non-medicated patients.

Radiotherapy of the head and neck region results in a markedly reduced salivary flow rate, acidic saliva, poor buffering capacity and abnormal electrolyte and protein content. The abnormal electrolyte and protein content can be due to contribution from their leakage from the plasma into saliva. The extent of salivary hypofunction depends on the volume of glandular tissue included in the field of radiation as well as to the total dose of radiation delivered. Hypofunction induced by doses of 30–50 Gray (Gy) may be reversible, whereas doses higher than 60 Gy usually induce irreversible salivary gland hypofunction and persisting xerostomia. Damage to the glandular tissue is caused by direct radiation effects on the acinar and duct cells, but also indirectly by injury of vascular structures resulting in increased capillary permeability, interstitial oedema and inflammatory reactions. Serous acinar cells are initially more affected by irradiation than mucous acinar cells and duct cells. Although the salivary glands are considered to be relatively resistant to irradiation because of their relatively slow cell division cycle, radiation induces acute changes in saliva flow rate and composition. However, results vary, and the long-term effects of the treatment on oral health are especially uncertain. Finally, patients undergoing chemo-

therapy may also experience similar changes in salivary flow rate and composition.

Systemic diseases and medical conditions

Numerous systemic diseases, and/or the medication used to treat them, are associated with impaired secretion of saliva and changes in its composition. Prominent examples are autoimmune diseases such as Sjögren's syndrome (see textbox) and inherited diseases like cystic fibrosis where changes in secretion are in part related to structural changes to the salivary glands. In neurological disorders like Bell's palsy (idiopathic paralysis of the facial nerve) and Holmes-Adie syndrome (autonomic dysfunction), compromised innervation of the glands results in salivary hypofunction. In inadequately-controlled insulin-dependent (type 1) diabetes or at the early onset of diabetes mellitus type 1 and 2, reduced salivary flow rate may occur as a result of dehydration due to polyuria. The salivary dysfunction may, however, also be related to diabetic autonomic neuropathy, and the associated sialosis (non-inflammatory salivary gland hypertrophy). Malnutrition, as well as eating disorders (bulimia and anorexia nervosa) of long duration reduce salivary flow, induce compositional changes of saliva and cause enlargement of the major salivary glands.

■ Symptoms and objective findings in salivary gland hypofunction

Reduced salivary secretion is usually associated with a sensation of a dry mouth that persists throughout the day. The dryness continues at night leading to disturbed sleep because of the need for regular sips of liquid. Furthermore, patients with salivary hypofunction, regardless of the cause, often have symptoms of burning mouth, difficulties in

Characteristics of Sjögren's syndrome
Definition:
Chronic inflammatory systemic auto-immune disease that principally causes dry eyes (keratoconjunctivitis sicca) and dry mouth (hyposalivation) due to by lymphocyte-mediated destruction of the glandular tissue. The syndrome has a primary and secondary form. The latter is usually associated with rheumatoid arthritis.

Demography:
All ethnic and racial groups, prevalence: 1–3%, 90% of the patients are women in the age of 40–60 years

Aetiology:
Unknown. Probably multifactorial. Including interactions between genetic, immunological, neuroendocrinological, and environmental factors

Symptoms:
Xerostomia, ocular dryness, arthralgia, myalgia, fatigue.

Clinical findings:
Hyposalivation, keratoconjunctivitis sicca, parotid enlargement, vasculitis, dry skin, Raynaud's disease, purpura, anemia and pharyngitis.

Diagnosis of the oral component:
Symptoms of oral dryness, sialometry (whole saliva), salivary scintigraphy, sialography, labial salivary gland biopsy (focal periductal lymphocytic infiltration of the salivary gland tissue). Supplement: sialochemical analysis of glandular saliva.

chewing and swallowing dry foods, difficulty in speaking, impaired sense of taste, acid reflux (heartburn) and halitosis. Removable dentures may cause discomfort due to the lack of mucosal lubrication. These distressing sequelae can significantly diminish the health-related quality of life. Permanently reduced salivary secretion commonly results in clinically evident changes in the oral soft and hard tissues. The oral mucosa in patients with hyposalivation is generally thin and pale and without the usual glistening appearance. Saliva frequently appears thick and foamy and can form whitish threads on mucosal surfaces. The dorsal part of the tongue looks dry and becomes lobulated with atrophy of the filiform papillae. In some cases, the tongue surface appears fissured. The most common symptoms and clinical signs related to permanently reduced salivary flow rate are shown in Table 4.

Salivary gland infections
Bacterial sialadenitis is a relatively rare condition, which occurs especially in elderly patients who have reduced salivary flow due to systemic diseases, medications or dehydration. The condition is usually characterized by acute tender swelling of the salivary gland, particularly the parotid gland, and in some cases fever and malaise. In medically or immunologically compromised patients, the infection may even become life-threatening due to sepsis. It is assumed that the reduced salivary flow allows ascending microbial colonization of the duct, which predisposes to the development of acute or chronic suppurative infection. Only limited information is available about the microflora of the salivary duct during salivary gland hypofunction, but the microflora in the excretory duct system appear to be more extensive and complex in patients with Sjögren's syndrome than in healthy individuals.

Table 4. Oral symptoms and signs often related to hyposalivation and xerostomia.

Oral mucosal dryness and soreness
Burning oral sensation
Difficulties in speech (dysphonia)
Difficulty in chewing dry food
Difficulty in swallowing dry food (dysphagia)
Difficulty in wearing removable dentures
Taste impairment (dysgeusia or hypogeusia)
Acid reflux, nausea, heartburn
Bad breath (halitosis)
Sensation of thirst
Dry, glazed and red oral mucosa
Lobulation or fissuring of the dorsal part of the tongue
Atrophy of filiform papillae
Dry, cracked lips
Increased activity of caries with lesions on cervical, incisal and cuspal tooth surfaces
Increased frequency of oral infections (e.g. recurrent oral candidiasis, angular cheilitis)

Additional non-oral symptoms may occur including dryness of the skin, throat, nose and eyes as well as constipation, weight loss and depression.

Mumps is an acute systemic viral infection caused by paramyxovirus. The parotid glands, which are primarily affected, become increasingly swollen and painful over a few days. As the glands swell, the patients often develop fever, headache and malaise. Mumps in adult males may result in the development of orchitis, an inflammation of the testicles, which can result in sterility. The disease can be prevented by the use of a vaccine giving long-life immunity. Mumps is the most common form of viral sialoadenitis, but parotitis may also be caused other viruses such as cytomegalovirus and Coxsackie A virus.

Sialoliths

Calcified masses within the salivary duct called saliva stones or sialoliths are a relatively common condition that affects as many as 1% of the population. Sialoliths occur more frequently in women than men and mostly in the submandibular duct. Most are asymptomatic and unilateral. The predisposing factors are changes in saliva composition, infection or inflammation in the ducts, or damage to the duct tissue.

Salivary gland tumours

Ranked according to occurrence salivary gland neoplasms or tumours may occur in 1) the parotid gland, 2) the minor glands, 3) the submandibular gland, and 4) very seldomly in the sublingual gland. The neoplasms can arise from both acinar and ductal cells as well as myoepithelial cells. The incidence of malignancy is low for the parotid gland, relatively high for the minor glands, and very high for neoplasms in the sublingual gland. Symptoms may include a lump in the mouth, swelling in the face, pain in the jaw or the side of the face, and weakness of the face muscles.

Saliva and oral microflora

Salivary gland hypofunction is associated with impaired antimicrobial capacity of saliva. Changes such as reduced oral tissue protein protection and lower saliva pH may favour an aciduric and acidophilic oral microflora, which increase the risk of dental caries and oral candidiasis. Thus, reduced salivary flow and/or altered salivary composition are associated with significant changes in the oral microflora including increases in acidophilic microorganisms such as *Streptococcus mutans*, *Lactobacillus*, and yeasts. High salivary *Lactobacillus* counts are strongly associated with low salivary secretion and the number of lactobacilli in saliva is positively correlated with caries activity.

Saliva and dental caries

Dental caries is the result of an interaction between many different variables such as oral hygiene, diet, oral microflora, and tooth morphology. Nevertheless, several clinical studies have shown that dental caries is a common consequence of salivary hypofunction. In patients with low saliva flow rates, carious lesions usually develop rapidly, especially in retention sites for dental plaque along the gingival margin and adjacent to dental restorations. Chronic hyposalivation may even result in early loss of natural teeth due to progressive caries. In patients with hyposalivation, the increased caries activity is mainly attributed to a reduction in oral clearance. Thus, reduction in salivary flow rates leads to impairment of the mechanical flushing and cleansing action of saliva, which results in slow elimination of oral bacteria, dietary sugars and dietary acids, as well as plaque accumulation on the tooth surfaces (Figure 6).

Saliva and tooth wear

Tooth wear occurs as a result of abrasion (pathologic wearing of teeth resulting from an abnormal habit or abnormal use of abrasive substances orally), attrition (physiologic wearing of teeth resulting from mastication) and erosion (irreversible loss of dental hard tissue due to a non-bacterial chemical process). The aetiology of each of these conditions is like dental caries, i.e., the result of interactions between a number of different variables, which make it difficult to make a clinical differential diagnosis between chemical and mechanical aetiology of tooth wear. The relationship between dental erosion and various salivary factors such as pH, buffer capacity, concentrations of calcium and phosphate, and mucins as well as unstimulated and stimulated salivary flow rates, have been investigated. However, only unstimulated salivary flow rate and saliva buffering capacity have been shown to be associated with the presence of dental erosion. Thus, patients with unstimulated

whole salivary flow rate of 0.10 ml/min or less have a higher risk of dental erosion than patients with higher unstimulated saliva flow rates.

Saliva and periodontal disease

A few studies have demonstrated a relationship between salivary flow and periodontal parameters such as pocket depth, gingival bleeding, dental plaque, and the extent of attachment loss. However, most studies do not support a causal relationship between periodontal diseases and reduced salivary flow rates even in patients with Sjögren's syndrome who have long-term reductions in saliva flow rates. However, impaired mechanical flushing and cleansing due to reduced salivary flow may accelerate accumulation of dental plaque that in turn may lead to gingivitis.

Saliva and gastrointestinal functions

Reduced salivary flow results in decreased bicarbonate concentration in the swallowed saliva and therefore decreased neutralization and clearance of gastric acid that enters the lower oesophagus as the result of normal reflux activity: this may increase the risk of developing gastro-oesophageal reflux and gastric ulceration. Furthermore, mucosal protection may be impaired because of diminished lubrication of the oral, oro-pharyngeal and oesophageal mucosa by salivary mucins. Salivary epidermal growth factor also plays an important role in the maintenance of oro-oesophageal and gastric tissue integrity. The biological effects of saliva influence the biology of the oesophagus through their effects on epidermal growth (including the healing of ulcers), inhibition of gastric acid secretion (through a feedback mechanism), and mucosal protection against intra-luminal factors such as gastric acid, bile acids, pepsin and trypsin, as well as physical, chemical and bacterial factors. Dysphagia is a common complaint in patients with hyposalivation and is assumed to be a consequence of oesophageal dysmotility and altered swallowing pattern due to reduced salivary flow as well as prolonged bolus formation. Moreover, salivary gland hypofunction may indirectly influence gastrointestinal functions by causing loss of appetite, fear of eating, special food preferences, weight loss, malabsorption and malnutrition.

Saliva and taste

Taste is a major stimulus for the secretion of saliva. At the same time, tastes are perceived only when saliva is present in the mouth because taste receptor cells respond only to dissolved substances (chapter 2). Furthermore, taste sensitivity is related to saliva composition as this fluid baths each receptor cell's oral surface. Complaints of taste disturbances including abnormal and impaired sense of taste are common among patients with Sjögren's syndrome and patients who have received radiotherapy and chemotherapy. In these patients, impairment of the threshold for perceiving taste as well as perception of the intensity of the four basic taste modalities has been reported.

function, past and current medication, general and oral diseases, trauma to the head, previous therapies including surgery, radiotherapy in the head and neck region and/or chemotherapy (Tables 3 and 4). A questionnaire including four questions may be useful in identifying patients with xerostomia and salivary gland hypofunction (Table 5). Dryness of the lips and buccal mucosa, inability to provoke salivary secretion by palpating the gland as well as total score of decayed, missing and filled teeth are additional predictive measures of salivary gland hypofunction. The level of oral dryness experienced by the patients may also be measured by different methods (Table 6).

Extra- and intra-oral examination

The second step in the evaluation of potential salivary gland dysfunction is a thorough facial and intraoral examination including inspection and palpation of the major and minor salivary glands, the major salivary duct orifices, the oral mucosa, the dentition, and the gingivae (see Table 4 for clinical signs).

Collection of saliva

The clinical examination should be followed by measurement of salivary flow rates. Stimulated and unstimulated flow rates can

■ Diagnosis of salivary gland hypofunction

History-taking and subjective measures of xerostomia

The procedure for identifying an individual with potential salivary gland dysfunction requires a careful and systematic evaluation. The first step is to take a detailed history of present symptoms, compromised oro-pharyngeal functions related to salivary hypo-

Table 5. Selected xerostomia related questions.

1. Does your mouth feel dry when eating a meal?
2. Do you have difficulties swallowing any foods?
3. Do you sip liquids to aid in swallowing dry foods?
4. Does the amount of saliva in your mouth seem too little, too much, or have you not noticed it?

Scientifically validated questions, which may be helpful in identifying patients with xerostomia and salivary gland hypofunction. The questions are mainly related to dry mouth experienced during mealtime and positive responds are highly predictive of salivary gland hypofunction.

Table 6. Methods for assessment of subjective symptoms of dry mouth.

A.	B.
Self-rating categorised questionnaire with 4 degrees of severity*:	Visual analogue scale (VAS)
0=I have no feeling of dry mouth	100 mm; Worst imaginable feeling of dry mouth
1=I have a slight feeling dry mouth	
2=I have a severe feeling of dry mouth	
3=I have an annoying feeling of dry mouth that makes speech difficult.	
Modified according to Beck's inventory scale, item 9.	0 mm; No feeling of dry mouth

An ordinal scale based on rank-ordered categories (A) and a visual analogue scale (B) representing magnitude estimation. Regarding the latter, the patients are asked to mark the point that best corresponds to their feeling of dry mouth on a 100 mm straight line. Verbal labels are assigned to both ends of the scale to indicate the extremes. 0 mm represents no feeling of oral dryness and 100 mm the worst imaginable feeling of oral dryness intensity. The methods may also be helpful in assessing the intensity of oral dryness over a time span or the effects of saliva stimulatory treatment.

be measured for whole saliva or individually for the parotid, submandibular/sublingual glands using various techniques. This chapter, however, deals with only one method for measurement of whole saliva secretion (i.e. the "draining method") for the following reasons: the method is relatively simple; it can easily be conducted in the dental office; it requires only a few tools (Figure 11); it is internationally accepted, it is the standard method for measuring unstimulated whole saliva flow rate (1993 European classification criteria for the diagnosis of Sjögren's syndrome), and is highly reproducible and reliable. Finally, the measurement of whole saliva provides a general assessment of salivary gland capabilities under basal and stimulated conditions.

Prior to the collection of saliva, the patient sits relaxed in a chair for a few minutes. The collection of unstimulated saliva is done without any masticatory or gustatory stimulus. Movements of the tongue, cheeks, jaws or lips should be avoided during the collection period. For comparisons of salivary gland function over time, collections in each patient should be carried out at the same time of day. The patient must be instructed to refrain from eating, drinking, smoking, and oral hygiene manoeuvres for at least 90 minutes prior to the collection.

Salivary flow rates exhibit large variations between healthy individuals. Despite the wide variation in normal whole saliva flow rates, it is generally accepted that unstimulated rates of 0.3–0.5 ml/min and stimulated rates of 1.0–1.5 ml/min are within the normal range. The diagnosis of hyposalivation is given when the unstimulated, whole salivary flow rate is 0.1 ml/min or less and when whole salivary flow rates stimulated by chewing paraffin are 0.5 ml/minute or less for women, and 0.7 ml/minute or less for men. Thus, the flow rates in hyposalivation are much lower than the "normal" values. If the flow rate measurements suggest salivary gland dysfunction, a more extensive and specialized investigation of the patient is indicated. In cases of medication-induced hyposalivation and/or xerostomia and polypharmacy, the patient's physician should be consulted to discuss the possibility of changing the medication to another with less adverse effects or, subject to the need to treat the underlying systemic disease adequately, changing the dose.

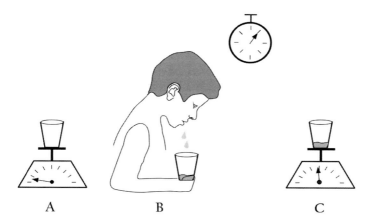

A   B   C

Figure 11. *Measurement of unstimulated and stimulated whole saliva flow rate.*
The tools required are a watch, a weight with two digits, a plastic cup, and for saliva stimulation 1 g of paraffin (inert chewing material) and a metronome. The patient is seated in a relaxed position with his/her head slightly tilted forward. After an initial swallowing action, the patient is instructed to allow saliva to passively drain from the lower lip into a pre-weighed plastic cup. The collection starts at time zero. At the end of the collection period, residual saliva is expectorated from the mouth into the cup. The saliva-containing plastic cup is reweighed, and the flow rate is calculated in g/min, which is almost equivalent to ml/min. Collection of stimulated whole saliva is performed after collection of unstimulated saliva following the same the procedure as described above with the exception of shorter collection time and application of a chewing stimulus. Every 30 seconds the patient should let the saliva drip into the pre-weighed plastic cup for a few seconds and then saliva collection continues. Measurement of the unstimulated whole saliva flow rate is usually performed for 15 minutes and chewing stimulated saliva for 5 minutes.

Sialochemistry

Saliva may also be collected for analysis of its composition (sialochemistry). The easy accessibility of salivary glands and their secretion has increased the interest in sialochemical analysis. Thus saliva can serve as an excellent tool for determination of various substances like hormones and drugs as well as for determination of infections of the oral cavity. For these purposes a number of chair side and handy test kits are available on the market. Nevertheless, when it comes to determination of the inorganic saliva composition it is important to keep the physiology of the salivary glands in mind. Thus, in contrast to many other bodily fluids, human saliva does not have a constant inorganic composition, because its inorganic composition is strongly influenced by the flow rate and stimulation intensity at which it is collected. It is therefore a prerequisite for inorganic sialochemistry that the methods of collection are in accordance with the methods described earlier in this chapter. Furthermore, determination of saliva pH, bicarbonate concentration and buffer capacity, requires closed systems to avoid loss of CO_2 and thus bicarbonate.

■ Management of oral sequelae of salivary hypofunction

First, the patient must be informed about the relationship between salivary hypofunction and the increased predisposition for oral disorders. The key concepts of preventive dental management include careful instruction of patients in oral hygiene, and regular (at least every 3-month) follow-up at a dental clinic including dental plaque control, dietary instruction and application of topical fluoride in order to reduce the caries activity. Sugar-free chewing gum containing fluoride may be useful. In these patients, the beneficial effect of fluoride on tooth substance is prolonged due to the low saliva flow rate and subsequently, reduced oral clearance. During meals, these patients should be advised to sip water when eating and swallowing. After the meal they should rinse their mouths thoroughly with water.

At present, due to the lack of controlled clinical trials, there is no consensus on which dental materials are the most appropriate for restorative treatment in patients with hyposalivation. The mouths of denture-wearers should be examined frequently to detect and treat possible mucosal ulcerations and denture stomatitis. If present, oral candidiasis should be treated with topical application of miconazole (2%) ointment or gel, nystatin ointment or oral suspension. Systemic treatment with fluconazole, ketaconazole or itraconazole should be reserved for refractory cases and immuno-compromised patients.

The stimulation of salivary secretion is dependent on the presence of residual functioning salivary gland tissue, and this is determined by measurement of whole saliva flow rate stimulated by chewing. Gustatory and/or masticatory stimulation with regular use of sugar-free sweets or sugarless chewing gum may increase secretion of saliva. Acupuncture therapy has been shown to increase salivary flow rates significantly in Sjögren's syndrome patients with remaining functional salivary gland tissue. Pharmacological sialogogues (e.g., pilocarpine and cevimeline) may also stimulate an increase in salivary secretion. These drugs are cholinergic agonists that stimulate muscarinic receptors. They should be prescribed only in collaboration with the patient's physician in order to avoid unexpected side effects such as the aggravation of heart disease or interactions with other drugs. Symptoms of oral dryness may be alleviated by the use of mouth gels, oral sprays or artificial saliva. Some of the latter products contain carbomethylcellulose, mucins or electrolytes. However, many patients prefer to take small sips of water rather than use these preparations.

Future perspectives

The most common use of saliva as a diagnostic tool is to predict a patient's future caries risk. For this purpose, a simple measurement of the unstimulated saliva flow rate is still the most reproducible and informative measure to perform (Figure 6). Although measurements of saliva's buffer capacity and saturation with hydroxyapatite were among the first caries-related measurements performed with saliva, there are problems with performing both these measurement for clinical purposes because of the diffusion of CO_2 out of the saliva, as discussed earlier. The possible role of the salivary proteins as indicators of caries risk and progression still needs to be determined. If it turns out that specific salivary proteins have an impact on caries risk and progression, modern molecular techniques for protein characterisation could be used as tools for individual caries treatment planning. Thus, the future challenge for salivary researchers is to understand the functions of the genes and their expression of proteins in the salivary glands and saliva.

Several inexpensive and user-friendly diagnostic analysis systems are now appearing for salivary-based diagnosis. There is strong interest in the development of such systems for routine monitoring of biomarkers of systemic diseases, since saliva collection is a non-invasive and painless procedure.

Whole saliva samples contain desquamated epithelial cells from the oral mucosa from which DNA can be extracted and used for gene characterization. This may be utilised, for example, for gene mapping for identification of systemic disease polymorphisms that will give further insight into the pathophysiology of the disease. Microarray chip technology now allows for the simultaneous evaluation of gene expression patterns for thousands of genes, which enables comparisons to be made of gene expression profiles between different patient groups. The combination of the identification of disease gene polymorphisms and the understanding of the expression of these genes will be important tools for new therapies not only for salivary gland diseases but also for systemic diseases.

As the glands serve both exocrine and some endocrine functions, one strategy behind the use of gene therapy in salivary glands is to utilise the fact that, in addition to secreting proteins into saliva, the salivary gland tissues secrete proteins into the blood circulation. Although this technology is at a relative primitive stage today, the future for using human parotid or submandibular glands as target organs for gene therapies using recombinant DNA technology in which the genetic material of the host's cells can be manipulated is promising. Access to the gland via cannulation and retrograde infusion (by viral or non-viral methods) is a relatively simple procedure due to the easy accessibility of the main excretory duct of these glands.

■ Selected references

Bardow A, Moe D, Nyvad B, Nauntofte B. The buffer capacity and buffer systems of human whole saliva measured without loss of CO_2. Arch Oral Biol 2000;45:1–12.

Dawes C. A mathematical model of salivary clearance of sugar from the oral cavity. Caries Res 1983;17:321–334.

Garrett JR, Proctor GB. Control of salivation. In: Linden RWA (ed). The Scientific Basis of Eating. Basel: Karger 1998;135–155.

Larsen MJ, Pearce EI. Saturation of human saliva with respect to calcium salts. Arch Oral Biol 2003; 48:317–322.

Lenander-Lumikari M, Loimaranta V. Saliva and dental caries. Adv Dent Res 2000;14:40–47.

Levine MJ. Development of artificial salivas. Crit Rev Oral Biol Med 1993;4:279–286.

Mandel ID. The functions of saliva. J Dent Res 1987; 66 (Spec Issue): 623–627.

Nauntofte B. Regulation of electrolyte and fluid secretion in salivary acinar cells. Am J Physiol 1992;263:G823–G837.

Navazesh M, Christensen CM. A comparison of whole mouth resting and stimulated salivary measurement procedures. J Dent Res 1982;61:1158–1162.

Pedersen AM, Nauntofte B. Primary Sjögren's syndrome: oral aspects on pathogenesis, diagnostic criteria, clinical features, and approaches for therapy. Expert Opin Pharmacother 2001;2:1415–1436.

Thaysen JH, Thorn NA, Schwartz IL. Excretion of sodium, potassium, chloride and carbon dioxide. Am J Physiol 1954;178:155–159.

CHAPTER 2

Taste and smell

Andrew I. Spielman and Jonathan A. Ship

Goals:
The goals of this chapter are to provide the oral health practitioner with an understanding of
- The cranio-facial anatomy and physiology of the chemosensory systems
- The role taste and smell play in providing adequate sensory input about the nature, quality and quantity of food
- The interactions between taste and smell dysfunction and oral, pharyngeal and systemic health.

Key words:

chemosensory system; taste cell; bitter; sweet; sour; salty; umami; fungiform; filiform; foliate; circumvallate papillae; taste stripes; olfactory system; olfactory receptor cell; olfactory bulb; olfactory nerve; taste disorders; olfactory disorders; ageusia; dysgeusia; hypogeusia; hypergeusia; anosmia; dysosmia; hyposmia; hyperosmia; halitosis; malodour.

▇ Introduction

All animals including humans respond to chemical stimuli through specialized chemosensory systems such as taste and smell. However, not all soluble and volatile chemicals are detected by these sensory systems. For instance, painful, irritating and pungent chemicals are detected by other sensory receptors in the trigeminal system. Other chemicals associated with sexual and social signals (pheromones) are detected by the vomeronasal organ in most mammals and reptiles.

The senses of taste and olfaction in lower animals can affect a variety of social behaviours such as feeding, mating and territoriality. In all animals, including humans, taste and smell provide an important tool for food selection, evaluation, and avoidance of potentially toxic compounds: these senses are thus important in nutrition and metabolism and the quality of life in general.

Receptors for taste and olfaction are located at the entry port of the digestive and respiratory systems, respectively. Unlike other sensory systems where stimuli have a very short-term effect, soluble and volatile chemicals that interact with specialized peripheral chemosensory receptors are subsequently ingested or inhaled with potential long-term effects on the host. Intake or inhalation of chemicals could have both beneficial and harmful effects. Because taste and smell are the last steps before acceptance or rejection, both act as screening mechanisms for potentially harmful compounds.

Chemosensory systems have a close anatomical and functional relationship with the oral cavity. Head, neck, and oral health professionals (including dentists) need to have a thorough understanding of the anatomy, physiology, biology and pathology of the chemosensory systems to provide appropriate diagnosis or referral and for therapy for patients who experience chemosensory disorders. These conditions affect primarily the elderly, the fastest growing segment of the population of the Western world. Chemosensory disorders have frustrated clinicians for decades. Our lack of knowledge of the aetiopathogenesis of taste problems has prevented development of new and significant treatment options. This lack of progress has multiple reasons. It is difficult to maintain cultures of human taste and olfactory cells that could provide an *in vitro* model to study taste and smell in health and disease. This has forced most biochemical, electrophysiological, molecular and genetic studies to be carried out in experimental animals even though there are no taste and/or smell disorder animal models.

A distorted sense of taste and smell has a significant negative impact on the quality of human life. Although millions of adults suffer from taste disorders (for terminology, see Table 1), such diseases do not evoke the same degree of public recognition as visual or hearing-impairments. This is due, in part, to a lack of awareness of the existence of taste disorders even among many health professionals, public health officials, lawmakers, and the general public.

Taste

Organization of the taste (gustatory) system

The peripheral gustatory system is exposed to a variety of physical, chemical and biological insults. Extreme hot, cold, irritating, acidic and non-sterile stimuli may have damaging effects on peripheral taste receptors. Therefore, unlike all other sensory systems that have peripheral neuronal receptors, the peripheral gustatory system has evolved to have receptor cells that are rapidly-renewing, specialized *epithelial* cells. This adaptation ensures rapid regeneration of taste receptor cells that become damaged. The peripheral organ in the gustatory system is the *taste papilla*. Visible to the naked eye, taste papillae in humans come in at least 4 different shapes and are located on the tongue (Figure 1A), soft and hard palate, pharynx, epiglottis and larynx. The largest of the four types, the circumvallate (CV) papillae, are located on the dorsal surface of the tongue between the anterior 2/3 and posterior 1/3 along a V shaped line (Figure 2). The number of CV papillae varies from species to species. There are between 3 and 13 papillae in humans. In other animals, their number varies from just one in rodents to 25 in cows.

On the postero-lateral border of the tongue are the foliate papillae, each of which is a pocket shaped invagination lined with taste buds. The invaginations protect the taste buds from direct physical damage.

The third type of papillae, the mushroom shaped fungiform papillae, cover the anterior dorsal surface of the tongue. Compared with other gustatory papillae, they are the largest in number with 50–200 in humans.

Finally, the extralingual papillae are located on the soft and hard palate, the larynx, epiglottis and pharynx, with the most prominent being the Taste Stripes (or "geschmackstreifen" from the original German term), located on both sides of the palatal midline at the transition of the soft and hard palate.

Table 1. Commonly used terms and definitions of chemosensory disorders[1].

Term	Definition
Gustation	
Hypogeusia	Diminished ability to detect gustatory stimulants
Hypergeusia	Increased sensitivity to gustatory stimulants
Dysgeusia	Distorted perception of gustatory stimulants
Taste Agnosia	The inability to identify a gustatory stimulant although properly perceived
Ageusia	The inability to detect gustatory stimulants
Olfaction	
Normosmia	Normal smell
Hyposmia	Diminished ability to detect olfactory stimulants
Hyperosmia	Increased sensitivity to olfactory stimulants
Dysosmia	Distorted perception of olfactory stimulants
Olfactory Agnosia	The inability to identify an olfactory stimulant although properly perceived
Anosmia	The inability to detect olfactory stimulants

[1]All of the conditions can be: *General* to all stimulants. *Partial* to some but not all stimulants. *Specific* to one or a few stimulants.

Interestingly, the most abundant and recognizable structures, the filiform papillae are non-gustatory (Figure 1A and 2). When overgrown and stained by beverages and food dye these thread-like papillae tend to provide a characteristic colour to the tongue. Similarly, excessive shedding of the papillae provides a "white coat" on the tongue. On the other hand, loss of the filiform papillae creates a dry and smooth appearance which is associated with a variety of oral and systemic conditions such as dry mouth, anaemia and Scarlet fever. The filiform papillae act like "Velcro®" to help secure food to the tongue so that the bolus can be moved around the oral cavity.

Within each taste papilla there are varying number of *taste buds* visible under transmission and electron microscopes. The number of taste buds varies from one papilla to the next. In humans, fungiform papillae contain 1–10 (Figure 1B), CV papillae contain 100–200, while foliate papillae may have from a few hundred to a few thousand buds.

The taste bud is the functional unit of the peripheral taste organ. It is onion-shaped and contains 50–100 continuously-maturing *taste receptor* and supporting cells (Figure 1D). Most of the taste cells in a bud are shielded from the oral cavity. Only the apical tip containing taste receptor proteins of a few taste cells is exposed to the oral cavity through a 3–5 micron wide opening, referred to as the *taste pore* (Figure 1C). Unlike any other sensory system, taste cells have a rapid turnover rate of 10.5 days, which is about twice as fast as the surrounding epithelial cells. The progenitor cells, also known as basal cells, are located in an epithelial layer at the base of the taste bud that corresponds to the germinal layer of the epithelium. As taste receptor cells continuously grow and mature, they migrate from the basal area of the bud toward the taste pore. Exposure of an individual receptor cell to taste stimulants is limited usually to a single meal. Within a few hours of a chemosensory experience, the exposed taste receptor cells are shed into the oral cavity and are washed away by saliva. The fungiform- and taste-stripe-containing taste buds are bathed in saliva from the bilateral major salivary glands (parotid, submandibular, sublingual). In contrast, taste buds in the circumvallate and foliate taste papillae are washed primarily by the saliva of the von Ebner's salivary glands located in the body of the tongue with openings into the trenches that surround these papillae.

The sensory pathway for taste involves a chain of neurons in series (Figure 2). *First order neurons* connect the periphery to the nucleus of the solitary tract where they synapse *second order neurons,* cross the midline and connect with the thalamus, while the *third order neurons* connect the thalamus to the cortex. The sensory pathway for taste involves neural connections with the salivary nuclei to activate a reflex pathway (see Chapter 1 on Saliva) and the perception of taste depends on the signals reaching the sensory cortex.

First order neurons: The peripheral epithelial taste receptor cells synapse at the taste bud level with the primary afferent neurons whose cell bodies within the three cranial

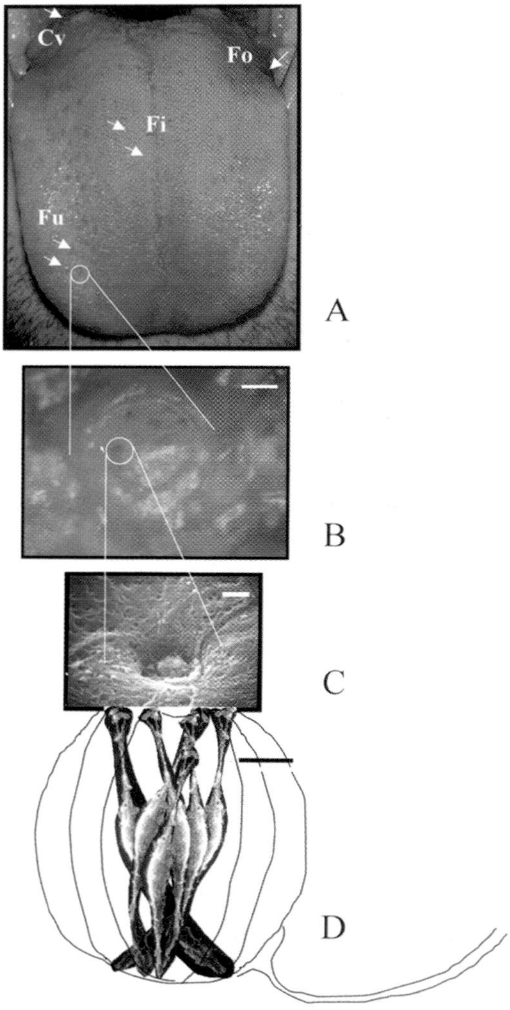

Figure 1. *Human tongue.*
A. The dorsal surface of the human tongue has three gustatory [fungiform (Fu), circumvallate (Cv) and foliate (Fo)] and one non-gustatory papillae [filiform (Fi)]. The foliate papillae are sheltered in the side of the tongue and hence are not visible.
B. A magnified view of a human fungiform papilla. Each fungiform papilla may contain 1–10 taste buds that communicate with the oral cavity through a taste pore. (Bar ~ 100 μm).
C. Magnified view of a taste pore. A scanning electron micrograph (SEM) of a rat fungiform papilla. The central pit represents the taste pore. Bar ~1 μm.
D. Underneath each taste pore in each fungiform papilla is a barrel-shaped taste bud that contains 50–100 taste cells. The SEM of a few mouse taste receptor cells are schematically assembled in a composite graphic representation of a taste bud. (Bar ~10 μm). The taste cells synapse with first order neurons belonging to the chorda tympani nerve (one such synapse is represented in the lower right corner of the taste bud). (Fig. A. – Reproduced with permission from Spielman and Lischka, Taste and Smell, Encyclopedia of Gastroenterology, Academic Press Inc. 2004, in press; Fig. C. – Spielman and Brand, Tongue and Taste, In: Encyclopedia of Human Biology, 1997, pp. 456–466; Fig D. – Spielman et al., Brain Research, 1989, 503:326–329).

Figure 2. *Gustatory receptors, innervation and central pathways.*
The human tongue is innervated by four branches of three cranial nerves: chorda tympani (VII) glossopharyngeal (IX), vagus (X) and the greater petrosal superficial nerves (VII). The central projections of the three cranial nerves end in the nucleus of the solitary tract of the rostral medulla. The cell bodies of the three cranial nerves are located in the geniculate ganglion of the facial nerve, the petrosal ganglion of the glossopharyngeal nerve, and the nodose ganglion of the vagus.

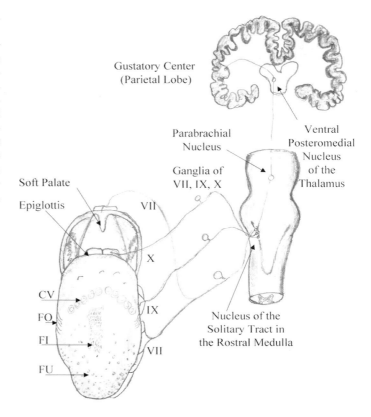

nerve ganglia: facial, glossopharyngeal and vagus. The anterior two-thirds of the tongue from the fungiform papillae and some of the foliate papillae are innervated by the facial (VII) nerve (*chorda tympani* branch) and have their cell bodies in the geniculate ganglion. The greater petrosal superficial nerve, another branch of the facial nerve, conducts chemosensory signals from the papillae located on the soft palate: the cell bodies of these neurones, like those of *chorda tympani* neurons, are located in the geniculate ganglion. Chemosensory input from the posterior one-third of the tongue is conducted along the glossopharyngeal nerve (IX) whose cell bodies are in the inferior glossopharyngeal ganglion (petrosal ganglion). In-

formation from taste receptors in the pharynx, epiglottis and larynx is transmitted along the vagus (X) nerve whose cell bodies lie in the inferior ganglion of the vagus (nodose ganglion). Central projections of the three nerve ganglia enter the brain stem and synapse with *second order neurones* in the *gustatory division of the solitary nucleus* of the medulla. Fibers ascend from the medulla and project to the *ventral posterior medial nucleus* of the thalamus. From the thalamus, *third-order neurons* project to the primary gustatory cortex, which is located in the insular and orbitofrontal regions of the parietal lobe. In contrast, in lower animals, gustatory connections from the nucleus of the solitary tract are mediated through the parabrachial nucleus to the hypothalamus and amygdala. This functional connection, however, does not exist in humans.

Taste physiology and clinical function

The sensation of taste can be elicited by a diverse group of chemical compounds. These range from simple ions such as iodine or potassium to complex carbohydrates such as sucrose octa-acetate. The traditional classification of taste in humans is based upon four basic taste qualities: sweet, sour, salty, and bitter. However, additional taste qualities and stimuli are known. Umami or savory taste, for instance, is elicited by the amino acid monosodium glutamate and monosodium aspartate, and is considered, along with fat, electric and metallic taste, as distinct taste qualities. These diverse stimuli use diverse signalling mechanisms.

Gustatory stimuli interact first with cell surface or intracellular taste receptor proteins. Generally, the specific *receptor proteins* both the ionotropic and the metabotropic receptor types, are located on the apical tip of the exposed taste receptor cells. Binding of the chemical to the receptor induces a change in the balance of ions across its cell surface membrane which leads to cell depolarisation and release of neurotransmitter from the receptor cell. The resulting depolarisation of the afferent fiber of the cranial nerve innervating the cell and generation of an action potential. Changes in the firing rate of this nerve fibre are conveyed to the primary gustatory cortex where the message is decoded into a perceptual modality.

During the last few years, a variety of taste receptor candidates, ion channels, ligand-gated channels, enzymes and G-protein-coupled receptors (GPCRs) have been identified for the five better known taste qualities: sour, salty, sweet, bitter, and the taste of the amino acid monosodium glutamate (umami or savory taste). The distribution of these receptors to most taste papillae demonstrates that there is no exclusivity of a particular area of the tongue to a specific taste quality. However, certain subtypes of taste receptors within a taste quality are predominantly located in one or another region of the tongue making that region more sensitive, but not exclusive, to a taste quality. For instance, the structure of the ENaC ion channel involved in salty taste reception is different in the back of the tongue vs. the front of the tongue. Similarly, certain, but not all bitter taste receptors are predominantly located on the taste buds of the circumvallate taste papillae and almost non-existent on the fungiform papillae. This distribution shows taste papillae-specific expression of certain taste receptors.

Sour taste: Sour taste is elicited by protons (H^+) and the intensity of the sour taste is proportional to the concentration of titratable acids in contact with the taste buds. This taste quality, along with bitter, is a protective or warning signal because protons may have a local effect on oral soft and hard tissue, or a systemic effect when acidity indicates spoiled food.

Several candidate receptors for sour taste have been identified, including amiloride-sensitive epithelial sodium channels (ENaCs), proton-gated channels (MDEG1, K^+ channels), hyperpolarization-activated cyclic nucleotide-gated channels (HCNs), H^+-gated ion channels, and the acid-sensing ion channels (ASICs). With such diverse putative receptors, it is not surprising that a number of different mechanisms are associated with the transduction of the sour taste signal, indicating the complexity of this sensory quality. Generally, all potential mechanisms for sour taste lead to an increase in intracellular positive charge that results in direct depolarisation of the receptor cells. Some of these mechanisms are supported by behavioural studies in which the administration of the epithelial sodium channel blocker amiloride to experimental animals reduced the normal aversive response to the presence of acids in their mouths. The specific signal transduction mechanisms for most of these receptors remain to be elucidated.

The mechanisms of salivation and gustation are tightly linked. Sour is the strongest stimulus for salivary secretion. As the salivary flow rates increase, higher levels of bicarbonates are secreted (Chapter 1), and these then buffer the protons and hence protect the oral tissues from damage. Humans grimace strongly when they experience sour tastes (that is, they screw up their faces, which you can easily demonstrate for yourselves). The grimace involves strong contractions of facial muscles that channel saliva onto the surface of the tongue and thus help to neutralize the protons. Sour stimuli such as lemon juice can have a pH of about 2. These concentrations are potentially injurious to intra-oral tissues, particularly enamel, and are in fact more acidic than is necessary to elicit a sour taste: hence buffering with saliva is a desirable outcome.

Salty taste: Like "sour", "salty" taste indicates the presence of ions which directly interact with ion channels. Unlike sour, however, salty is an essential detector of minerals and provides an important mechanism for ion homeostasis. The most important ions for the stimulation of the salty taste are sodium and chloride.

In rodents, an amiloride-sensitive epithelial sodium channel (ENaC) on the receptor cell membrane allows for sodium influx while the detection of chloride appears to be mediated by a paracellular transport. In humans, ENaC is less prominent. Additional, as yet been unidentified mechanisms may also be involved in human salty taste.

Sweet taste: Sweet taste in humans is elicited by a variety of compounds including sugars and sugar derivatives, D-amino acids, some of the small L-amino acids (glycine, and L-alanine), artificial sweeteners such as cyclamate, saccharine, aspartame, sucralose, and very high potency sweeteners. Unlike sourness, sweetness is associated with high-calorie foods: because they taste desirable, humans (and animals) seek out sweet-tasting foods, with some adverse consequences for metabolic balance in Western societies in particular.

The mechanism of sweet taste detection is mediated by G-protein coupled receptors (GPCRs) A candidate sweet receptor, the T1R3, was cloned and found to be functional only in the presence of another taste receptor, T1R2, as a heterodimer. Both receptors are expressed in about twenty percent of the taste cells located in the posterior, lateral and anterior taste buds of the tongue. The mechanism by which sweet taste is transduced has been previously elucidated. T1R3/T1R2 receptors are probably coupled through an increase in cGMP and activation of a cyclic-nucleotide-gated channel that leads to depolarization of the receptor cells through an influx of calcium. Interestingly, artificial sweeteners use a different pathway (the IP3 pathway) which is similar to that used in the transduction of taste elicited by many bitter compounds.

Bitter taste: Detection of potentially harmful, even toxic compounds is one of the primary roles of bitter taste. This gustatory response can be evoked by a large and diverse array of compounds ranging from ions (such as potassium) to complex artificial (denatonium), or naturally-occurring compounds (caffeine, strychnine, quinine). Many poisonous substances have a bitter taste; hence the aversive response that bitter tastes evoke has a potential survival benefit. This is reflected in the threshold for the perception of bitterness which is the lowest of all the taste qualities. In addition, there are more receptors for bitter taste than for any other taste quality, and the range of mechanisms for the transduction of bitter taste is believed to be the most diverse of all the taste qualities.

Like sweet taste, bitter taste transduction involves primarily G-protein coupled receptors as cell surface binding sites for many bitter stimulants. A family of 50 to 80 membrane-associated bitter taste receptors, termed T2Rs, was recently identified in rodents and humans. In humans, T2Rs are encoded in 24 genes and located on three chromosomes. It is assumed, although not yet verified, that all T2Rs are bitter responsive.

Bitter taste receptors are coupled through gustducin, a taste tissue-enriched G protein α subunit, and associated $\beta 3$ and $\gamma 13$ subunits to the cyclic nucleotide and the phosphoinositide signal transduction pathways. Gustducin activates one or more phosphodiesterases, reducing the levels of cyclic nucleotides (cAMP and cGMP) leading to opening of a cyclic nucleotide-gated cation channel and cell depolarization. The $\beta 3/\gamma 13$ activates Phospholipase C$\beta 2$ that releases two second messengers: inositol trisphosphate (IP$_3$) and diacylglycerol (DAG). The former releases intracellular calcium leading to cell depolarization. The specific interplay of these two second messengers, reduction of cyclic nucleotides and increase of IP$_3$ and DAG, are not known; nor is it clear which

of these is the leading event in causing depolarization.

A number of additional mechanisms have been described for bitter compounds including inhibition of potassium channels, inhibition of phosphodiesterases, and inhibition of several types of protein kinases. The scope of this chapter precludes a detailed description of these mechanisms.

Umami (amino acid) taste: A taste quality specific for monosodium glutamate (MSG) has been named "umami", from the Japanese word for delicious (*umai*). This taste is synergistically enhanced in the presence of 5' ribonucleotides, especially inosine 5'-monophosphate (IMP) and guanosine 5'-monosphosphate (GMP). MSG and glutamate, the excitatory neurotransmitter, are almost identical. It was therefore reasonable to expect that receptors might be related. A truncated form of the brain glutamate receptor mGluR4 has been found in the taste system and is one of a number of candidate receptors for umami. The signal transduction mechanism for umami which uses the mGluR4 receptor is assumed to be similar to that located in the brain, and a reduction in the level of cAMP leads to a closure of an unspecified cation conductance. One problem with this mech-

In aquatic animals, other amino acids act as taste stimulants. Catfish for instance shows sensitivity to L-arginine, L-alanine and glycine. The L-arginine receptor is a ligand-gated non-selective cation channel and is primarily located on the barbell, two large projections on both sides of the face close to the oral cavity.

anism is that the mGluR4 receptors are generally inhibitory. Since tasting MSG probably requires an excitatory response from the taste cell, the actual role that an inhibitory receptor like mGLuR4 plays in transduction of the taste of MSG is open to question.

Recently, a completely different receptor type for MSG has been proposed, one that has little homology with other known glutamate receptors. This receptor is a dimer of two of the receptor proteins of the T1R family, namely T1R1/T1R3. This dimer is similar to the proposed sweet receptor, except that one monomer of the dimer pair is different. For sweet taste the dimer is T1R2/T1R3. One interesting feature of the T1R1/T1R3 receptor for MSG is that its response to glutamate is enhanced by the ribonucleotides. This synergism between glutamate and the ribonucleotides is a hallmark of umami taste, and the observation that IMP enhances the T1R1/T1R3 dimer lends credence to the suggestion that T1R1/T1R3 is the major receptor for umami taste.

Japanese cuisine has taken advantage of appropriate combinations of foods to maximize this synergistic effect. The combination of pork, chicken, black mushroom, sea bream, etc. which contain nucleotides, and tomatoes, cauliflower, celery, carrots, and mushroom that are rich in MSG, lead to an enhanced taste for glutamate via this synergistic culinary effect.

As explained before, it was assumed for many years that specific regions of the tongue are tuned for specific taste qualities. However, it is now clear that all three gustatory nerves (VII, IX, X) carry all taste stimuli. In fact, many single nerve taste afferent fibres are broadly tuned to carry information about multiple types of gustatory stimuli.

Opposed to regional variations in sensitivity are individual variations in taste. In mice, genetic variations in perception of bitter and sweet taste are well documented. Such genetic variation, although not as widespread is also true in humans with the best studied being "taste blindness" or insensitivity to phenylthiocarbamide (PTC). From mouse genetic studies we know that the difference among individuals is located on the periphery, most likely in the structure of a receptor or one of the signal transduction components. The molecular basis of PTC taste insensitivity is not fully understood but likely to be associated with a peripheral receptor or signalling molecule.

Repeated exposure to the same taste quality induces a process called *adaptation*, a decreased response to the same concentration of a stimulus. That is, taste cells respond only at a higher threshold. This phenomenon is relatively slow in taste. It may take seconds before taste cells adapt to a particular stimulus. Taste cells threshold can be reset (lowered) by exposure to water.

Saliva-taste interaction

Gustatory function at the peripheral level requires three factors: a molecule that elicits taste, a taste receptor cell, and an aqueous environment usually provided by saliva. Saliva plays a critically important role in taste function, and there is a mutual interaction between taste and salivation: saliva affects taste perception and various gustatory stimuli influence salivary composition (see Chapter 1 for more information on the various roles of saliva). Saliva contributes to tasting ability in several ways: first, as a solvent of food, second, as a carrier of taste-eliciting molecules, and third, through its composition. Accordingly, when salivary output is affected adversely (due to oral or systemic conditions, medications, or head and neck radiotherapy), taste function can be concomitantly affected.

The effect of saliva on taste

Saliva's primary role in taste function is to dissolve the taste stimulus and carry it to the taste buds. This capacity is diminished when there is inadequate salivary production, particularly in response to gustatory stimuli. Taste stimuli play a major role in salivation, by affecting output quantitatively and qualitatively. For example, sour taste increases salivary flow-rates and bicarbonate levels, the major buffering agent in saliva. As a consequence, an increase in salivary pH has a diminishing effect on sour taste perception. Lower salivary flow rates lead to lower sour taste recognition thresholds and conversely, individuals with higher salivary flow rates have higher sour taste thresholds. Thus, variations in salivary flow rates may partly explain individual differences in sour taste sensitivity.

Salivary composition, taste thresholds, and adaptation

Saliva itself contains sweet, sour and bitter compounds (e.g., glucose in trace amounts, NaCl, and urea), which are not perceived in normal individuals because of a continuous exposure to salivary stimulation and taste cell adaptation. The sour, sweet or salty taste of these compounds are perceived only when host threshold levels are exceeded.

Saliva – a dynamic ionic environment of taste cells

The taste pore of each taste papilla is either directly or indirectly bathed by saliva which provides the ionic environment in which transduction of the taste signal occurs. The ionic composition of saliva depends on its flow-rate, and is different from the interstitial fluid that surrounds the rest of the unexposed

taste cell. The dual ionic environment of taste cells, especially at the apical membrane, is critically important during the process of gustation. Taste cells, like most excitable cells, have a negative resting potential across the membrane. Unstimulated parotid and submandibular saliva contains Na^+ in the range of 1–3 mmol/l. This is almost identical to intracellular Na^+ levels. When parotid saliva is stimulated (flow rate of $\sim$1 ml/min), sodium concentrations increase to approximately 35 mmol/l, and they can even reach over 100 mmol/l at very high flow rates, approaching the levels of interstitial sodium. Under similar stimulation circumstances, salivary potassium concentrations fall from a high level of 24 mmol/l to $\sim$13 mmol/l, and thus remain well below the intracellular levels of the taste cells, but still at a much higher level that that of the interstitial fluid. Therefore, changes in the salivary electrolyte concentrations upon stimulation affect the cation gradients across the taste cell membrane and consequently the membrane potential and the opening of the cation channels clustered on the apical membrane. These events are important not only for the depolarization but also for the mechanism of repolarization following taste receptor-mediated depolarization.

In summary, there are parallel mechanisms in healthy persons between taste transduction and salivary function.

Diminished salivary flow rates and taste perception

Local and systemic disorders that affect salivary output have been shown to affect the sense of taste. A common example is the radiation of the head and neck that is used for the treatment of cancer. Radiation has deleterious effects on both taste cells and salivary glands and thus directly or indirectly affects gustation. Other diseases and medical problems affect the composition of saliva (e.g., adrenergic blocking agents) which could then influence taste. While no specific salivary constituent has been directly connected to gustatory disorders, it has been hypothesized that certain salivary electrolytes and minerals contribute to normal taste sensation. One mineral that was traditionally implicated in taste dysfunction was zinc, however it is now accepted that zinc supplementation is not a useful method for treating dysgeusia (i.e., the distortion or absence of the sense of taste).

Salivary proline-rich proteins and bitter taste

Salivary proline-rich proteins (PRPs) represent 70% of the proteins and the largest single family in human parotid saliva. An early study reported a genetic link between PRPs and the ability to taste the bitter compounds quinine, raffinose undecaacetate, and cycloheximide in mice. However, the decoding of the murine genome has revealed that there is no link between these two sets of genes, except closely sharing some of the same chromosomes.

■ Disorders of gustation

The gustatory system is remarkably resilient to damage and to age-related disorders. This is due primarily to the bilateral and nearly redundant system of cranial nerves (VII, IX, X) that subserve taste function. In addition, the trigeminal nerve (cranial nerve V) that innervates the soft tissues in which the taste buds are imbedded relays thermal, tactile, and pain sensation to the brain that augments the sensation and interpretation of taste function. For instance chilli pepper activates a number of sensory and chemosensory receptors. Cold beer activates: pain, temperature and taste receptors. Many oral and systemic conditions, topical oral medicaments, oral traumatic events, and the treatment of systemic diseases (medications, radiotherapy, chemotherapy) affect the gustatory system. Commonly-used topical oral medicaments, such as anti-plaque mouth-

Saliva and chemical communications

All animals, including humans, respond to chemicals in the environment through a process termed chemoreception. In lower animals, chemical signalling is the most important means of communication. Animals release chemicals through body secretions or odours that influence other animals' behaviours. There are a large number of potential sources of chemical signals such as urine, faeces, genital discharge, secretions from the accessory organs, and saliva. Secretions may be applied either onto the body or into the environment. One salivary molecule that is associated with chemical signalling has been identified, named pheromaxein. This is a pheromonal steroid-binding protein from submandibular glands and saliva of the miniature wild boar. Pheromaxein acts as a carrier for 16-androstenes, which is abundantly secreted by the submandibular gland of the male boar primarily when it is aroused by the presence of estrous females or alien boars. Therefore, the combination of smell and taste, in conjunction with chemicals released through body secretions or odors, plays a major role in animals' behavior including suckling and mating.

rinses, toothpastes, and gels are associated with taste alterations (Table 2). Iatrogenic injury during or subsequent to dental treatments and the use of local anaesthetics can cause taste disorders. Other trauma such as exposure to excessively hot food or liquids or chemical burns are common. Metal restorations of teeth are commonly reported to cause a transient metallic taste in some patients. Complete and partial dentures can block access to taste receptor cells and produce a transient gustatory alteration. Intra-oral infections and inflammatory conditions such as candidiasis, gingivitis, periodontal disease, dental caries, dentoalveolar infections, herpetic lesions, pulpal necrosis, traumatic lesions, vesiculobullous diseases (e.g., pemphigus, pemphigoid, lichen planus) and burning mouth syndrome can all contribute to unpleasant tastes or altered taste function (Table 3).

Losses in gustatory function are not a common consequence of aging, and most changes in taste perception occur later in life than olfactory dysfunction. Taste-specific (i.e. sweet, salty, sour, bitter) changes have been reported, yet it appears that global changes in gustation do not occur as a result of the aging process. Further, there is no evidence that numbers of papillae and taste buds decrease over time. However, numerous older adults are treated for systemic conditions that may affect the gustatory system either directly or indirectly. For example, many medications taken by elderly patients directly affect taste perception and inhibit salivary output impairing gustation. Head and neck cancer treatment (surgery, chemotherapy, radiotherapy) causes short and long-term damage to the anatomical and nerve pathways responsible for transmitting taste sensation.

Many older adults complain of taste losses, but they are typically due to problems with olfaction. Age- and disease-related losses in olfaction play a large role in diminished gustatory function. Any condition that results in a compromised environment for the mediators of chemosensation (e.g., tongue, saliva, oral and nasal mucosa, neural pathways, neurotransmitters) will result

Table 2. Oral products and medications commonly used in dentistry that are associated with chemosensory disorders.

Drug or oral product	Taste disorder	Smell disorder
Amphotericin B	✓	
Ampicillin		✓
Azathioprine	✓	
Benzocaine	✓	✓
Carbamazepine	✓	✓
Chlorhexidine	✓	✓
Ciprofloxacin		✓
Dexamethasone	✓	✓
Doxycycline		✓
Hydrocortisone	✓	✓
Isotretinoin	✓	
Lidocaine	✓	✓
Metronidazole	✓	
Sodium lauryl sulfate	✓	✓
Tetracaine	✓	
Tetracycline	✓	✓

Table 3. Oral conditions associated with chemosensory disorders.

Burning mouth syndrome
Candidiasis, denture stomatitis
Dento-alveolar infections
Drugs in saliva
Galvanism
Gingival and periodontal diseases
Oral mouthrinses, dentifrices, gels
Removable prosthodontic appliances
Salivary hypofunction
Soft tissue lesions
Trauma (burns, lacerations, chemical damage, anaesthetic, surgical)
Viral infections

in altered taste and smell perception at any age.

Salivary function plays an integral role in the generation and maintenance of taste sensations (see above). Accordingly, salivary hypofunction can result in altered taste perception or elevation of detection thresholds. Numerous medical problems (e.g., Sjögren's syndrome, diabetes, Alzheimer's disease), prescription and non-prescription medications (e.g., anticholinergics, antihypertensives, antipsychotics, antihistamines), head and neck radiotherapy for the treatment of cancers, and chemotherapy cause salivary dysfunction. The extent to which salivary hypofunction affects gustation is still under debate. Nevertheless, it is hypothesized that in the absence of saliva there is a diminished ability to transport stimuli to taste buds, and an increased risk of developing oral-pharyngeal microbial infections that will alter taste perception. Saliva may also act as a reservoir for medications or their metabolites resulting in an unpleasant taste.

Numerous medical problems and their treatment with medications and chemotherapy have been associated with altered taste sensation. Infections (e.g., influenza, sinusitis, herpes zoster, Human Immunodeficiency Virus or HIV), trauma (e.g., motor vehicle accident), and head and neck surgery can result in temporary or permanent damage to the nerves subserving taste sensation. Endocrine and metabolic disorders, including diabetes and hypothyroidism, have been associated with altered taste sensation. For example, diabetic neuropathies have been shown to increase taste thresholds. Finally, there is some evidence that genetics may determine the number of taste buds in an individual that could cause variable gustatory ability and perhaps even predisposition to or increased risk of developing taste disorders.

The effect of medications on the gustatory system may be transient, modifiable, or chronic. For example, 0.12% chlorhexidine rinse has been reported to produce a reversible peripheral impairment of taste sensation, in particular salty and bitter taste. While some medications cause alterations of specific tastes (sweet, bitter, salty, sour), others will increase taste or recognition thresholds. Drugs that have been associated with total loss of taste include local anesthetics (lidocaine), antineoplastics (bleomycine), and anti-rheumatics (penicillamine) (Table 2). The mechanisms behind these effects are complex and not yet clearly defined, but medication-induced taste dysfunction can occur at any of the transport, sensory, or processing levels of the gustatory system.

Finally, little is known regarding pollutants and their affect on the gustatory system. Environmental pollutants range from airborne chemicals, to metallic particles, to dust. Some pollutants such as insecticides can actually bind to the tongue altering taste bud morphology and consequently function.

Olfaction

Organization of the olfactory system
Thousands of volatile compounds in the environment can be detected by the sense of smell. The olfactory sensory neuroepithelium that mediates detection of such diverse compounds is located on the superior and middle turbinate (nasal conchae, Figure 3b). The olfactory neuroepithelium is made up of olfactory receptor neurons (ORNs), supporting (sustentacular) cells and mucous secreting cells that belong to the Bowman's glands. The ORNs are primarily bipolar neurons that detect the volatile compounds (Figure 3A). The dendritic processes of these neurons extend beyond the mucosa, cross the bony structure at the roof of the nasal

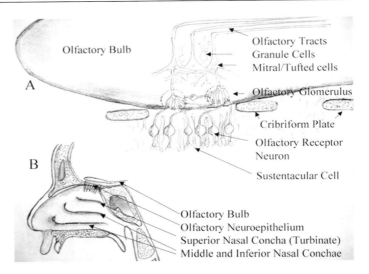

Figure 3. *Organization of the olfactory system.*
A. Olfactory neuroepithelium and the olfactory bulb.
B. Peripheral olfactory organ. Figure **A** represents a magnified image of the olfactory neuroepithelium, cribriform plate and olfactory bulb connections depicted in Figure **B**. Olfactory receptor neurons are located in the neuroepithelium around the superior and middle nasal conchae (turbinates). Axons of the olfactory neurons cross the cribriform plate (part of the ethmoid bone) and synapse in olfactory glomeruli. Second order neurons from the olfactory glomeruli synapse with the dendrites of the mitral/tufted cells. The axons of the mitral/tufted cells form the olfactory tracts connect to the olfactory cortex (not shown in the figure, described in the text).

cavity, the cribriform plate (ethmoid bone) and synapse with the olfactory glomeruli in the olfactory bulb.

At the apical end of the olfactory neuron, the receptor cells exhibit a knob-like structure that contains the olfactory receptor proteins and the proteins that participate in the signal transduction apparatus.

The turnover rate of the dividing basal cells that develop into mature functional olfactory neurons is 30–90 days. The non-sensory epithelium contains mucous secreting Bowman glands that cover the mucosa. The nasal (nonolfactory) mucosa is innervated by the infraorbital (second) branch of the trigeminal nerve.

■ Olfactory physiology

One of the largest family of related genes for olfaction was discovered in the early 1990s.

These putatively encode for several hundred, possibly one thousand different olfactory receptor proteins. To detect and distinguish thousands of different volatile structures, the olfactory system developed into a complex system of numerous olfactory receptors. These proteins, similar to those described for bitter and sweet taste, belong to the G-protein coupled, 7-transmembrane-spanning receptor family of proteins. While many of these sequences are conserved and appear similar to each other, the extracellular domains have highly variable regions that correspond to the exposed regions of the membrane receptor, considered as the putative odorant-binding domains. Once all olfactory receptors are functionally expressed, it remains to be seen whether these regions account for odorant binding. In humans, there are at least 350 functional olfactory receptor genes.

Olfactory signal transduction involves a specific cell surface receptor, an olfactory receptor cell-specific G protein (G_{olf}), adenylyl cyclase, production of cAMP and activation of ion channels that lead to cell depolarization and generation of an action potential. Unlike the gustatory system, the axons of the olfactory receptor neurons form the olfactory nerve, which extends through the cribriform plate and synapse in the olfactory bulb with second order neurons, mitral and tufted relay neurons of the glomeruli, in the outer layer of the olfactory bulb. The organization of these relay neurons forms a functional odour map that is related to the general chemical features of odorant structure. Activation of a specific region of the olfactory neuroepithelium by a specific odorant will stimulate a group of neighbouring olfactory relay neurons in the olfactory bulb thus defining that particular odorant. This is reflected in the pattern of parallel activation of these relay neurons. From here, the signals are further sent via output axons that form the olfactory tracts to the primary olfactory cortex, parts of the amygdala and the anterior region of the parahippocampal gyrus. The primary olfactory cortex projects information to the hypothalamus, the hippocampus, the rest of the amygdala and the thalamus.

Clinical function

The sense of smell allows humans to detect thousands of volatile compounds in the environment, some at a concentration of a few parts per trillion. Olfaction plays a major role in identifying and evaluating the flavour of food. It allows humans to detect odours in the environment (cooking odours, flowers, and odours that signal danger) that enrich and protect their quality of life. It also probably plays a major role in social behav-

iours such as interpersonal communications and the selection of mates.

When taste and smell, as well as other senses (temperature, pain, and touch) interact, they produce the sensation of flavour. Flavour is not the simple sum of all of the various sensory inputs, but a complex integration of them all. A common example is when a person experiences a cold or allergic rhinitis. Typically, the person experiences a dramatic reduction in smell and overall appreciation of food. The symptoms are most often interpreted as a loss of taste, yet the vast majority of these individuals have experienced a reduction of smell, rather than taste.

The texture and temperature of food influence taste and smell as well. The flavour of ice-cream is connected with its fat content (which contribute to the perception of both texture and taste), its sweetness (taste), its volatile flavour chemicals (smell), and its temperature. Similarly, the enjoyment of beer is dependent upon the inter-relationships of bitterness (taste), carbonation (activating mechanical and nociceptive fibres of the trigeminal system), the fluid nature (texture) and temperature. Enjoyment of hot and spicy food is dependent on the interaction of pain and temperature systems, as well as taste and smell. Most spicy foods contain hot chilli peppers: the "hotness" comes largely from the chemical capsaicin, which induces the sensation of pain. (hence one should be careful never to rub one's eyes after cutting up chillies!)

Although removed from the day to day interaction with a dentist, olfaction is an essential component in tasting, through the retronasal route. The inability to taste food is often confused with taste disorder and reported first to a dentist, hence the importance of understanding normal and abnormal olfaction.

Disorders of olfaction

Olfaction is entirely dependent upon neural function at peripheral receptor sites and centrally in the olfactory nerve (cranial nerve I), and is especially at risk from any disease or event with neurological sequelae. The most common cause of changes in the sense of smell is upper respiratory infection, which also alters gustation. These frequent viral and bacterial infections alter or block peripheral receptor sites. Non-respiratory bacterial or viral infections acute dentoalveolar infections, HIV, and candidiasis can adversely affect olfaction.

Aging has significant deleterious influences on olfaction: these are often complicated by medical problems and the medications taken for them. Detection and recognition thresholds for smell are raised in elderly individuals. The glomeruli of the olfactory bulb deteriorate with age, and alterations in the olfactory epithelium and the reduction in protein synthesis that occurs with normal aging may contribute to diminished smell perception and identification. Olfaction can be further compromised by medications, chemotherapy, radiotherapy, and systemic diseases commonly encountered in the elderly.

Head trauma also results in a diminished sense of smell due to the location and fragility of the olfactory neurons and the susceptibility of the cribriform plate to fracture. Tumours and surgical procedures that affect olfaction-related structures in the brain or nasal cavity are associated with smell loss. Similarly, neurological disorders such as epilepsy, Parkinson's disease, Huntington's chorea, and Alzheimer's disease impair olfaction. For example, patients with Alzheimer's disease develop problems with smell perception since many of the same anatomical and neural structures destroyed by this dis-

ease are involved in olfaction. Furthermore, the limbic system in Alzheimer's disease is adversely affected resulting in poor re-

The vomeronasal organ
The vomeronasal organ (VNO) detects pheromones or sexual hormones in most mammals, including New World primates, rodent and reptiles. Pheromones are substances that elicit a behavioral, developmental or endocrine response. The VNO consists of small bilateral invaginations or pits on the anterior medial sides of the nasal cavity close to the vomer. The VNO pits are covered by a neuro-epithelial lining, containing neurons unresponsive to olfactory stimuli. Interestingly, there is controversy about the status of a VNO in humans. There appears to be evidence of a VNO, but there is no evidence of functional connections with higher centres. The human olfactory mucosa expresses receptors that have significant homology to known rodent VNO receptors, yet no appropriate human counterpart has been isolated and its ligands are unknown. In humans, one documented phenomenon may simulate a pheromonal effect: menstrual synchrony. Women who live in the same space for several months develop synchronized menstrual cycles. The nature and mechanism of menstrual synchrony is mediated through specific apocrine gland secretion-containing proteins, ASOB1 and ASOB2. Similar to odorant-binding lipocalins, these proteins carry small aliphatic acids, 3 methyl-2-hexenopic acid.

cognition, identification, and recall of odorants.

Other diseases may have indirect effects on the sense of smell because of treatments and/or medications used to treat the disease. Numerous medications cause olfactory changes, including cardiovascular (nifedipine), anti-thyroid (methylthiouracil), antibacterial (streptomycin), and analgesic (codeine) drugs (Table 2). Chronic use of inhaled corticosteroids alters the respiratory tract flora and leads to unpleasant smells. Radiation, chemotherapy, and hemodialysis regimens can also interfere with olfactory pathways. Environmental pollutants (e.g., acrylates, petrochemicals) have been reported to alter neurotransmitters, damage the structures involved in olfaction, or accumulate in the olfactory bulbs. These losses may be transient or chronic.

Oral malodours

Oral sources of olfactory problems are also common (Table 3). Halitosis, gingivitis, poor oral hygiene, and periodontal diseases cause abnormal smell sensations. The most common oral malodour, *halitosis*, which is defined as bad breath originating from the mouth is caused by volatile sulphur compounds (VSCs; e.g., hydrogen sulphide, methyl mercaptan, dimethyl sulfide, but also by non-sulphur containing acids, cadaverine and putrescine). The dorsum of the tongue is the major reservoir for microbes, with the gingival sulcus also housing bacteria producing VSCs. The source of the VSCs is usually gram-negative anaerobic bacteria, which can produce objectionable volatile compounds that make up the "oral bouquet".

Several factors can result in a shift from gram-positive to gram-negative bacteria in the oral cavity: alkaline salivary pH, diminished salivary flow, and inflammatory diseases (i.e., gingivitis, periodontitis, major aphthous stomatitis, herpetic gingivostomatitis). The odour-producing compounds in the oral-pharyngeal region are inspired into the lungs and then expired, producing the unpleasant smell. Unpleasant smells can also be experienced when externally produced odiferous foods are ingested or when tobacco is inhaled.

Several systemic diseases also produce halitosis. Pulmonary infections involving gram-negative anaerobic bacteria (tuberculosis, pneumonia), obstructions (foreign bodies), tumors (lung cancer), and the production of pus (tonsillitis, empyema, bronchiectasis) can all contribute to the emission of foul odours from the nasal cavity, sinuses, nasopharynx, pharynx, and lungs. Gastrointestinal diseases such as hiatus hernias, gastro-oesophageal reflux, and pyloric stenosis permit the release of gastric odours into the oral cavity. Achalasia is a swallowing disorder in which there is a failure of the contents of the oesophagus to empty into the stomach; these patients experience halitosis when food debris and saliva are trapped and decay in the oesophagus. Gastric ulceration, infection, carcinoma, and mal-absorption can also contribute to oral malodors. Diabetic ketoacidosis produces oral malodors, and patients with diabetes are also at increased risk of infections and poor wound healing, which predisposes them to odour-producing periodontal diseases and other intra-oral infections. Hepatic and renal failure, leukaemias and other blood dyscrasias, can all produce malodors. Finally, trimethylaminuria (TMAU) or fish-odour syndrome is an inherited recessive disorder where the absence of one or several forms of the flavin-mono-oxygenase enzyme in the liver leads to a failure to metabolize choline in the diet. This leads to accumulation in the blood, breath, sweat, and urine of an intermediary bacterial breakdown product (trimethylamine or TMA), which smells like rotten fish. The incidence of this disorder in some populations, (e.g., Anglo-Celtic Britons) may be as high as 1%.

■ Conclusion

A variety of chemicals act on chemosensory systems. The primary binding site for these stimuli is a large number of recently identified cell surface receptors that are coupled with diverse signal transduction mechanisms. Taste and smell interact with other sensory systems, in particular temperature, texture and pain. Together, they provide an overall assessment of the chemosensory and somatosensory properties of food that enable communication and nutritional intake, protect the human host from potentially toxic compounds, and contribute significantly to a person's quality of life.

■ Selected references

Ackerman BH, Kasbekar N. Disturbances of taste and smell induced by drugs. Pharmacother 1997; 17(3):482–496.

Adler E, Hoon MA, Mueller KL et al. A novel family of mammalian taste receptors. Cell 2000;100:693–702.

Bartoshuk LM, Gent J, Catalanotto FA, Goodspeed RB. Clinical evaluation of taste. Am J Otolaryn 1983; 4(4):257–260.

Cullen MM, Leopold DA. Disorders of smell and taste. Med Clin N Amer 1999;83(1):57–74.

Getchell TC, Doty RL, Bartoshuk LM, Snow JB, Jr. Smell and Taste in Health and Disease. New York: Raven Press; 1991.

Lindemann B. Receptors and Transduction in Taste. Nature 2001;413:219–225.

Margolskee RF. Molecular mechanisms of bitter and sweet taste transduction. J Biol Chem 2002; 277(1): 1–4.

Mombaerts P. Seven-transmembrane proteins as odorant and chemosensory receptors. Science 1999;286: 707–711.

Mori K. Nagao H. Yoshihara Y. The olfactory bulb: coding and processing of odor molecule information. Science 1999;286:711–715.

Preti G, Spielman AI, Wysocki CJ. Vomeronasal Organ and Human Chemical Communications, In: Encyclopedia of Human Biology, Second Edition, Vol 8., Dulbecco editor, Academic Press; 1997. p. 769–783.

Schiffman SS. Taste and smell losses in normal aging and disease. J Am Med Assoc 1997;278(16):1357–1362.

Schild D, Restrepo D Transduction mechanisms in vertebrate olfactory receptor cells. Physiol Rev 1998;78: 429–466.

Ship JA, Chavez EM. Special Senses: Disorders of Taste and Smell. In: Silverman S, Jr., Eversole LR, Truelove EL, editors. Essentials of Oral Medicine. 1st ed. Hamilton, Canada: BC Decker; 2001. p. 277–288.

Spielman AI. Gustatory function and dysfunction. Crit Rev Oral Biol Med 1999;9:267–291.

Thermosensation

Greg K. Essick and Mats Trulsson

Goals:
- To discuss the characteristics of the different types of low-threshold and high-threshold thermoreceptors that innervate the orofacial region.
- To understand the receptor responses to sustained temperatures and to changes in temperature that occur when foods and objects come into contact with the tissues.
- To describe why humans can detect small differences in temperatures.
- To describe how sensitivities to warmth and to cold vary among sites in the mouth and on the face.
- To describe clinical examples of altered temperature perception in the orofacial region.

Key words:
Thermoreceptors; face; mouth; trigeminal; thermal sensitivity; temperature; warm; cool; heat pain; cold pain.

◼ Introduction

A cool drink of water, a hot cup of coffee, a warm glass of flavoured milk. Qualitatively different adjectives such as cool, hot, and warm describe our perception of a single dimension of stimulation, that of temperature or thermal energy. In much the same way that different wavelengths of light result in subjectively different colours, different temperatures result in subjectively different sensations due to several types of receptors that are sensitive to different temperatures. Signals from temperature-sensitive receptors, or *thermoreceptors*, in the orofacial region contribute greatly to our enjoyment of foods. The signals also result in reflexes and behaviours that prevent us from consuming substances that can burn or freeze our alimentary canals or can adversely alter core body temperature and homeostasis.

Orofacial thermoreception results in qualitatively diverse percepts of temperature as the result of the operation of complicated central neural mechanisms along the thermosensory pathways to the cortex. Many thermally sensitive neurons in the central system receive inputs from more than one type of thermoreceptor in the tissues, and these inputs can be inhibitory as well as excitatory. As a result of non-linear processing of signals from the different thermoreceptors, novel patterns of stimulation that are rarely encountered outside the laboratory can result in unexpected sensory experiences. Study of these percepts provides a means to improve our understanding of brain mechanisms underlying temperature perception. For example, in normally innervated skin, slightly warmed areas are made to feel hot by cooling the adjacent skin sites, producing sensations of so-called "synthetic heat". Moreover, application of alternating hot (40 °C) and cold (20 °C), but non-painful, stimuli across the skin can result in burning or stinging pain. These observations demonstrate that perceptual mechanisms in the brain combine inputs from different types of thermoreceptors in complicated ways. Disruption of the normal balance of inputs by novel patterns of stimuli in the laboratory results in temperature percepts that are not predicted by the sensations evoked by the individual components of the stimuli. A similar disruption in the balance of inputs from different classes of thermoreceptors might explain why about 10% of patients with injuries to the trigeminal nerve report pain or discomfort in the absence of noxious stimulation of the tissues. Of particular note are those nerve-injured patients who exhibit cold hyperalgesia, which is an unpleasant, increased sensitivity to cold (see also Chapter 4). These patients experience burning, painful cold sensations in the face or mouth to cool temperatures that are not uncomfortable to normal individuals.

Stimulation of thermoreceptors

At rest and under normal conditions, depending on the ambient temperature, the resting baseline temperature of the facial skin averages about 33–34 °C: this is slightly warmer than the skin of the fingers, hand and forearm (30–33 °C). The skin overlying the lateral chin (due to the facial artery) and of the scalp is warmer than other facial areas, and temperatures intraorally are higher than those extraorally. The mucosal surface of the lips approximates 34–35 °C and the tongue 36–37 °C, with all intraoral tissues becoming warmer when the mouth is closed. When an external object such as food is brought into contact with the soft tissues of the mouth or face, thermal energy is transferred between the object and tissue, causing the temperature of the tissue either to decrease (with cooler foods) or to increase (with foods of higher temperature). The changes in tissue temperature, if sufficient in magnitude and rate of change, evoke or alter activity in the different types of thermoreceptors. These receptors are either lightly myelinated or unmyelinated axons that terminate predominantly in the basal and deeper layers of the epithelium. The transfer of energy to their receptor terminals depends on the thickness of the epithelium, the degree of keratinization, and the present amount of saliva. For example, heat is transferred less effectively, in turn, to receptors in the hairy skin of the lips, the vermilion, and the inner mucosal surfaces of the lips due to the increase in the thickness of the epithelium. The relatively poor thermal conductivity of the thicker mucosa, however, is offset in part by the presence of saliva, which increases sensitivity to changes in temperature. Keratin provides a highly effective thermal barrier. Due to a higher degree of keratinization, the mid-dorsal surface of the tongue is less sensitive to thermal changes than is, e.g., the tip of the tongue.

The terminal endings of thermoreceptors are characterised by receptor channels that respond to thermal energies of specific magnitudes. These channels control the passage of ions across the cell membranes and thereby the development of depolarising receptor potentials. When the receptor potentials are large enough to exceed the axon's firing threshold, they initiate action potentials that are conducted to the brain. There is much interest in the identification and characterization of the different receptor channels on different types of thermoreceptors. To date, channels that respond to temperatures above 41 °C (the vanilloid receptor subtype 1, VR1), to temperatures above 50 °C (the vanilloid receptor-like type 1, VRL-1), and to temperatures within the range of about 8 to 28 °C (the cold-menthol receptor type 1, CMR1) have been discovered. As their names imply, the channels are opened not only by thermal energy associated with the specified temperature ranges, but also by chemical compounds. Vanilloid compounds such as capsaicin, the hot component of chilli peppers, are highly effective in activating the high temperature channels and in decreasing the threshold temperature at which heat pain is first felt, from about 43 °C to 33 °C (the resting temperature of the skin) in the extreme case. Similarly, menthol and related "minty-tasting" compounds increase sensitivity to cold. As a result, temperature that are usually mildly cool (25 °C to 28 °C) feel cold, and lower temperatures feel colder than they do in the absence of the compounds. The development of highly specific agonist and antagonists of the receptor channels should enable control of temperature perception purely by chemical means. This gives rise to the common descriptions of curries as being "hot", and food substances such as mints being "cool" in the mouth.

Perception of temperature

At rest, the temperature of our body surface, face and mouth is rarely noticed. Our sense of temperature completely adapts over the range of normal resting temperatures of the skin and oral mucosa, i.e., from about 29 to 37 °C. A change in temperature within this range, results in a different baseline or adapting temperature that ceases to be perceived within a minute or so. For example, when an initially cool object is held against the skin of the face, it will soon cease to feel cool. This adaptation occurs within the central nervous system as the thermoreceptors respond to the new temperature with different intensities and patterns of neural discharge. In contrast to changes in temperature within the range from 29 to 37 °C, decrements in temperature below 29 °C evoke persisting sensations of cool, cold and cold pain, depending on the final temperature of the tissues. Similarly, increments in temperature above 37 °C evoke persisting sensations of warmth, heat, or heat pain. Because the resting temperature of the tongue approximates the upper limit of the range of temperatures over which adaptation occurs, the tongue often feels slightly warm when the mouth is kept closed.

As temperatures become more extreme, heat sensations in turn assume sharp/pricking/stinging and burning/throbbing qualities. Cold sensations often assume tickling, painful pricking, and aching/burning/numbing qualities. Temperatures that possess potential for tissue damage occur above about 45 °C and below about 15 °C, where these noxious qualities are first felt. However, the temperatures at which individuals first report thermal sensations as unpleasant or painful differ substantially among subjects in the same way that the criteria for reporting pain differ from subject to subject, as well as from day to day for the same subject (see also Chapter 4). Intense aching and burning pain is often felt at about 50 °C and 0 °C, temperatures that destroy soft tissues if maintained for more than short periods of time. Painfully hot stimuli can damage the skin quickly and are detected quickly on their contact with the skin. In contrast, noxious cold stimuli tend to cause damage more slowly. Ten or more seconds may be required before pain is perceived.

Perceived and preferred temperatures of foods

The perceived temperature of food depends on both its temperature and its physical and textural properties. High-fat, semi-solid foods tend to have low thermal conductivities and high viscosities and often are perceived as warmer than low-fat foods, or water, at the same temperature. Moreover, differences in the temperature of high-fat foods are less easily discerned. Water is perceived to be cooler than food at the same temperature partly because it spreads more easily and quickly within the oral cavity. The perceived temperature of food is also affected by the manner in which it is manipulated in the mouth. Measurement of intraoral temperatures during mock ingestion of foods has shown that the temperature of the tissues rarely attains that of hot and cold foods at intake. For example, the temperature of steaming hot coffee at the palate or facial surface of the mandibular molars is 20 °C cooler than in the cup. Oral manipulative strategies, such as sipping air, are employed to lower the temperature to safer levels. The transient thermal spikes above the heat pain threshold and below the cold pain thresholds, respectively, contribute to the enjoyment of foods. This is evidenced by the loss of enjoyment and complaints of habitual coffee drinkers treated with maxillary full dentures made of acrylic polymers. The acrylic insulates the palatal tissues from the enjoyed challenges of hot coffee at temperatures that exceed normal pain thresholds. Dentures fabricated with thin metal bases

may cause a different problem for coffee drinkers because temperatures that exceed the pain threshold may be transferred more effectively and maintained against the tissues for uncomfortably long periods of time.

The temperature of the mouth also affects the perception of foods that are ingested. For example, the temperatures of high-fat foods are more difficult to discriminate when placed in a pre-warmed mouth (heated by rinses of hot water) than in a pre-cooled mouth. However, the effect of mouth temperature is less than one might predict. This probably reflects the ability of the thermosensory system to adjust to changes in environmental conditions. During respiration, the oral mucosa is exposed to core body temperatures (air from the lungs at about 37 °C) and environmental temperatures that can range from < -20 °C (freezing winter weather) to > 40 °C (blistering summer weather). As a result, temperature gradients from the oropharynx to the face change dramatically across the seasons of the year and various geographic locations. To protect the alimentary canal from tissue-damaging temperatures, the thermosensory system must take into account these often-extreme differences in oral temperatures resulting from environmental conditions.

The thermosensory system also serves in the selection process for foods and drinks that help maintain a constant core body temperature and homeostasis, e.g., hot foods are typically preferred during cold weather. However, the rules that govern thermal effects on preference and drinking behaviour are poorly understood. To illustrate, individuals rate water as most pleasurable for drinking when it is at about 5 °C. However, the temperature at which water is selected for drinking is higher, about 15 °C. The preferred temperature of semi-solid and solid foods is also related to its effect on the foods' flavour and texture. For example, higher temperatures increase the release of volatile odour molecules, which reach the olfactory mucosa retronasally. Higher temperatures also decrease the viscosity of many foods. Decreased viscosity facilitates the entry of flavour molecules into the saliva and taste buds. Moreover, it has recently been shown that warm stimuli applied to the tongue directly evoke the taste of sweet. Cool stimuli evoke tastes of sourness or saltiness.

Orofacial thermoreceptors

Classification

With a few minor exceptions, the temperature-sensitive afferents supplying the orofacial region are remarkably similar to those that have been characterized physiologically in other parts of the human and animal body. The afferents are classified as low-threshold thermoreceptors (including warm and cold fibres) or high-threshold thermoreceptors (including thermo-nociceptors and high-threshold cold receptors). The low-threshold thermoreceptors signal information about temperature and changes in temperature that possess little, if any, potential for tissue damage, i.e., temperatures roughly within the range of about 15 to 45 °C. In contrast, the high-threshold thermoreceptors signal information about temperatures and changes in temperature that have potential to damage tissue, i.e., temperatures greater than about 45 °C and less than about 15 °C. Although they sometimes respond to temperature within the low-threshold range of 15 to 45 °C, high-threshold thermoreceptors respond maximally to higher and/or lower temperatures.

Recordings from neurones in the infraorbital nerve in monkeys and from nerves supplying the hand/arm and leg in animals and humans provide evidence for at least two different types of low-threshold thermoreceptors and three types of high-threshold thermoreceptors. All of these thermally sensitive afferents are thinly-myelinated Aδ fibres (conduction velocity >2.5 m $\cdot$ s^{-1} but usually <25 m $\cdot$ s^{-1}) or unmyelinated C-fibres (conduction velocity <2.5 m $\cdot$ s^{-1}). That is, action potentials from thermoreceptors travel much more slowly to the central nervous system than those from the low-threshold mechanoreceptors supplying the same skin sites.

Methods to study thermosensation

The responses of different thermosensitive afferents have been studied in both animal and human experiments. In experimental animals, the peripheral nerve is usually cut under general anaesthesia, and individual axons are teased out carefully from the skin-side of the cut nerve. These are then placed on electrodes so that the signals (action potentials) that travel along them can be recorded. Sometimes the nerve is not cut and a microelectrode is placed directly on ganglion cells. In human studies, a microelectrode is inserted through the skin into a nerve to record the activity of single afferent fibres. The thermoreceptors are then stimulated by radiant heat from a light bulb that is projected onto the skin supplied by the nerve. This distinguishes thermally sensitive afferents from other afferents such as mechanoreceptors. Warm fibres are identified by an immediate increase in discharge to the warmth, and cold fibres by a decrease in their on-going discharge. Thermo-nociceptors respond to intense radiant heat, whereas, warm fibres cease to respond or respond unreliably to intense heat. Many high- threshold thermoreceptors also respond to ice.

After identification of the receptor, the borders of the skin area supplied by the afferent (its receptive field) is mapped with miniature metal probes that are heated or cooled. A computer-controlled, thermal contact stimulator is often used to study the response characteristics of the isolated afferent quantitatively. The active component of the stimulator is a cylindrical probe, the end of which is flat, typically about 1 cm^2 in area, whose temperature is controlled by a computer. The end is placed in light but positive contact with the receptive field at the baseline temperature under investigation. Temperature "ramps" (i.e., changing at a constant rate) from the baseline temperature are produced while the ramp rate ($°C \cdot s^{-1}$), the target temperature, and the duration of the target temperature are controlled. The different classes of thermoreceptors respond differently to these stimulus parameters.

Receptive fields

Orofacial thermoreceptors are found to have small receptive fields, which are often single spots on the skin or mucosa of about 300 μm in diameter. The receptive fields of thermo-nociceptors tend to be larger (2–4 mm^2) than those of warm and cool fibres. Multispot receptive fields are occasionally observed. These findings are consistent with perceptual studies conducted on human subjects in the early 1900s which showed that thermal sensitivity is not continuous across the skin, but punctate in nature. That is, the skin is a mosaic of thermally-sensitive spots surrounded by thermally-insensitive areas. More recent studies, however, have shown that the spots do not necessarily correspond to the receptive fields of single thermoreceptors.

Low-threshold thermoreceptors

The orofacial region is better equipped to process information about cooling than information about warming. The tissues are

supplied with a notably higher density of cold fibres than of warm fibres. In addition, cold fibres conduct action potentials about three times faster, on average, than warm fibres. Most textbooks state that cold fibres conduct only along Aδ-fibres and warm fibres conduct only along C-fibres. However, there is mounting evidence that humans also possess Aδ and C, warm and cold fibres, respectively.

In addition to their sensitivity to thermal energy, warm fibres discharge in response to mechanical stimuli that apply about 0.01 N of force (i.e., the force resulting from 1 gram weight) or more to the receptive fields. The threshold forces are 10 to 100 times greater in magnitude than the force required to stimulate low-threshold mechanoreceptors in the same skin areas. To activate cold fibres by mechanical stimulation requires even greater forces that risk tissue damage. These findings, particularly for the warm fibres, suggest that the texture of food interacts with the encoding of information about temperature at the most peripheral level of the thermosensory system. They may explain why temperature differences are more difficult to discern for some foods than others. It has also been shown that cooling of the skin alters the response of slowly-adapting low-threshold mechanoreceptors that encode information about texture (Chapter 6).

Warm and cold fibres innervating the face are identified by their on-going activity at the normal resting temperatures of the orofacial tissues (Fig. 1). At the resting temperature of the facial skin (33 °C), activity in the cold fibres substantially exceeds that of the warm fibres; however, at the higher temperature of the tongue (37 °C in the closed mouth), both classes discharge at about the same rate. Although the different resting temperatures of the tissues evoke different levels

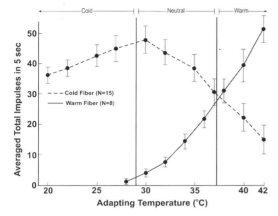

Figure 1. Responses of 8 warm fibres (solid curve) and 15 cold fibres (dashed curve) in the primate maxillary skin to constant temperatures. Each point represents the mean (±1 standard error of the mean) number of total impulses evoked by 5 seconds of exposure to the temperature indicated on the abscissa. Each number is based on the average value from a 90 second period of constant temperature stimulation after the skin had equilibrated to the temperature. The vertical lines demarcate temperature ranges over which humans perceive persisting cold or cool sensations (Cold), perceive neither cool nor warm sensations after a short period of adaptation (Neutral), and perceive persisting warm or hot sensations (Warm). (Modified from Sumino R, Dubner R. Response characteristics of specific thermoreceptive afferents innervating monkey facial skin and their relationship to human thermal sensitivity. Brain Research Reviews 1981;3:105–122. Copyright © 1981. Reprinted with permission of Elsevier/North-Holland Biomedical Press.)

of discharge activity in the warm and cold fibres, the combinations result in the same perception of a neutral (neither warm nor cool) resting temperature due to adaptation in the central nervous system as noted above. However, temperatures greater than 37 °C and less than about 29° evoke a persisting perception of warmth and cold, respectively.

Warm fibres

Above 37 °C, the discharge activity of warm fibres increases in proportion to temperature

while the activity in cold fibres decreases in similar fashion (Fig. 1). One subgroup of warm fibres reaches maximum firing rates at temperatures of about 40 to 45 °C (Fig. 2). These afferents either do not respond, respond poorly, or respond less intensely to higher, tissue-threatening and tissue-damaging temperatures. Moreover, exposure to

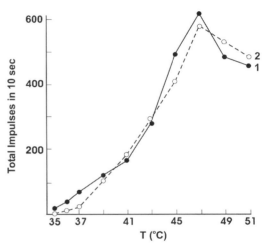

Figure 2. Responses of a warm fibre in the primate maxillary skin to different levels of thermal stimulation before and after desensitisation by noxious heat. The ordinate shows the total impulse count in 10 seconds after the onset of sudden increments from an adapting skin temperature of 35 °C to the final temperatures shown on the abscissa. Curves 1 and 2 represent the first and second series of trials, one trial at each temperature in order of ascending temperatures. After exposure to the noxious temperatures of the first series of trials (curve 1, temperatures above 45 °C), the responses to warming temperatures were depressed (curve 2, temperatures less than 41 °C), indicating desensitisation of the receptor to warming stimuli. Note that there was no on-going discharge at 35 °C during the second series (curve 2) compared with the first series (curve 1). (Modified from Sumino R, Dubner R, Starkman S. Responses of small myelinated "warm" fibres to noxious heat stimuli applied to the monkey's face. Brain Research 1973;62:260–263. Copyright © 1973. Reprinted with permission of Elsevier Scientific Publishing Company, Amsterdam.)

higher temperatures compromises their ability to respond subsequently to lower temperatures near their thresholds. These warm fibres become desensitised as illustrated in Fig. 2. A second subgroup of warm fibres reaches maximum firing rates for temperatures in the noxious range, about 50 °C (not shown in figures). These fibres respond to noxious temperatures only for the first few seconds of exposure. Like the first subgroup, the second subgroup of fibres becomes desensitised and they function thereafter as high-threshold thermoreceptors, responding only to higher temperatures. The activity of these warm fibres probably contributes to the stinging quality of hot stimuli.

Cold fibres

Cold fibres, also known as low-threshold cold receptors (LCR), are maximally active at about 30 °C (Fig. 1). They signal information about increasing intensities of coolness down to about 20 °C. Paradoxically, cold fibres discharge less intensely (rather than more intensely) as temperature is decreased to 20 °C. However, the pattern of action potentials changes, becoming periodic and burst-like in nature. The number of action potentials per burst increases as the temperature decreases from 30 °C to 20 °C. It has been suggested that the increasing discharge intensity within the bursts signifies the increasingly cold nature of the stimuli. Cold fibres respond poorly to temperatures less than 20 °C. Below this temperature, a second group of receptors discharge and encode information about cold. These receptors are high-threshold cold receptors (HCRs; Fig. 9) and will be discussed later.

Sensitivity to rapid changes in temperature and perceptual correlates

The low-threshold thermoreceptors are highly sensitive to rapid changes in temperature. Hence, they are particularly well suited to signal information about the temperature of objects that touch the face and lips, and of foods that enter the mouth. Their response to a change in temperature depends on the initial (baseline) temperature of the tissue, the rate of temperature change, and the new (target) temperature. This is illustrated for a warm fibre in Fig. 4A. From a baseline temperature of 35 °C, the temperature of the receptive field was increased in different trials at 1, 2 and $5 °C \cdot s^{-1}$ to new, warmer temperatures of 36, 38 and 40 °C. A burst of activity was evoked upon initiation of the change. The magnitude of the burst increased with both the rate of change and the target temperature. The rate of change had an additive effect only for the larger increments in temperature. Although not shown in Fig. 4, the fibre's response to the target temperatures would have gradually re-

> Most low-threshold cold fibres cease to respond to temperatures greater than about 40 °C. However, a proportion of the cold fibres also respond to higher, tissue-threatening and tissue-damaging temperatures (Fig. 3). This discharge underlies *paradoxical cold*, the sensation of cold that sometimes accompany painfully hot stimuli. In contrast to the warm fibres, exposure of cold fibres to high temperatures does not compromise their ability to respond to the lower temperatures at which they are most sensitive. Rather, cold fibres become sensitised and discharge more readily to heat, thus increasing the likelihood of paradoxical cold sensations (see also Chapter 4).

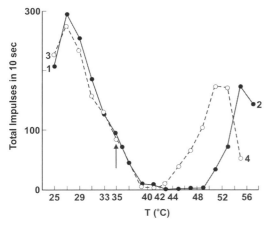

Figure 3. Responses of a cold fibre in the primate maxillary skin to different levels of thermal stimulation before and after sensitisation by noxious heat. The ordinate shows the total impulse count in 10 seconds after the onset of sudden decrements or increments from an adapting skin temperature of 35 °C to the final temperatures shown on the abscissa. Points above the vertical arrow represent the on-going response of the receptor to the 35 °C adapting temperature. Curves 1–2 and 3–4 represent the first and second series of trials, one trial at each temperature in order of ascending temperatures. After exposure to the noxious temperatures of the first series of trials (curve 2, temperatures above 50 °C), the cold fibre's threshold to heat was lowered from 49 °C (curve 2) to 43 °C (curve 4) and responses to the higher temperatures were greater than those observed before exposure to the noxious temperatures. The lower threshold and more intense responses in curve 4, compared with curve 3, illustrate sensitisation of the cold fibre by noxious heat stimulation. (Modified from Dubner R, Sumino R, Wood WI. A peripheral "cold" fibre population responsive to innocuous and noxious thermal stimuli applied to monkey's face. J Neurophysiol 1975;38:1373–1389. Copyright © 1975. Reprinted with permission of the American Physiological Society, Bethesda, MD.)

turned to the steady state levels shown in Fig. 1.

Cold fibres respond similarly to decrements in temperature. Fig. 4B shows the responses of a cold fibre. From a baseline adapting temperature of 35 °C, the tempera-ture of the receptive field was decreased at 1, 5 and 8 °C · s^{-1} to new, cooler temperatures of 33, 30 and 27 °C. Cold fibres recorded intraorally, e.g., from the tongue exhibit similar behaviours. For both warm and cold fibers, the initial burst of activity increases in magnitude with the rate of temperature change, suggesting that smaller changes in temperature might be required for one to detect warmth and cool at faster rates. In contrast to this prediction, the rate of temperature change has little effect on one's ability to detect warmth and cool for rates exceeding 0.2 °C · sec^{-1}. Moreover, suprathreshold increments or decrements in temperature are perceived to be of the same magnitude for different rates of temperature change exceeding this lower limit.

The effect of the adapting skin temperature on the response of warm and cold fibres to rapid changes in temperature is complex. In general, thermoreceptors respond poorly to changes in temperature from adapting temperatures at which they are least sensitive. That is, warm fibres are less able to signal increments in temperature at 30 °C (a "cool" temperature for warm fibres) than they are at 35 °C. Cold fibres are less able to signal decrements in temperature at 40 °C (a "warm" temperature for cold fibres). Consistent with these findings, human subjects have more difficulty detecting increments in temperature that feel warm from a baseline temperature <30 °C than at higher baseline temperatures (Fig. 5). In addition, a given increment (e.g., 5°) feels less warm from lower, than from higher baseline temperatures. Similarly, subjects have more difficulty detecting decrements in temperature that feel cool from a baseline of 40 °C than at lower baseline temperatures (Fig. 5). A given decrement feels less cool from higher than from lower baseline temperatures.

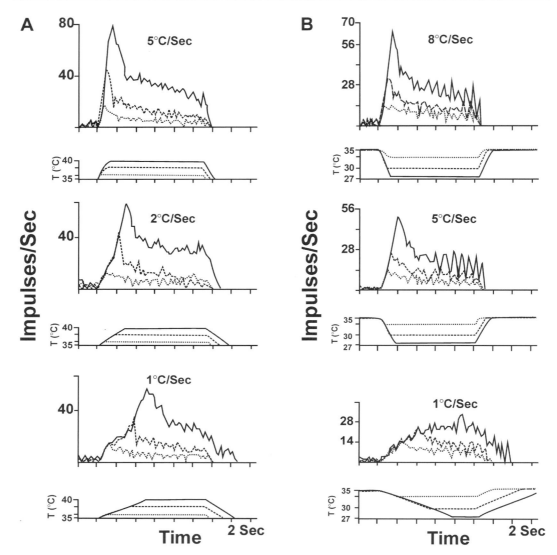

Figure 4. Sensitivity of low-threshold thermoreceptors in the primate maxillary skin to rapid changes in temperature. **A**, Responses of a warm fibre to rapid increments in warmth. Superimposed plots of the discharge rate (impulses/second) versus time are shown for increments of 1, 3, and 5 °C from an adapting skin temperature of 35 °C. Temperature was changed at $5 °C \cdot s^{-1}$ (top), $2 °C \cdot s^{-1}$ (middle), and $1 °C \cdot s^{-1}$ (bottom). Actual magnitudes and rates of the temperature shifts are shown below each plot of the discharge rates. **B**, Responses of a cold fibre to rapid decrements in temperature at rates of 1, 5, and $8 °C \cdot s^{-1}$. Figure format parallels that of part A. (Modified from Sumino R, Dubner R. Response characteristics of specific thermoreceptive afferents innervating monkey facial skin and their relationship to human thermal sensitivity. Brain Research Reviews 1981;3:105–122. Copyright © 1981. Reprinted with permission of Elsevier/North-Holland Biomedical Press.)

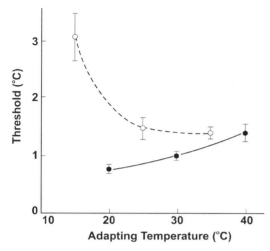

Figure 5. The minimum change in temperature for detecting warming and cooling depends on the baseline temperature of the skin (abscissa of graph). Shown on the ordinate are the threshold increments in temperature at which five male subjects detected warmth (○, dashed curve) and the threshold decrements in temperature at which they detected cold (●, solid curve) on the maxillary skin. Note that increments are more readily detected at the warmer temperatures and decrements are more readily detected at the cooler temperatures. These trends parallel the greater sensitivity of warm fibres to increments in temperature at warm temperatures and the greater sensitivity of cold fibres to decrements in temperature at cool temperatures. (Modified from Davies SN, Goldsmith GE, Hellon RF, Mitchell D. Facial sensitivity to rates of temperature change: neurophysiological and psychophysical evidence from cats and humans. Journal of Physiology 1983;344:161–175. Copyright © 1983. Reprinted with permission of The Physiological Society, Cambridge University Press.)

In contrast to detecting warmth and cool, subjects are able to detect a given temperature change (but not its direction) equally well at 30 and 40 °C. This is because at 30 °C, increments in temperature evoke bursts of activity in warm fibres, but also depress the on-going activity in cold fibres. At 40 °C, decrements in temperature evoke bursts of activity in cold fibres, but also decrease the on-going activity in warm fibres. Thus,

changes in temperature are signalled by changes in the discharge activity of both populations of thermoreceptors. However, greater changes in the discharge of warm and cold fibres are required to perceive warmth and cool, respectively, than are required to perceive only a change in temperature.

High-threshold thermoreceptors

In contrast to low-threshold thermoreceptors, high-threshold thermoreceptors do not exhibit on-going activity at the normal resting temperatures of the orofacial region. However, the more sensitive high-threshold thermoreceptors begin to discharge at hot and cold temperatures that are not injurious to tissues or painful to most individuals. High-threshold thermoreceptors include the thermo-nociceptors and the high-threshold cold receptors (HCRs).

High temperatures and heat pain

The most prevalent high-threshold thermoreceptor is the C-fibre polymodal nociceptor (CPN). These afferents are responsible for the burning, often intolerable, quality of noxious hot and cold stimuli. Their receptive fields tend to be single spots on the skin about 2–4 mm² in area. CPNs also respond to strong mechanical stimuli, having thresholds that are 10 to 1000 times higher than those of the low-threshold mechanoreceptors supplying the same areas of skin or mucosa. Many CPNs also respond to endogenous mediators of inflammation and noxious chemical agents.

The response of CPNs to high temperatures has been studied in the primate face. Most CPNs have thresholds between about 40 and 45 °C, temperatures that are very hot but usually not painful (Fig. 6). With an increase in temperature, the onset of pain and its growth in intensity depend on the pro-

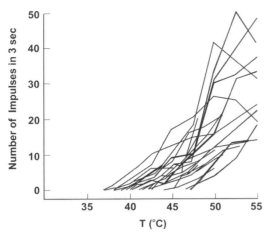

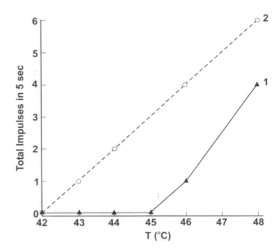

Figure 6. Responses of 22 CPNs in the primate maxillary skin to different levels of thermal stimulation. The ordinate shows the total impulse count in 3 seconds after the onset of sudden increments from an adapting skin temperature of 35 °C to the final temperatures shown on the abscissa. Roughly 50% of the CPNs fired at least 1 action potential to temperatures as low as 41 °C, indicating that many nociceptors become active at temperatures that are not perceived as painful. (Modified from Beitel RE, Dubner R. Response of unmyelinated (C) polymodal nociceptors to thermal stimuli applied to monkey's face. Journal of Neurophysiology 1976;39:1160–1175. Copyright © 1976. Reprinted with permission of the American Physiological Society, Bethesda, MD.)

Figure 7. Responses of a CPN in the primate maxillary skin to different levels of thermal stimulation before and after sensitisation by noxious heat. The ordinate shows the total impulse count in 5 seconds after the onset of sudden increments from an adapting skin temperature of 35 °C to the final temperatures shown on the abscissa. Curves 1 and 2 represent the first and second series of trials, one trial at each temperature in order of ascending temperatures. After the data for curve 1 were collected, the receptive field was exposed for 30 seconds to noxious heat at 48 °C. The noxious heat sensitised the receptor, lowering its threshold from 46 °C to 43 °C and increasing its response to all suprathreshold temperatures (compare curve 2 to curve 1). (Modified from Beitel RE, Dubner R. Response of unmyelinated (C) polymodal nociceptors to thermal stimuli applied to monkey's face. Journal of Neurophysiology 1976;39:1160–1175. Copyright © 1976. Reprinted with permission of the American Physiological Society, Bethesda, MD.)

gressive recruitment of less sensitive CPNs and higher rates of discharge in those that are active. CPNs discharge with progressively increasing intensities into the range 50 to 55 °C. In contrast to warm fibres, the discharge of CPNs is relatively unaffected by the rate (°C · s^{-1}) at which temperature increases or by the baseline temperature of the receptive field. The impact of changes in the baseline adapting temperature has been particularly difficult to study because temperatures only a few degrees above the threshold can sensitise CPNs to subsequent stimuli (Fig. 7). The sensitised CPNs respond more vigorously to reapplication of the same stimuli and re-

spond to temperatures that were subthreshold prior to sensitisation. As a result, temperatures that normally produce sensations of warmth, instead evoke burning pain. Maximal sensitisation of CPNs lowers their thresholds into the range of the normal resting temperatures of the tissues, resulting in continuous burning pain. Very high temperatures (i.e., >55 °C), however, desensitise and deactivate CPNs. At these higher temperatures, a second class of thermo-nociceptors, the Aδ heat nociceptors (AHN; not illustrated in figures), continues to discharge and underlies intense heat pain that results in escape behaviours. The AHNs respond more vigorously in general to noxious heat than CPNs. They are sensitised by the higher temperatures that desensitise and deactivate the CPNs. Like the CPNs, the AHNs also respond to noxious mechanical stimuli.

Sensitivity to rapid increments in temperature and perceptual correlates

Although CPNs discharge fewer action potentials, they are usually more sensitive to changes in temperature than warm fibres. A similarly high sensitivity to changes in temperature is exhibited by the AHNs. The higher sensitivity of CPNs and AHNs compared to warm fibres is thought to explain why human subjects detect changes in the temperature of painful heat more readily than of warmth (Fig. 8). For example, on the face, the smallest temperature difference that subjects can detect is about 0.3 °C at 47 °C, a painfully hot temperature. However, the smallest temperature difference that can be detected at 39 °C, which is a moderately warm temperature, is about 0.5 °C. The higher sensitivity to painful heat compared to warmth serves well the need to escape from noxious stimuli to avoid the risk of burning.

Receptors for low temperatures

High-threshold cold receptors (HCRs) have been identified in the primate hand and foot. It is assumed that they also exist in the orofacial region and signal information about cold temperatures lower than those to which the low-threshold cold fibres (LCRs) respond. The HCRs in primates exhibit on-going discharge activity over the range 0 to 15 °C, in contrast to the LCRs which exhibit

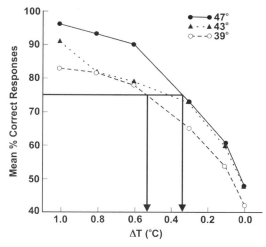

Figure 8. The ability of human subjects to distinguish differences in temperature on the maxillary skin is better at higher, noxious temperatures than at lower, warm temperatures. Shown is the mean percentage of trials (ordinate) on which three subjects correctly detected the differences in temperature shown along the abscissa at 39 °C (warm; *dashed lines*), 43 °C (hot; *dotted lines*), and 47 °C (painfully hot; *solid lines*). The subjects were instructed to choose the hotter of two stimulator probes positioned on opposite sides of the philtrum of the lip. Note that the curve obtained for painfully hot stimuli (solid lines) is shifted to the right of the curve obtained for warm stimuli (dashed lines), indicating a higher performance level for the noxious stimuli. The differences reported correctly on 75% of the trials defined the threshold difference. Extrapolation of the thresholds at 39 °C (left arrow) and at 47 °C (right arrow) is illustrated. (Modified from Bushnell MC, Taylor MB, Duncan GH, Dubner R. Discrimination of innocuous and noxious thermal stimuli applied to the face in human and monkey. Somatosensory Research 1983;1:119–129. Copyright © 1983. Reprinted with permission of the Taylor and Francis Group.)

on-going activity over the range 20 to 40 °C (see Fig. 1). Some receptors of both types likely respond steadily to temperatures within the intervening range, 15 to 20 °C. However, it is the HCRs that underlie our sense of sustained cold for temperatures at and near the freezing point.

Sensitivity to rapid decrements in temperature and perceptual correlates

In addition to signalling information about very cold, sustained temperatures, HCRs also reliably encode information about decrements in temperature from baseline skin temperatures as high as 30 °C (Fig. 9). As shown in the figure, the number of impulses signals the magnitude of cooling. Although both LCRs and HCRs encode information about cooling at temperatures above 15 °C, only the HCRs encode information at temperatures below 15 °C. This probably explains why human subjects detect changes in mildly-to-moderately cool temperatures much more readily than of cold-to-very cold temperatures (Fig. 10). For example, on the face subjects detect minimal differences of about 0.3 °C at 22 °C, a moderately cool tem-

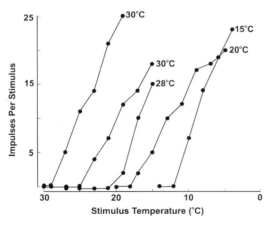

Figure 9. Responses of 5 high-threshold cold fibres (HCRs) supplying the primate or feline upper or lower limb to different levels of thermal stimulation. The ordinate shows the total impulse count in 5 seconds after the onset of sudden decrements from the baseline skin temperatures listed beside each curve to the final temperatures shown on the abscissa. (From LaMotte RH, Thalhammer JG. Response properties of high-threshold cutaneous cold receptors in the primate. Brain Research 1982;244:279–287. Copyright © 1982. Reprinted with permission of Elsevier Biomedical Press, Amsterdam.)

perature. Thirty-fold greater differences (i.e., 9 to 10 °C) are required for their detection at 6 °C, a decidedly cold temperature. The higher sensitivity to differences in temperatures that are mildly cool serves well the thermosensory system's function in processing information about foods and objects that differ only slightly in temperature from the orofacial tissues.

Cold and pain

Although HCRs respond to temperatures that are close to freezing, their discharge does not result in pain, so they are not considered to be nociceptors. However, decrements in temperature from baseline skin temperatures as high as 20–25 °C activate nociceptors as well as HCRs. Thus, cold pain is a blended percept of cold and pain: cold from activation of cold thermoreceptors plus pain from activation of nociceptors. These nociceptors include a subset of the CPNs, and possibly a subset of AHNs, that respond to noxious heat stimuli. At least half of the CPNs that respond to noxious heat and mechanical stimuli also respond to cooling (Fig. 11). Those that respond to cooling do not differ from those that fail to respond in terms of their conduction velocities or sensitivities to noxious heat and mechanical stimuli. However, the responses to nearly-freezing temperatures are only a fraction (10–50%) of the responses to noxious heat. The reduced discharge is probably due, in part, to blockage by the low temperatures of the conduction of action potentials in the superficially-located unmyelinated C-fibres.

The perception of the responses from nociceptors to temperatures as high as 20–25 °C are normally suppressed and become manifest only at lower, nearly freezing temperatures and upon prolonged exposure to above freezing temperatures. This suppression occurs within the central nervous system and

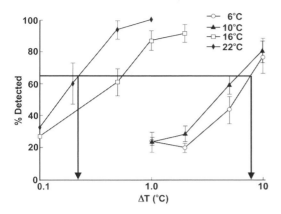

Figure 10. The ability of subjects to distinguish differences in temperature on the maxillary skin is better at cool-to-cold temperatures than at lower, nearly freezing temperatures. The subjects were instructed to report a decrease in the temperature of a stimulator probe positioned above the nasolabial fold. The mean (± 1 standard error of the mean) percentage of trials (ordinate) on which five subjects correctly detected differences in temperature (abscissa) is plotted for baseline temperatures of 22 and 16 °C (cool-to-cold temperatures), and 10 and 6° °C (very cold temperatures). Note that small differences that are detected well at cool and cold temperatures (curves to the left) are poorly detected or not detected at temperatures that approximate the freezing point (curves to the right). The difference reported correctly on 62.5% of the trials defined the threshold difference. Extrapolation of the thresholds at 22 °C (left arrow) and at 6 °C (right arrow) is illustrated. Note that the abscissa is scaled logarithmically. (From Chen C-C, Rainville P, Bushnell MC. Noxious and innocuous cold discrimination in humans: evidence for separate afferent channels. Pain 1996;68:33–43. Copyright © 1996. Reprinted with permission of the International Association for the Study of Pain and Elsevier Press.)

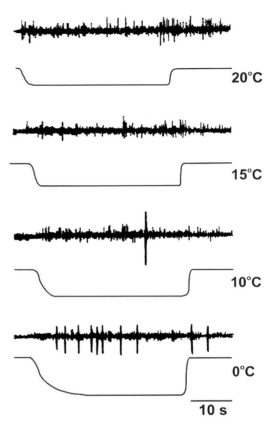

Figure 11. Many CPNs respond to noxious cold as well as to noxious heat. Recordings from a single CPN in human skin to four graded ramps of low temperature from a baseline skin temperatures of 30 °C are shown. The CPN first responded to a temperature of 10 °C, 23 seconds after the onset of stimulation (see third pair of tracings). With temperatures lower than 10 °C, the response latencies were shortened and the discharge frequencies were higher. (From Campero M, Serra J, Ochoa JL. C-polymodal nociceptors activated by noxious low temperature in human skin. Journal of Physiology 1996;497.2:565–572. Copyright © 1996. Reprinted with permission of The Physiological Society, Cambridge University Press.)

is produced by the concurrent discharge of the cold receptors. Only when the activity in the nociceptors is great enough to overcome the inhibition mediated by cold receptors is cold pain perceived. Cold hyperalgesia occurs after some nerve injuries. In these cases, it is thought that myelinated afferents (often LCRs and HCRs) are damaged to a greater extent than unmyelinated axons (often CPNs). Due to the decreased inhibition, burning pain sensations occur in response to temperatures that are only moderately cold (Fig. 12). Burning pain sensations are also produced in the arms and legs by ischemic

A

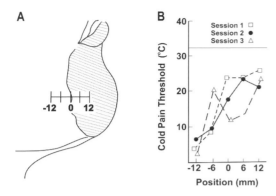

B

Figure 12. Cold hyperalgesia in a 25-year-old male patient following injury to the inferior alveolar and mental nerves during orthognathic surgery. A, Schematic illustration of the five locations at which sensitivity to cold was measured with a thermal stimulator. Adjacent sites were separated by 6 mm. The site at "0" was located at the skin border over which the patient reported a loss in sensation to pinprick. B, The threshold temperatures (i.e., the highest temperatures) at which the subject reported an uncomfortable (stinging, pricking or burning) cold sensation are shown. The thresholds were measures for the five sites on each of three different days, shown by the three curves. More laterally on the chin, only temperatures near 0 °C were reported as painfully cold. In contrast, cool temperatures evoked painful sensation within the pinprick-impaired area (shaded). (Modified from Essick GK, Patel S, Trulsson M. Mechanosensory and thermosensory changes across the border of impaired sensitivity to pinprick after mandibular nerve injury. Journal of Oral and Maxillofacial Surgery 2002;60:1250–1266. Copyright © 2002. Reprinted with permission of the American Association of Oral and Maxillofacial Surgeons.)

nerve blocks that preferentially eliminate the discharge of myelinated afferents, and by novel patterns of thermal stimuli that suppress the activity of central neurons that receive input from cold receptors. There is evidence that these central neurons can be suppressed by heating the skin with hot (40 °C) stimuli alternated with cold (20 °C) stimuli presented across the skin. The result is a sensation of "heat" accompanied by burning and stinging (the so-called "heat grill illusion", or "synthetic heat"). The same areas of the human brain that respond to noxious heat stimulation and whose levels of activation correlate with the magnitude of the heat-evoked pain are activated by these novel patterns of innocuous stimulation.

■ Orofacial thermal sensitivity

The orofacial region is covered by epithelial tissue that varies notably in thickness, degree of keratinization, and level of hydration. These biophysical factors affect the thermal conductivities of the epithelia and thus the ease with which thermal energy is transferred to the molecular receptor channels on the underlying terminal endings of the thermoreceptors. The density of innervation by nerve endings, many of which are thermoreceptors and nociceptors, also varies considerably in different orofacial structures. As a result of variations in the thermal conductivities of the tissues, their baseline resting temperatures, and their innervations, the sensitivity to thermal challenges differs substantially in different sites in the mouth and on the face.

The spatial variations among orofacial sites in sensitivity to warming and cooling were first studied in the 1980s. Briefly, aluminium rods were heated or cooled in water baths of constant temperatures. The stimulus rod was dried and brought into contact with the test site for 3 seconds. The temperature of the rod before placement on the tissue and the change in tissue temperature produced by the rod were determined. The temperatures of the rod ranged from 37 to 44 °C for warming and from 10 to 27 °C for cooling and were not uncomfortable or painful. The change in tissue temperature produced by the stimulus depended on both the resting temperature and thermal conductivity of the epithelium as well as the temperature of the aluminium rod. Subjects assigned numbers to the sensations of warmth or of cold that were in proportion to the relative intensities of the sensations.

Thermal sensitivity of the lower lip

Fig. 13 shows the ratings of the sensations produced by warming and cooling stimuli obtained at three sites across the lower lip: the facial surface ("hairy"), the glabrous vermilion surface ("glabrous"), and the inner mucosal surface ("mucosal"). Study of the lower lip provided a means to evaluate and compare thermal sensitivities across facial, transitional, and oral epithelia covering the same structure. Sensitivity to warmth was found to vary 3-fold across the lip. As shown in Fig. 13A, ratings of warmth on the facial surface were 2–4 times higher than ratings on the mucosal surface for the same changes in tissue temperature. It is rather remarkable that the difference in sensitivity from outside to inside the mouth approximates the maximum difference reported elsewhere over the body surface from head to foot! A higher sensitivity of hairy skin compared to glab-

rous skin has also been observed on the upper and lower limbs. The thicker epidermis of glabrous skin is thought to absorb more thermal energy than does hairy skin. As a result, higher temperatures are required to attain the same critical firing rates from the glabrous skin receptors.

The relatively poor sensitivity to warming of the labial mucosa was found in subsequent studies to extend to the buccal mucosal and to the masticatory mucosa of the hard palate and alveolar ridge (Fig. 15A), indicating that the intraoral mucosa is less well-equipped to respond to warmth than extraoral sites. The two-limbed nature of the psychophysical functions for warmth in Fig. 13A is relevant to previous findings reported in this chapter. The higher slopes at the greater increments in temperature suggest that subjects better detect differences in stimuli that are hot than those that are warm. This observation parallels the finding that subjects' thresholds for detecting changes in the temperature of hot and painfully hot stimuli are lower than for warm stimuli (Fig. 8).

Figure 13. A, Perceived warmth on the hairy facial skin, the vermilion, and the oral mucosa of the lower lip as a function of $+\Delta T$, the increase in skin temperature produced during stimulation with a heated rod. B, Perceived cold on the same locations as a function of $-\Delta T$, the decrease in skin temperature produced during stimulation with a cooled rod. Twenty young adult subjects participated in each of the experiments. (Modified from Green BG. Thermal perception on lingual and labial skin. Perception & Psychophysics 1984;36:209–220. Copyright © 1984. Reprinted with permission of Psychonomic Society Publications.)

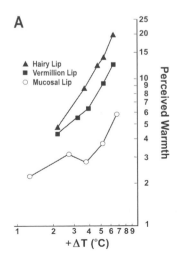

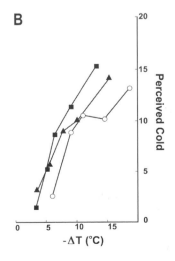

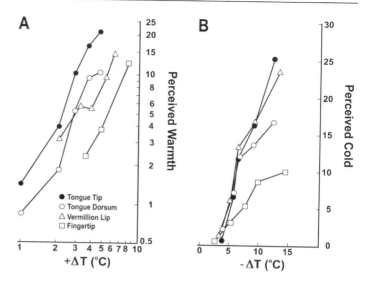

Figure 14. A, Perceived warmth on the tip and dorsum of the tongue, the vermilion of the lower lip, and the fingertip as a function of +ΔT, the increase in skin temperature produced during stimulation with a heated rod. B, Perceived cold on the same locations as a function of -ΔT, the decrease in skin temperature produced during stimulation with a cooled rod. Fifteen young adult subjects participated in each of the experiments. (Modified from Green BG. Thermal perception on lingual and labial skin. Perception & Psychophysics 1984;36:209–220. Copyright © 1984. Reprinted with permission of Psychonomic Society Publications.)

In contrast to warmth, differences in sensitivity to cold across the lower lip were much less pronounced (Fig 13B). The mucosal surface of the lip was only slightly less sensitive to cold than the vermilion and facial surface. Like warmth, the psychophysical functions for cold were two-limbed in nature. However, higher slopes were observed at the smaller changes in temperature. This observation parallels the finding that subjects' thresholds for detecting changes in the temperature of mildly to moderately cold stimuli are lower than for very cold, nearly freezing temperatures (Fig. 10).

Thermal sensitivity of the tip and dorsum of the tongue

The same procedures have been used to study sensitivity of the tip and dorsum of the tongue to warming and cooling stimuli. The vermilion of the lower lip and the fingertip was also studied. Increments in temperature on the tip of the tongue felt twice as warm as the same increments on the dorsum of the tongue (Fig. 14A). In contrast, the dorsum of the tongue was as sensi-

tive as the tip to cold except at the colder temperatures (Fig. 14B). All three oral or perioral sites were found to be substantially more sensitive to both heating and cooling than the fingertip. Remarkably, the same increments in temperature were perceived to be six times warmer on the tongue tip than on the fingertip. Cold temperatures also felt much colder on the tongue and lips than on the fingertip.

Thermal sensitivity of extraoral versus intraoral sites

In other experiments, subjects rated the warmth and cold of stimuli applied to twelve sites on the face and in the mouth. The stimuli were applied by a device that maintained the temperature constant throughout the 5-second exposure period. The warm stimuli were about 39, 43 and 45 °C and the cold stimuli about 14, 19 and 24 °C. Of all sites tested, the intensity of warmth was greatest on the peri-nasal skin, the same region of the body surface that is most sensitive to touch (see Chapter 6). With the exception of the tip of the tongue, discrete extraoral sites were more sensitive to warmth than discrete intraoral sites (Fig. 15A). The tip of the tongue was equally sensitive to warmth as sites on the face. Subsequent experiments showed that the tip of the tongue was also as sensitive to noxious heat as the facial skin. However, the dorsum of the tongue and oral mucosa were substantially less sensitive to noxious heat.

In contrast to warmth, sensitivity to cold varied little among extra- and intra-oral sites. That is, sites inside and outside the mouth were about equally sensitive to cold (Fig. 15B). The high degree of intraoral sensitivity to cold appears to complement the high degree of intraoral sensitivity to mechanical stimulation (see Chapter 6).

In the experiments whose results are described above, the stimuli were either clearly warm/hot or cool/cold. Investigators have also evaluated perioral thermal sensitivity using threshold testing methods. Briefly summarized, a thermal probe with contact area of 1 cm^2 was positioned on the test site. The temperature of the probe, initially at the resting temperature of the skin or mucosa, increased or decreased at a constant rate until the subject signified that warmth or cool had been detected, respectively. Thresholds for heat pain and cold pain were determined in a similar manner. Based on the thresholds, the upper and lower vermilion were found to be the most (and equally) sensitive sites on the face to both warmth and cool as

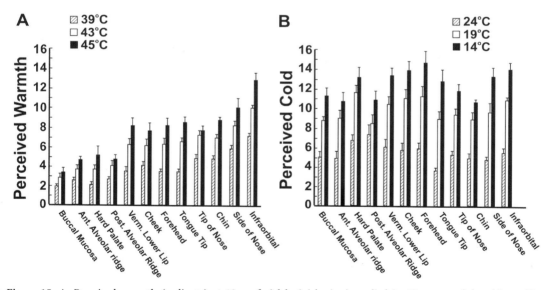

Figure 15. A, Perceived warmth (ordinate) at 12 orofacial loci (abscissa) studied in 20 young adult subjects. The data are arranged from left to right according to the mean perceived intensity reported for the three warm temperatures. The estimates were normalized so that the mean rating for each subject at the infraorbital site became "10". Shown are mean values (+1 standard error of the mean). **B,** Same as Fig. A, but for cold temperatures. The sequence of orofacial locations is the same as that used for warmth in order to illustrate the difference in the spatial pattern of sensitivity for warmth and cold. (Modified from Green BG, Gelhard B. Perception of temperature on oral and facial skin. Somatosensory Research 1987;4:191–200. Copyright © 1987. Reprinted with permission of the Taylor and Francis Group.)

well as to noxious heat and cold. All sites were more sensitive to cooling than to warming. Moreover, sensitivity decreased with distance from the mouth, more so for warmth than for the other three sensations. These findings suggest that sensitivity to barely detectable levels of thermal stimulation does not necessarily predict sensitivity to larger, suprathreshold levels of thermal stimulation.

Whole mouth thermal sensitivity

Other studies have sought to evaluate whole mouth thermal sensitivity. Subjects sipped a 20-ml sample of warmed or cooled liquid, expectorated, and assigned a number or verbal descriptor to rate the intensity of the warmth or cold, respectively. It was predicted that the mouth would be more sensitive to cooling than to warming because the mouth is more uniformly sensitive to cold than to warmth when tested with a thermal probe (Fig. 15). Moreover, the mouth is equally sensitive as the face to cold but less sensitive than the face to warmth. In contrast to the prediction, it was found that the mouth as a whole was more sensitive to differences in increments in temperature (i.e., warming) than to differences in decrements in temperature (i.e., cooling). This finding

Burning mouth syndrome is characterized by a painful, burning sensation of the oral mucosa in the absence of any implicating pathology or relevant laboratory findings. Most often affected are the anterior tongue (sides and tip), the hard palate and the lower lip. The bilateral pain is either constant throughout the waking hours or re-develops slowly over the course of each day. The condition is most frequently found in postmenopausal women with an increased prevalence of personality disorders. Patients often report burning, tingling, and numb sensations similar to individuals who have experienced injuries to the trigeminal nerve. However, in contrast to patients with pain resulting from nerve injury (i.e., neuropathic pain), patients with burning mouth syndrome do not have discrete somatosensory or thermal deficits in the affected areas. A decreased tolerance to noxious thermal stimuli applied to the tongue tip has been reported.

Other studies have shown that patients exhibit abnormal responses to brief laser pulses applied to painful intraoral sites as well as to sites that are seemingly unrelated to the syndrome, e.g., to the hand. Many patients with burning mouth syndrome also have distortions and persistence of taste sensations. Treatments that reduce the burning pain often lessen the taste dysfunction. Based on this and other observations, it has recently been hypothesized that patients with burning mouth syndrome have defective central nervous system regulation of pathways that process nociceptive (pain) and gustatory (taste) information from the mouth. Such dysfunction might result from viral infections of the gustatory or somatosensory nerves in the tongue, or from hormonal changes. Additional studies are needed to evaluate these potential etiological factors.

suggests that the thermal sensitivity of small discrete areas in the mouth or on the face does not necessarily predict sensitivity to whole-mouth or to whole-face thermal stimulation. Sensitivity measured at discrete sites may underestimate sensitivity across larger areas over which the central nervous system integrates temperature information. In addition, the finding for whole mouth stimulation might be attributed to the higher baseline temperatures of the intraoral tissues. As discussed previously in this chapter, sensitivity to warmth is greater, and sensitivity to cold is less, at higher baseline temperatures such as those found in the mouth, than at lower baseline temperatures.

The higher sensitivity of the whole mouth to warming than to cooling was observed independently of whether the liquid was unflavoured (water) or flavoured (coffee) and whether the subject held or swished the liquid during the stimulus period. Interestingly, the oral cavity warmed most of the liquids during swishing, yet the results were similar to those obtained when the subjects simply held the liquid in the mouth, without swishing, prior to expectoration. This suggests that perceptually relevant information about temperature is extracted when a liquid first enters the mouth and its temperature differs most greatly from those of the oral tissues.

Without the benefit of fire and refrigeration (which are comparatively recent on the evolutionary scale!), most edible objects in one's natural surroundings are slightly cooler than the tissues. Differences in their thermal conductivities result in differences in the extents to which the oral and lingual mucosa are cooled by the objects. These thermal cues no doubt contribute to the identification, discrimination and enjoyment of food substances. There is also some evidence that cooling of the teeth contributes to intraoral sensations of cold. However, most studies conclude that all natural stimuli (including cold, heat, and osmotic challenges applied to exposed dentinal tubules) result in sensations of only pain. The stimulation of pulpal afferents clearly dominants subjects' perception and ratings of intraoral cold intensity when the mouth is exposed to low, noxious temperatures. Cold, and to a lesser degree hot, liquids and foods produce sharp dental pain when brought into contact with sensitive dentin. The intensity of the pain correlates with the discharge activity evoked in pulpal Aδ-fibre nociceptors. These nociceptors are thought to be mechanoreceptors, not high-threshold thermoreceptors. They respond to the mechanical movements of fluid in the dentinal tubules produced by the thermal gradients rather than to the temperature changes *per se* (see Chapter 5).

◼ Summary

Foods that enter the mouth and objects that touch the face often have temperatures that differ from the orofacial tissues. The resulting transfer of thermal energy evokes discharges in, or alters the on-going discharge activity of different classes of thermoreceptors supplying the epithelia. Low-threshold warm and cold thermoreceptors (fibres) respond to the resting temperatures of the tissues and to changes in temperature that will not damage tissues. In contrast, high-threshold thermoreceptors, such as C-fibre polymodal nociceptors, respond to more extreme changes in temperature that can burn or freeze the tissues. High-threshold cold receptors respond to temperatures lower than those to which the low-threshold cold fibres respond. The different classes of thermoreceptors differ in their response properties, and explain humans' capacity to distinguish between thermal stimuli at very high to very low temperatures. Exposure of thermoreceptors to very high, noxious temperatures can sensitise or desensitise them, changing the threshold temperature to which the thermoreceptors respond and the magnitude of their responses to higher temperatures.

Cold stimulates the low-threshold cold fibres, high-threshold cold receptors and nociceptors. Activity in cold fibres and high-threshold cold receptors inhibits inputs from the nociceptors *via* central neural mechanisms. Burning pain is perceived when the inhibition is insufficient to block the effects of the nociceptive inputs. Individual orofacial sites are better equipped for sensing cold than warmth, although whole mouth sensitivity is greater for differences in warmth than for differences in cold. Discrete intraoral and extraoral sites are about equally sensitive to cold. In contrast, with the exception of the tip of the tongue, discrete intraoral sites are less sensitive to warmth and noxious heat than extraoral sites. The tip of the tongue is the most thermally-sensitive intraoral site, contribu-

ting to its role in the identification, discrimination and enjoyment of foods.

■ Selected references

Bushnell MC, Taylor MB, Duncan GH, Dubner R. Discrimination of innocuous and noxious thermal stimuli applied to the face in human and monkey. Somatosen Res 1983;1:119–129.

Chen C-C, Rainville P, Bushnell MC. Noxious and innocuous cold discrimination in humans: evidence for separate afferent channels. Pain 1996;68:33–43.

Engelen L, De Wijk RA, Prinz JF, van der Bilt A, Janssen AM, Bosman F. The effect of oral temperature on the temperature perception of liquids and semisolids in the mouth. Eur J Oral Sci 2002;110:412–416.

Green BG. Thermal perception on lingual and labial skin. Percept Psychophys 1984;36:209–220.

Green BG, Gelhard B. Perception of temperature on oral and facial skin. Somatosen Res 1987;4:191–200.

Kenshalo DR. Psychophysical studies of temperature sensitivity. In: *Contributions to Sensory Physiology*, edited by W. D. Neff. New York: Academic Press, 1970, vol. 4, pp. 19–74.

Sumino R, Dubner R. Response characteristics of specific thermoreceptive afferents innervating monkey facial skin and their relationship to human thermal sensitivity. Brain Res Rev 1981;3:105–122.

Zuker CS. A cool ion channel. Nature 2002;416:27–28.

Orofacial pain

Peter Svensson and Barry J. Sessle

Goals:
- To understand the complexity of the neurobiological and psychosocial aspects of acute and chronic orofacial pain.
- To know how to diagnose, assess and manage the most common types of orofacial pain.
- To identify the less common types of orofacial pain and to appreciate the importance of referral and coordination of pain diagnosis and management with pain specialists.

Key words:
Nociception; physiology; psychology; mechanisms; diagnosis; classification; assessment; management.

Introduction

Pain has always been very important in dental practice. Even today toothaches remain one of the most common reasons for people to seek dental treatment; however, there are now many complaints about types of orofacial pain other than toothaches. Population-based studies indicate that 1–2% of the population may suffer or have suffered from face pain within the last 6 months, 8% of the population from musculoskeletal pain in the orofacial region (the so-called temporomandibular disorders or TMDs) and 10–12% from toothache. Furthermore, women seem to suffer more frequently than men from many of the chronic types of orofacial pain. Acute pain can also be produced by many dental procedures, which unfortunately prevents many people from obtaining optimal dental care. Furthermore, there are

many acute pain conditions seen in the dental office that require immediate control and management and, as age-based demographics change, dentists will see increasing numbers of chronic orofacial pain conditions. Dentists will require good diagnostic skills and knowledge about pain and its control since management approaches for acute pain conditions will differ markedly from those for chronic pain.

Acute pain is a sign that something is wrong and has a significant value to the person as an alert signal. Acute pain is particularly important as a learning signal that should help to avoid future situations in which tissue damage may occur. However, in chronic pain conditions, this signal and learning value is lost and pain may become a disease or disorder in itself. This latter type of pain is not protective and has no clear biological meaning and yet it is associated with severe emotional or health-related stresses. These stresses are likely to affect the patient by reducing their quality of life such as loss of appetite, libido and sleep disturbances and even leading to psychological disturbances. However, they may also affect the patient's family and friends, and even the attending clinician who can become frustrated that no "cure" seems to work. Moreover, pain in the face and mouth has special biological, emotional and psychological meaning to the patient because of the special role of the orofacial region in basic drives such as eating, drinking, speech and, sexual behaviour, and in expression of emotions.

In addition to the emotional and social consequences of pain to the patient and others, orofacial pain, especially when chronic, will become an increasing socio-economic burden as the population changes with more people being middle-aged or elderly, the age span in which many chronic pain conditions are prevalent. There is therefore a strong need for greater education and dissemination of knowledge in order to diagnose and manage orofacial pain conditions more efficiently, and dentists must be aware of their special responsibility and obligation to help their patients with orofacial pain complaints.

Unfortunately, there has been a limited focus on orofacial pain in the teaching programs in many dental schools. Despite the prevalence of pain in dental practice, this topic is often only a minor component of curricula. Even today, many health care providers continue to think that pain is a "hardwired" system with a one-way transmission of "pain signals" from an injured site to the brain, and that pain is simply one of the cardinal symptoms of inflammation. Pain can be simply a part of the inflammatory response and the consequences of tissue in-

jury, but it can also be much more complex and indeed can often be considered a complex disease or disorder in itself.

■ Definition and classification of pain

It is useful to consider first how to classify pain, because management will vary widely between acute pain conditions such as toothache and persistent pain problems such as those in the temporomandibular joint (TMJ). The most widely accepted definition of pain is provided by the International Association for the Study of Pain (IASP):

> "Pain is an unpleasant sensory and emotional experience with actual or potential tissue damage, or described in terms of such damage".

This definition captures the most salient features of pain and points out that pain is more than the outcome of a tissue-damaging (noxious) stimulus. The main issue is that pain is always a subjective sensory experience, that is, there are no objective means to detect pain, and that pain first will become pain when the subject says it is pain. The obvious limitations of the definition are then related to the person's ability to say that a stimulus or condition is painful or not: this is not possible, for example, for a pre-verbal child or baby, or a person in coma, or some mentally handicapped people, and certainly not for animals. In such situations, one must depend upon the behaviour and the responses of the subject which may include crying, facial expressions and reflex withdrawal responses.

Various theories of pain have been suggested. For example, it was previously postulated that pain is a specific sensation analogous to vision and touch, with a hard-wired line from a "pain receptor" to the brain (specificity theory). Other theories proposed that excessive stimulation involving several types of receptors would lead to summation of signals and pain (intensive or summation theory), and another that the pattern of signals produced by the noxious stimulus would be important for the recognition of pain (pattern theory). Since many different afferent fibres project to the same neurones in the brain, it was suggested that nociceptive and other afferent fibres also could influence each other and modify the perception of pain (sensory interactive theory). The latter theory was later refined with special emphasis on the potential inhibition of nociceptive transmission by large mechanoreceptive fibres (gate control theory). Today it is known that not all elements of the gate control theory as originally proposed are correct, but this theory has had a huge impact on the understanding of pain and its control because it provides a good general framework of pain and its complexity.

Pain is best thought of as a complex and multidimensional experience, and there are a variety of behavioural responses associated with both acute and chronic pain. The sensory-discriminative component of pain is related to the person's ability to tell if there is a little pain, moderate pain or very severe pain (monitoring the intensity of pain); where the pain is coming from, e.g., a tooth, the tongue, the TMJ, etc., (pain localisation); and what kind of pain it is, e.g. "diffuse cramping" pain from muscles, "sharp" or "shooting" pain from a tooth, or "burning" pain from the oral mucosa (pain quality). Clearly, pain also involves an emotional re-

sponse because it is unpleasant and associated with suffering (the so-called affective component of pain). Furthermore, the person will automatically compare the pain with previous painful experiences and interpret it in relation to the actual situation (cognitive component of pain). For example: "I need to go the dentist to have my toothache fixed and then I will be alright" or "I have now had this jaw pain for so long and nothing has helped me and I am feeling so depressed". Still another component of the pain experience is the motivational component, which is the conscious or unconscious drive state for a person to initiate, sustain or direct behaviour in a certain manner. This may vary substantially from an acute pain situation which is a warning signal that something is wrong and requires dental or medical treatment, to a situation where chronic orofacial pain can be the reason and even the excuse for the person in pain not to participate in social or work activities, a situation referred to as "secondary gain".

A particular useful way to think about pain is formulated in the so-called bio-psycho-social model, which encapsulates much of the complexity of pain (Fig. 1). Pain is rarely a question about simply the presence of nociceptive activity (nociceptive pain) or its absence (psychological pain) but rather a complex relationship where the same nociceptive activity can be interpreted and expressed by one person very differently from other persons and be associated with quite different response, and illness behaviour (sick role).

In practical terms, the IASP has classified pain according to its duration (acute or chronic). Often the distinction between acute and chronic is set to 6 months but this is rather arbitrary and it may be more relevant to distinguish between pain which

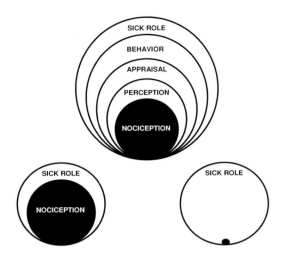

● **Figure 1.** Bio-psycho-social pain model modified after Dworkin (2001). In some patients, the nociceptive component will constitute a significant part of the pain problem (lower left), whereas in other patients the nociceptive component is relatively small compared to the sick role (lower right).

subsides within few weeks after an injury, and pain which lasts beyond the normal tissue healing time. Instead of chronic pain, the term *persistent pain* is now often used. Furthermore, pain can be classified according to the region affected (head, face and mouth; cervical region, thoracic region, etc.), and divided into organ systems (musculoskeletal, visceral, cutaneous-subcutaneous, nervous, respiratory, cardiovascular, etc.). The temporal characteristics are also important to consider to classify the pain (single episode, continuous, intermittent, paroxysmal etc.). Finally, the aetiology of pain can be used to classify pain (genetic-congenital, trauma, infection, inflammatory, degenerative, psychological). IASP has used these characteristics to classify more than 50 fairly localised pain syndromes in the head and face (Table 1). The International Headache Society has developed another classifi-

cation system which also can be relevant for dentists. Currently, there is no universal classification system, and different names and criteria are sometimes used to label similar pain conditions.

From a clinical perspective, it is important to know if pain is located in the skin, mucosa, tooth or muscle, but from a physiological point of view this may not be so important if it is the result of similar pathophysiological mechanisms even in different tissues. Thus, the underlying mechanisms of pain can share many common characteristics but the clinical presentation may differ between different tissues and regions. Therefore, it is a matter of current discussion in the pain field whether it is possible to classify pain according to the mechanisms involved in addition to the classification of the symptoms. Table 2 lists the classification based on current knowledge of pain mechanisms, which will be discussed later in this chapter.

Finally, it makes sense from a clinical dental perspective to distinguish between spontaneous pain and procedural pain (also known as iatrogenic, or "physician-induced" pain). The latter is often transient: obvious examples include the pain occurring during dental scaling, drilling in a deep dental cavity, application of orthodontic appliances etc., but may also involve tissue injury pain (post-operative pain). Procedural pain can usually be predicted: if so, appropriate prevention is possible and mandatory.

It is important for dentists to understand the modern concept of pain and to appreciate both the neurobiological and psychosocial components. The current classification of pain is based primarily on its signs and symptoms, but one should seek to elucidate its underlying mechanisms because this understanding will also facilitate its control and management.

Table 1.

Neuralgias	Musculoskeletal pains	Primary headaches
• Acute herpes zoster	• Acute tension-type headache	• Carotidynia
• Geniculate neuralgia (VII)	• Chronic tension-type headache	• Chronic paroxysmal hemicrania
• Glossopharyngeal neuralgia (IX)	• Crushing injury of head or face	• Classic migraine
• Hypoglossal neuralgia (XII)	• Rheumatoid arthritis of the	• Cluster headache
• Post-herpetic neuralgia	temporomandibular joint	• Common migraine
• Secondary neuralgias	• Temporomandibular disorders	• Hemicrania continua
• Short-lasting, unilateral,	(TMDs)	• Mixed headache
neuralgiform pain with		• Post-traumatic headache
conjunctival injection and		• Temporal arteritis
tearing (SUNCT)	**Pains in the ear, nose and oral**	
• Tolosa-Hunt syndrome	**cavity**	
• Trigeminal neuralgia		**Psychological pains**
	• Atypical odontalgia and facial	
	pain	• Associated with depression
	• Burning mouth syndrome	• Delusional or hallucinatory pain
	• Cracked tooth syndrome	• Hysterical, conversion or
	• Diseases of the jaw	hypochondriacal pain
	• Dry socket	
	• Frostbite of face	
	• Gingival disease	
	• Maxillary sinusitis	
	• Odontalgia	
	• Otitis media	

Examples of pain conditions that occur in the head and face. Some are extremely rare (e.g. Tolosa-Hunt syndrome) and are most likely to be seen only by neurologists or other pain specialists. Others are very common (acute tension-type headache, TMDs and odontalgias) in everyday dental practice. Note that the groupings are based on a mixture of e.g. regions, tissues and pain mechanisms. Modified from Merskey, H. and Bogduk, N. (Eds.) Classification of chronic pain. IASP Press: Seattle, 1994.

■ Basic neurobiology of orofacial pain

Primary afferent properties and peripheral sensitisation

General features

The orofacial tissues are innervated almost exclusively by branches of the trigeminal (V) sensory nerve. Chapter 6 describes the V primary afferent fibres that terminate in these tissues in sense organs (receptors) that are quite complex in their structure, and that respond to tactile stimulation (e.g. low-threshold mechanoreceptors) or to proprioceptive stimuli such as stretch or tension (e.g. proprioceptors). Other primary afferents may terminate as free nerve endings, many of which respond to noxious stimuli and are termed *nociceptors*. These so-called nociceptive afferents are generally smaller in size and slower-conducting than the A-beta or A-delta afferents that convey tactile or proprioceptive information into the central nervous system (CNS). Nociceptive afferents are either small-diameter, myelinated (A-delta) primary afferent fibres or even smaller (and even slower-conducting) unmyelinated (C) afferent fibres. It is important to note that not all of the A-delta and C-fibre afferents conduct nociceptive information: some

Table 2.

Transient pain	Tissue injury pain (Inflammatory pain)	Nervous system injury pain (Neuropathic pain)
Nociceptor specialisation*	Primary afferent <ul><li>Sensitisation</li><li>Recruitment of silent nociceptors</li><li>Alteration in phenotype</li><li>Hyperinnervation</li></ul> CNS mediated <ul><li>Central sensitisation recruitment, summation and amplification</li></ul>	Primary afferent <ul><li>Acquisition of spontaneous and stimulus-evoked activity by nociceptor axons and cell bodies at loci other than peripheral terminals</li><li>Phenotype changes</li></ul> CNS mediated <ul><li>Central sensitisation</li><li>Deafferentation of second order neurons</li><li>Disinhibition</li><li>Structural reorganisation</li></ul>

* Specialisation refers to specific membrane and neurochemical properties of nociceptors and associated afferent nerve fibres that allows them to be differentially activated by different types of brief noxious stimuli (e.g. mechanical, heat or chemical).

Suggested classification of pain according to underlying mechanisms. Modified from Woolf et al. Towards a mechanism-based classification of pain? Pain 1998;77:227–9. Note that similar mechanisms may be at work in both tissue and nervous system injury pain.

are associated with receptors that respond to cooling, warming or even tactile stimuli (Chapters 3 and 6).

The nociceptive afferents convey sensory information as action potentials from the nociceptors into the CNS and thereby provide the brain with sensory-discriminative information about the spatial and temporal qualities of the noxious stimulus. The frequency of the nerve impulses and the duration of the nerve impulse discharge of the nociceptive afferent fibres provide the peripheral basis for coding the intensity and duration of the noxious stimulus. In the case of localisation of the stimulus, the important peripheral feature is the receptive field of the fibre, i.e. the area of skin, mucosa or deep tissue from which the afferent fibre and its associated receptors can be excited by a threshold stimulus. The area of a receptive field of a nociceptive afferent fibre is usually less than 1 mm^2, and the threshold for its excitation from the receptive field is very high and in the noxious range. Note that nociceptive stimuli particularly in superficial tissues also activate other receptors such as mechanoreceptors that code for touch, and these play an important role in determining the location and quality of the sensation perceived. In tissues that have no touch receptors, such as tooth pulp and muscles, nociceptive stimuli give rise to a different quality of pain sensation.

How are the nociceptive afferents activated by a noxious stimulus? The tissue damage produced by the noxious stimulus causes the release of chemical mediators from surrounding tissues (e.g. prostaglandins, bradykinins) that activate free nerve endings. Their activation may result in the production of action potentials in the A-delta and/or C-fibre afferents, which are

Figure 2. Mechanisms involved in activation of the peripheral endings of nociceptive afferents and in afferent sensitisation. **A.** A noxious stimulus, such as intense pressure, causes cell damage and release of potassium (K^+) and the synthesis of substances such as the prostaglandins (PG) and bradykinins (BK); PG enhances the sensitivity of the endings to BK and other substances. **B.** Indirect activation of the afferents may occur. Action potentials generated in the endings of a nociceptive afferent travel not only toward the CNS, but also into collaterals in which they bring about the release of the neuropeptide Substance P (SP). SP produces vasodilation, oedema, and release of histamine (H) and serotonin (5-HT) from adjacent cells. **C.** The rise in H and 5-HT levels in the peripheral tissues sensitises the endings of other nearby nociceptive afferents. (From Fields, H.L.: Pain. New York, McGraw-Hill, 1987.)

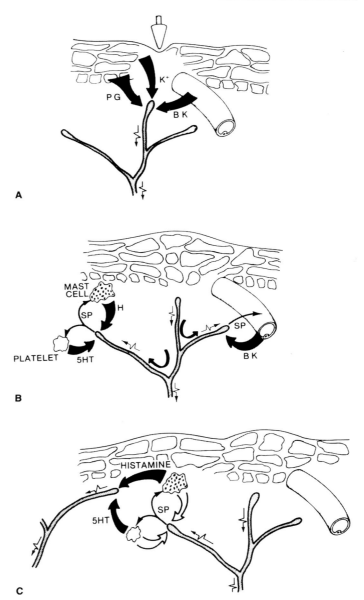

conveyed into the CNS and may elicit the perception of transient or acute pain (Fig. 2A).

However, a number of factors and chemical mediators influence the excitability of the nociceptive afferent endings. These are outlined in Fig. 3, and include damage to peripheral tissues which often results in inflammation and may also involve products released from blood vessels or from cells of the immune system. Substances synthesised in and released from the afferent fibres

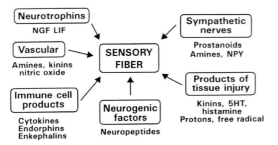

Figure 3. A variety of factors and chemical mediators can influence excitability of nociceptive endings. Recent research has also shown that additional neurogenic factors include the excitatory amino acid glutamate. (From Dray A. Agonists and antagonists of nociception. In: Jensen, T.S., Turner, J.A. and Wiesenfeld-Hallin, Z (Eds.) Proceedings of the 8th World Congress on Pain. Progress in Pain Research and Management, Vol. 8. IASP Press: Seattle, p.279–292, 1997.)

themselves may influence the excitability of the nociceptive afferents. Examples include the neurotrophins such as nerve growth factor, and neuropeptides such as substance P and calcitonin gene-related peptide (CGRP). Under certain conditions, substances such as noradrenaline that are released from sympathetic efferents innervating the tissues may also modulate the excitability of the nociceptors. In some situations, the tissue damage may lead to abnormal nerve changes that are associated with so-called ectopic or aberrant neural discharges. These are important in certain pain conditions (see Clinical presentation of orofacial pain, later in this chapter).

Increased excitability of the nociceptors may occur at the site of injury in many cases of tissue damage or inflammation. This is termed *nociceptor or peripheral sensitisation.* The processes and chemical mediators involved in producing peripheral sensitisation include the products of tissue injury as well as the release of neurochemicals (e.g. neuro-

peptides such as substance P and CGRP) that are synthesised in the primary afferent cell bodies of nociceptive afferents and are released from the afferent endings (Fig. 2). These neuropeptides may cause platelets, macrophages, mast cells and other cells of the immune system to release inflammatory mediators such as histamine, serotonin (5-HT), bradykinin and cytokines. Release of the neuropeptides and these inflammatory mediators results in oedema (swelling), redness, and local temperature increases which, along with pain, are the cardinal signs of inflammation. This process has been termed neurogenic inflammation, because it arises from nerves themselves. The chemicals also act on the nociceptive afferent endings and contribute to the peripheral sensitisation. Sensitised nociceptors exhibit spontaneous activity, lowered activation thresholds, and increased responsiveness to subsequent noxious stimuli. These changes appear to contribute, respectively, to the spontaneous pain, allodynia and hyperalgesia (see Glossary) that are features of many chronic or persistent pain conditions (Table 3).

The chemicals may also diffuse through the peripheral tissues and act on the endings of adjacent nociceptive afferents (Fig. 2), and thus contribute to the size of the

The earliest physicians did not of course understand the basis for acute inflammation but nevertheless described its classical signs which were referred to as *dolor* (pain), *calor* (warmth), *rubor* (reddening), *tumour* (swelling, and *functio laesa* (decreased function).

Table 3. Pain features that may be accounted for by peripheral sensitisation of nociceptive afferent.

Nociceptive Afferent	Pain Features
• Decreased activation threshold	• Allodynia
• Increased suprathreshold responsiveness	• Hyperalgesia
• Involvement of adjacent afferent endings	• Pain spread
• Spontaneous activity	• Spontaneous pain

painful area and pain spread (Table 3). The increased afferent barrage into the CNS from this increased nociceptor activity may also lead to functional changes in central nociceptive processing that contribute to persistent pain. Central processes such as *central sensitisation* (see below) especially seem to be involved in so-called secondary hyperalgesia which refers to increased sensitivity to noxious stimuli well beyond the site of tissue injury. In contrast, peripheral processes involving *peripheral sensitisation* of nociceptive afferent endings at the injury site can account for the increased pain sensitivity at the site of injury (primary hyperalgesia).

These effects of tissue damage and inflammation are important factors in many painful conditions that dentists are called upon to treat, such as pulpitis and mucositis. Furthermore, knowledge of the chemical mechanisms involved in the activation or sensitisation of the nociceptive afferents has led to the development of therapeutic agents targeting specific peripheral mechanisms. For example, common non-steroidal anti-inflammatory drugs (NSAIDs) including salicylates such as aspirin, as well as many newly developed analgesics such as COX-2 inhibitors, have their principal analgesic and anti-inflammatory actions in peripheral tissues (see Pain therapy). They can reduce inflammation associated with tissue injury, modulate nociceptive afferent excitability, and alter the hyperalgesia associated with short-term orofacial pain conditions.

Additional receptor mechanisms have been discovered recently in peripheral nerve endings that are involved in pain. They include the vanilloid VRI (or TRPVI) receptor that responds to protons (H^+), heat, and chemicals such as capsaicin, the ingredient in chilli (hot) peppers that produces pain. Chemical mediators long thought to be involved in nociceptive transmission or modulation within the CNS (e.g. the excitatory amino acid glutamate, and opioid-related substances such as enkephalins) can also act peripherally on the nociceptive afferents. For example, glutamate is synthesised by primary afferent cell bodies. It can excite nociceptive afferents supplying craniofacial musculoskeletal tissues and produce a transient pain in humans by activating *glutamate receptors* (N-methyl-D-aspartate [NMDA] and non-NMDA receptors) located on the afferent endings. In contrast, the opiate drug morphine can depress the activity of these afferents by interacting with opioid receptors on the nociceptive afferent endings. The multiplicity of peripheral chemical mediators involved in peripheral nociceptive activation, sensitisation and related events (e.g. inflammation) are all potential targets for the development of new and more effective therapeutic approaches to pain control.

Specific orofacial nociceptive afferents
The *tooth pulp* is a highly vascular and richly innervated tissue that is exquisitely sensitive to stimulation. Dentine is also very sensitive despite its very sparse innervation. The properties of the afferent fibres supplying pulp and dentine and their role in pulpal

pain and dentine sensitivity are outlined in Chapter 5.

The *periodontal ligament* contains free nerve endings associated with A-delta and C-fibre nociceptive afferents that may respond to mechanical, thermal and/or chemical stimuli. The different classes of receptors are in general similar to nociceptors in other tissues. Some periodontal afferents branch to innervate the pulp of an adjacent tooth: the significance of this is unclear, but this could be a substrate for the spread or referral of pain to adjacent teeth (see below).

A-delta and C-fibre nociceptive afferents also exist in the *oral mucosa* and are sensitive to a variety of noxious stimuli. Their responsiveness may also be influenced by biomechanical factors in the tissues.

The *cutaneous tissues* of the orofacial region have a dense nerve supply, especially in the perioral region. These include 3 major classes of nociceptive afferent fibres: (1) high-threshold mechanoreceptive afferents that respond best to strong mechanical stimuli (most of these conduct in the A-delta range, although some may have conduction velocities in the A-beta and C-fibre ranges); (2) A-delta mechano-thermal nociceptive afferents that are excited by strong thermal and mechanical stimuli (Chapter 3 and 6);

and (3) C-polymodal nociceptive afferents that are excited by intense mechanical, thermal and chemical stimuli.

Nerve terminals penetrate into the *corneal* epithelium and respond to a wide range of mechanical, thermal and chemical stimuli, all of which cause pain in man. Despite their low thresholds, these receptors are capable of evoking pain.

A-delta and C-fibre afferents also supply the TMJ and masticatory muscles. These small-diameter afferents and analogous afferents in spinal systems may respond to a wide range of peripheral stimuli that cause pain in humans, e.g. heavy pressure, algesic chemicals such as capsaicin, mustard oil, and glutamate, and inflammatory agents. Ischemia may also stimulate small-diameter muscle afferents if it is prolonged and associated with muscle contractions.

Finally, small-diameter afferent fibres supply cranial blood vessels as well as the dura mater overlying the cerebral hemispheres, and many of these can be activated by noxious stimuli. The modulation of the cerebrovascular afferents by peripheral neurochemical processes (e.g. 5-HT) may be important in the initiation and control of certain types of headaches such as migraine.

▪ Brainstem nociceptive transmission

Organisation and neuronal properties

The primary afferent cell bodies of most trigeminal (V) primary afferents innervating cutaneous, intraoral (e.g. mucosa, tooth pulp), deep (e.g. joint, muscle) and cerebrovascular tissues lie in the V ganglion. Their axons project from the ganglion to the peripheral tissues. The neuronal cell bodies also project centrally into the brainstem where they makes connections with neur-

Interestingly, sex differences have been found in some of these peripheral actions of glutamate and morphine, suggesting that peripherally based physiological mechanisms may contribute to the sex differences in prevalence of many chronic pain conditions. This is discussed further under the heading of Clinical presentation of orofacial pain.

ones especially in the V brainstem sensory nuclear complex. Each component of the V brainstem complex also receives neuronal projections from other brainstem or higher brain centres that constitute part of the substrate for the modulatory influences on V brainstem complex neurones that are described later in this chapter.

The V brainstem complex consists of the V main sensory nucleus and the V spinal tract nucleus, and the latter is subdivided into three subnuclei: oralis, interpolaris and caudalis (Fig. 4). Whereas subnucleus caudalis has a laminated structure similar to the dorsal horn of the spinal cord, the structure of the other 3 components of the V brainstem complex is more uniform, although subdivisions of each can be distinguished in some species. The neurones in each nucleus/subnucleus are somatotopically arranged (Fig. 5), with the dorsal part of the main sensory nucleus and the 3 subnuclei com-

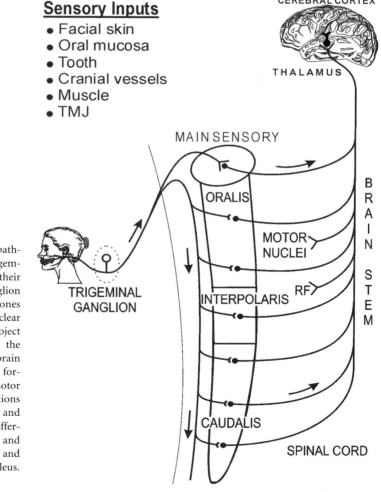

Sensory Inputs
- Facial skin
- Oral mucosa
- Tooth
- Cranial vessels
- Muscle
- TMJ

CEREBRAL CORTEX

THALAMUS

MAIN SENSORY

ORALIS

MOTOR NUCLEI

INTERPOLARIS   RF

TRIGEMINAL GANGLION

CAUDALIS

SPINAL CORD

BRAINSTEM

Figure 4. Major somatosensory pathway from the face and mouth. Trigeminal (V) primary afferents have their cell bodies in the trigeminal ganglion and project to second-order neurones in the V brainstem sensory nuclear complex. These neurones may project to neurones in higher levels of the brain (e.g. in the thalamus) or in brain stem regions such as the reticular formation (RF) or cranial nerve motor nuclei. Not shown are the projections of some cervical nerve afferents and cranial nerve VII, IX, X, and XII afferents to the V brain stem complex and the projection of many V, VII, IX, and X afferents to the solitary tract nucleus. (From Sessle, 2000.)

prised mainly of neurones with a receptive field in the orofacial region supplied by the mandibular branch of the V nerve. The ventral part contains neurones with ophthalmic receptive fields, and the area between the dorsal and ventral parts contains neurones with maxillary receptive fields. Neurones with an oral or perioral receptive field are usually located in the most medial part of each nucleus and subnucleus. However, this inverted, medially-facing somatotopic or topographical pattern of representation of the face and mouth may be different in subnucleus caudalis, with perioral regions represented in the rostral part of the subnucleus and more lateral regions of the face represented more caudally.

Most evidence favours the view that subnucleus caudalis is the principal brainstem relay site for V nociceptive information. Transection of the V spinal tract at the rostral pole of subnucleus caudalis in humans is a neurosurgical procedure called V tractotomy that was used in earlier times for the relief of the excruciating pain of V neuralgia. This transection also produces a marked reduction in the patient's ability to perceive noxious stimuli applied to the face, and analogous lesions in experimental animals reduce behavioural, autonomic and muscle reflex responses to noxious facial stimuli. This suggests that the caudalis lesion interferes with the relay of nociceptive signals from the small-diameter nociceptive primary afferents and second-order neurones in subnucleus caudalis. Indeed, the great majority of the small-diameter (A-delta and C-fibre) primary afferents carrying nociceptive information from the various orofacial tissues (see Primary afferent properties and peripheral sensitisation) terminate in caudalis. The laminated structure and morphological cell types in this subnucleus resemble the dorsal horn of the spinal cord,

which is critically involved in nociceptive transmission. These small-diameter afferents terminate in caudalis laminae I, II, and V and VI, whereas the larger A-fibre primary afferents conducting low-threshold mechanosensitive (tactile) information terminate primarily in laminae III-VI of caudalis and in the more rostral components of the V brainstem complex. Furthermore, increases in immunocytochemical markers of neuronal activity, such as so-called Fos protein, occur in caudalis neurones following noxious stimulation of craniofacial tissues. In addition, electrophysiological recordings of the activity of brainstem neurones in animal experiments have revealed that many neurones in caudalis can be activated by cutaneous nociceptive inputs.

The nociceptive neurones in subnucleus caudalis are predominantly located in its superficial (I/II) and deep (V/VI) laminae. They have been categorised as either nociceptive-specific (NS) or wide dynamic range (WDR) (Fig. 6). The NS neurones receive small-diameter nociceptive afferent inputs from A-delta and/or C fibres, and are excited only by high-intensity orofacial stimuli (e.g. pinch, heat) applied to a localised orofacial receptive field. WDR neurones in contrast receive not only A-delta and/or C-fibre inputs but also the large-diameter A-fibre inputs that transmit non-noxious (e.g. tactile) information. Thus, WDR neurones can be excited by both noxious and non-noxious stimuli, and they have a large receptive field with both low-threshold and high-threshold areas, whereas the receptive fields of NS neurones are purely nociceptive, and generally smaller. Both types of nociceptive neurones nonetheless increase their firing frequency progressively as the intensity of noxious stimulation is gradually increased or as more of the receptive field is stimulated. Our ability to localise, detect, discriminate and

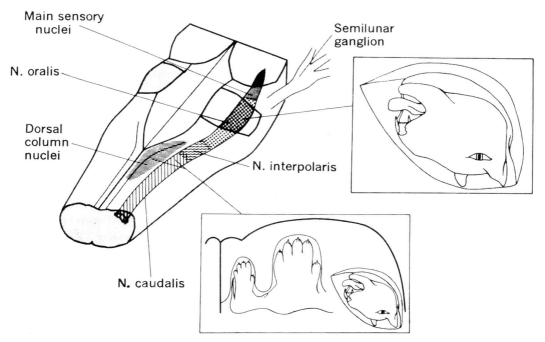

Figure 5. Schematic of the inverted representation of the face and mouth (of a cat, in this instance) in the different subdivisions of the V brainstem nuclear complex. Each area of the ipsilateral face is represented at all rostrocaudal levels within the V brainstem complex. The projections of ipsilateral limbs and trunk to the dorsal column nuclei are also shown. (From Mountcastle, V.B. Medical Physiology. Mosby, St. Louis, Vol.1, 1974.)

grade the intensity of noxious stimuli in the orofacial area is dependent on these receptive field and response properties of the caudalis NS and WDR neurones, many of which project to the thalamus where their information about the noxious stimulus is relayed to the somatosensory cerebral cortex (see Thalamo-cortical nociceptive transmission).

Some caudalis NS and WDR neurones respond to stimulation of only a cutaneous or mucosal receptive field and thus appear to contribute to our ability to localise, detect, and discriminate superficial noxious stimuli. However, very few appear to be activated specifically by peripheral afferents from other tissues, such as those supplying tooth pulp, cerebral blood vessels, TMJ or jaw muscle: indeed the majority of the NS and

WDR neurones can be excited by one or more of these afferent inputs as well as by cutaneous or mucosal afferent inputs (Fig. 7). The presence of a cutaneous receptive field as well as a deep receptive field (e.g. in tooth pulp, TMJ, muscle) in most of these neurones, plus the efficacy of deep nociceptive afferent inputs in inducing an expansion of both cutaneous and deep receptive fields (see Neuroplasticity and central sensitisation), contribute to the common clinical observations of poor localisation and referral of pain from these deep tissues, or from one tooth to another tooth (see Clinical presentation of orofacial pain).

Low-threshold mechanosensitive neurones also occur in subnucleus caudalis and other components of the V brainstem com-

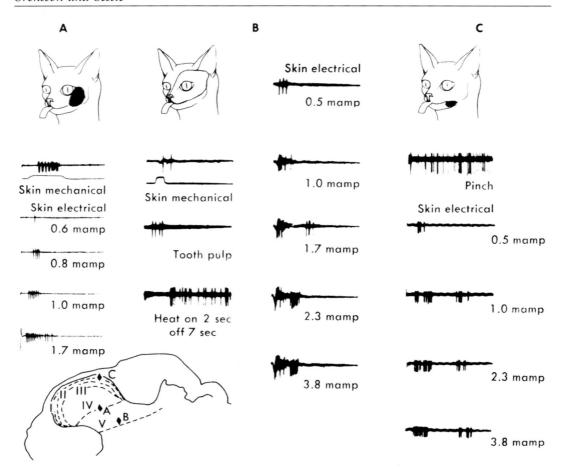

Figure 6. Examples of three classes of neurones found in trigeminal subnucleus caudalis. As illustrated from these data derived from studies in cats, a neurone may be a low-threshold mechanosensitive neurone A. a wide dynamic range nociceptive neurone B, or a nociceptive-specific neurone C. Records in A were obtained from a single low-threshold mechanosensitive neurone that was activated only by light tactile (mechanical) stimulation of the area of facial skin outlined. It discharged to mechanical stimulation of the skin and to increasing intensity levels of electric stimulation of skin; however, even at high intensities, only a single burst of action potentials was elicited. This neurone was located in lamina IV of subnucleus caudalis as illustrated below. The wide dynamic range neurone shown in B was activated by tactile stimulation of area of skin outlined as well as by electric stimulation of the canine tooth pulp, pinch (not shown), and noxious levels of radiant heat applied to the skin. Note that with increasing intensity levels of electric stimulation of the skin, late as well as early bursts of impulses were evoked. The late discharge probably reflects inputs from nociceptive afferent fibres, and the early burst reflects inputs from faster-conducting "tactile" afferent fibres. This neurone was located in lamina V of subnucleus caudalis. The nociceptive-specific neurone shown in C was located in lamina 1 and could only be excited by noxious stimulation of the skin (e.g. pinch). The early burst of impulses produced by high-intensity electric stimulation of skin probably reflects inputs from small myelinated (A-δ) nociceptive afferent fibres, and the later burst reflects inputs from unmyelinated (C) nociceptive afferent fibres. Time duration of records: A, 50 ms; B, 100 ms (except heat record: 10 s); C, 200 ms (except pinch record: 10 s). Record to pinch in C is at twice the gain for skin electric records. (From Sessle BJ. Pain. In: Roth GI & Calmes R (Eds) Oral Biology; St Louis, Mosby, 1981, pp 3–28).

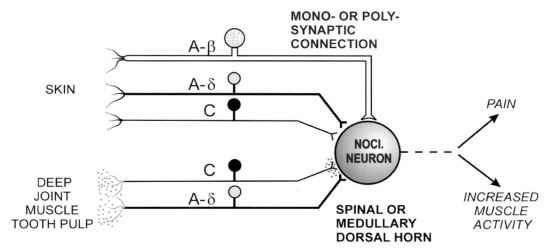

Figure 7. Convergence of afferent inputs onto nociceptive neurones in trigeminal subnucleus caudalis (medullary dorsal horn) or its analogous structure in the spinal cord. Some afferents are excited only by superficial afferent inputs from skin (or mucosa), others by superficial and one or more of the deep afferent inputs (e.g. from joint, muscle, tooth pulp). (From Hu, J.W. Cephalic myofascial pain pathways. In: Olesen, J. and Schoenen, J. (Eds.) Tension-type Headache: Classification, Mechanisms, and Treatment. Raven Press: New York, p. 69–77, 1993.)

plex. They are innervated by large-fibre afferents (e.g. A-beta) and so are responsive to light tactile stimulation of a localised receptive field in the facial skin or mouth but not to noxious stimuli. The low-threshold mechanosensitive neurones provide the brainstem substrate for the localisation, detection and discrimination of touch and send their detailed information about the tactile stimulus to higher brain regions such as the thalamus from where the information is passed on to the cerebral cortex.

The V nociceptive primary afferents release excitatory amino acids (e.g. glutamate) and neuropeptides (e.g. substance P, CGRP) in caudalis (Fig. 8). Thus, these neurochemicals are released not only from the peripheral endings of V nociceptive primary afferents but also from their central endings. The release of glutamate leads to the activation of caudalis nociceptive neurones by a process involving 2 different ionotropic glutamate receptors (i.e., that gates ion channels directly) for glutamate, N-methyl-D-aspartate (NMDA) and AMPA receptors (alpha-amino-3-hydroxy-5-methyl-4-isoxazole-propionic acid), as well as metabotropic glutamate receptors (i.e., that gates ion channels indirectly through the action of G-protein-coupled receptors which utilize intracellular second messengers) (Fig. 8). These different types of glutamate receptors have different physiological characteristics and actions. Activation of the AMPA receptor is rapid and short-lived. In contrast the NMDA receptor has a longer period of activation and is important in the processes called "wind-up" and "central sensitisation". Recent studies have shown that NMDA receptor antagonists in particular can block these nociceptive phenomena in caudalis, which has led to the view that NMDA antagonists might be useful analgesics in, for example, neuropathic pain conditions.

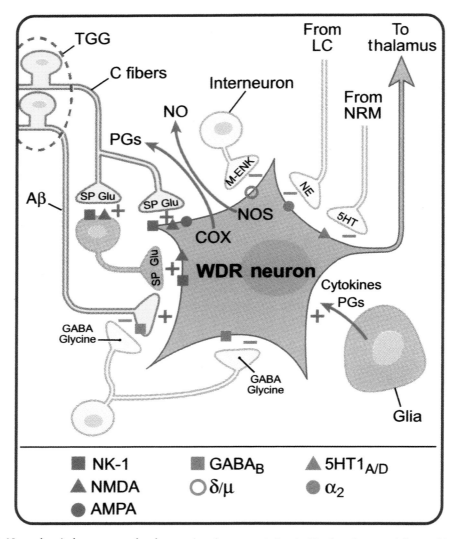

Figure 8. Neurochemical processes related to nociceptive transmission in V subnucleus caudalis. In this example, activation of nociceptive fibres leads to the release of glutamate (Glu) and substance P (SP), which are conveyed across a synapse to a wide dynamic range (WDR) neurone which projects to the thalamus. Glutamate binds and activates either NMDA or AMPA receptors, while substance P binds and activates the neurokinin 1 (NK-1) receptors. The afferent fibres can activate the WDR neurone directly, or indirectly *via* contacts onto excitatory interneurones. Several intracellular signal transduction pathways have been implicated in modulating the responsiveness of the nociceptive neurones, including the protein kinase A (PKA) and protein kinase C (PKC) pathways. The neurones can themselves modulate nearby cells by synthesis and release of prostaglandins (PGs) *via* cyclo-oxygenase (COX) and nitric oxide (NO) *via* nitric oxide synthase (NOS). Glia can modulate nociceptive processing by release of cytokines and prostaglandins. Descending terminals of fibres originating in regions such as the nucleus raphe magnus (NRM) or locus coeruleus (LC) can release serotonin (5HT) or noradrenaline (NE). The major proposed receptors for these neurotransmitters are also depicted. Drugs that alter these receptors or neurotransmitters have potential as analgesics. GABA, γ-aminobutyric acid. (From Hargreaves, K.M. and Goodis, H.E. (Eds.) Seltzer and Bender's Dental Pulp. Chicago: Quintessence, 2002, pp. 500.)

The neuropeptide "substance P" is also an important contributor to nociceptive mechanisms. Like glutamate, it also occurs not only in the peripheral endings of small-diameter primary afferents but is also concentrated in primary afferent terminals in the CNS, such as those of subnucleus caudalis (Fig. 8). Noxious orofacial stimulation may cause the release of substance P within caudalis: this then acts on the caudalis nociceptive neurones through so-called neurokinin receptors to produce a long-latency, sustained excitation of the nociceptive neurones that can be blocked by substance P antagonists.

The anatomy, physiology and neurochemistry of subnucleus caudalis are similar to the dorsal horn in the spinal cord, an area that is critical in spinal nociceptive transmission. Indeed, because of its close functional and structural similarity with the spinal dorsal horn, caudalis is now often termed the "medullary dorsal horn". However, different parts of subnucleus caudalis *per se* may have different functional roles since its rostral and caudal portions appear to be differentially involved in the autonomic and muscle reflex responses to noxious orofacial stimulation. Furthermore, caudalis may not be the only component of the brainstem complex with a nociceptive role. More rostral components of the V brainstem complex (e.g. subnuclei interpolaris and oralis) have NS and WDR neurones, and lesions of rostral components may disrupt some orofacial pain behaviours. These neurones have cutaneous receptive fields that are usually localised to intraoral or perioral areas, and many can be activated by tooth pulp stimulation. The receptive field and response properties of these rostral neurones, coupled with the effects of rostral lesions, suggest that the more rostral components may play some role in intraoral and perioral nociceptive processing.

■ Projections from the trigeminal brainstem sensory nuclear complex

Neurones in all components of the V brainstem complex project to the thalamus either directly or indirectly via polysynaptic pathways that involve the reticular formation. Some of the projections to the reticular formation, as well as projections to the cranial nerve motor nuclei, provide part of the central substrate underlying autonomic and muscle reflex responses to orofacial stimuli (see Nociceptive reflex and behavioural responses). Some neurones have only intrinsic projections, i.e. their axons do not leave the V brainstem complex but instead terminate within it. The neurones in lamina II of caudalis, the *substantia gelatinosa*, are of particular note in this respect. Most of their axons terminate locally within the V brainstem complex and release neuromodulatory substances such as enkephalin or gamma-aminobutyric acid (GABA). The substantia gelatinosa also receives inputs from fibres originating in other areas in the brain in addition to orofacial afferent inputs, and is one of the main sites in which these peripheral afferents and brain centres modulate somatosensory transmission. There are also intrinsic projections that connect different components of the V brainstem complex, e.g. many caudalis neurones project to and influence the activity of neurones in subnucleus oralis.

■ Thalamocortical nociceptive transmission

The thalamic regions that receive and relay orofacial somatosensory information from the brainstem are the ventrobasal complex (or ventroposterior nucleus) and the so-called posterior group of nuclei and the medial thalamus. As in the brainstem, glutamate is important in the transmission of the somatosensory signals, in this case from the terminals of the axons of the brainstem neurones to the thalamic neurones. Most of the ventrobasal thalamic neurones are low-threshold mechanosensitive neurones that are somatotopically organised so that neurones receiving and relaying tactile information from the face and mouth are concentrated in the medial portion of the ventrobasal thalamus (the nucleus ventralis posteromedialis, VPM) while neurones in the lateral portion of the ventrobasal thalamus relay somatosensory information from the trunk, neck and limbs. Most of these low-threshold mechanosensitive neurones faithfully relay the detailed somatosensory information they receive via the brainstem to the overlying somatosensory areas of the cerebral cortex; in contrast, analogous neurones in the posterior group and medial thalamus are generally much less specific in the information which they relay.

Nociceptive neurones also occur in these thalamic regions. Their properties in humans as well as experimental animals are generally similar to those described for NS and WDR neurones in the subthalamic relays such as subnucleus caudalis, including the convergence onto them of cutaneous and deep afferent inputs. Most NS and WDR neurones in the ventrobasal thalamus have receptive field and response properties and connections with the overlying somatosensory cerebral cortex that indicate a role in the sensory-discriminative dimension of pain. In contrast, nociceptive neurones in the more medial nuclei of the thalamus are considered to be involved more in the affective or motivational dimensions of pain, and are connected with other higher brain areas

(e.g. hypothalamus, anterior cingulate cortex) that also participate in these functions or in neuroendocrine responses related to pain.

NS and WDR neurones are also found in the so-called primary somatosensory area SI of the somatosensory cerebral cortex. These neurones respond to noxious stimuli in a manner that suggests a role for the somatosensory cortex in the localisation and discrimination of noxious stimuli (i.e. the sensory-discriminative dimension of pain), including intensity coding of noxious thermal stimulation of the face or tooth pulp. Nociceptive neurones also occur in other cortical regions such as the anterior cingulate cortex which has been implicated in the affective or motivational dimension of pain. Brain imaging studies in humans have also shown the differential involvement of somatosensory cortex and other cortical areas in different dimensions of the pain experience.

■ Nociceptive reflex and behavioural responses

As noted above, many of the neurones in the V brainstem complex project to brainstem or higher brain centres involved in reflex or more complex behavioural responses to noxious stimuli. For example, they are involved in the brainstem circuits underlying the reflex changes in blood pressure, heart rate, breathing, and salivation that can be evoked by noxious orofacial stimulation. The subnucleus caudalis appears to be crucial for autonomic (including adrenal) responses in cardiac, adrenal or respiratory function evoked by noxious orofacial stimuli. Caudalis neurones are also crucial in the prolonged reflex co-activation of jaw-opening and jaw-closing muscles that can be evoked by noxious stimulation of musculoskeletal tissues (e.g. TMJ) in animals but not humans, and in more complex pain-avoidance behaviours that are evoked by noxious stimulation of orofacial tissues. Some neurones in the rostral components of the V brainstem complex are involved specifically in the reflex circuits underlying in the jaw-opening reflex in animals.

Several behavioural paradigms have been developed to study the effects of noxious orofacial stimuli in humans. These include changes in autonomic function (e.g. heart rate), muscle reflexes, and facial expression, as well as the more subjective indicators of pain recorded by the human subject on a visual analogue scale, McGill Pain Questionnaire (MPQ), etc. (see Assessment of orofacial pain). Behavioural models of orofacial pain in animals have also recently been developed to replicate neuropathic or inflammatory pain (e.g. by chronic constriction injury of the infraorbital nerve or by the application of inflammatory irritants such as formalin or mustard oil to facial skin, tooth pulp and musculoskeletal tissues).

High-threshold reflex effects can be evoked in several orofacial muscles, with the jaw-opening reflex being the most extensively studied in animals. Until recently, the experimental methods employed have typically used transient stimuli that evoke brief reflex responses. More recently, algesic chemicals (such as hypertonic saline, capsaicin, glutamate, or mustard oil) have been injected into rat TMJ, jaw muscles, or tooth pulp to elicit more prolonged nociceptive effects. This stimulation activates neurones in subnucleus caudalis, which, through their connections with brainstem reflex centres such as the V motor nucleus, can result in prolonged increases in jaw muscle electromyographic (EMG) activity of the jaw-opening and jaw-closing muscles (Fig. 9). This

demonstrates the close interplay between sensory and motor pathways. Furthermore, central NMDA receptors appear to be involved in the EMG changes reflexly evoked in the rat jaw muscles by the application to orofacial tissues of mustard oil or glutamate, as they are in the neuroplastic changes in subnucleus caudalis (see below), since the evoked EMG activity may be blocked by NMDA antagonists and related compounds administered systemically or directly to subnucleus caudalis. Furthermore, a central opioid depressive effect may be "triggered" into action by noxious orofacial stimulation. These observations suggest that nociceptive afferent inputs evoke central NMDA-dependent neuronal activity in subnucleus caudalis, with associated neuromuscular changes, but that these neural changes are limited by the recruitment of central opioid mechanisms.

The reflex effects of noxious orofacial stimuli on masticatory muscle activity, and especially on their postural activity, have particular significance in the underlying pathophysiological mechanisms in many musculoskeletal disorders manifest as pain, such as TMDs and tension-type headaches. There is, however, no consensus at the moment on whether the EMG activity of these muscles increases, decreases or remains unchanged during orofacial pain, and a number of factors have been proposed to account for the disparity between experimental and clinical pain data. Even when increased jaw EMG activity does occur in humans, its relatively small magnitude suggests it may have little clinical significance. This contrasts with the robust and prolonged jaw EMG increases induced reflexly by algesic stimuli in animals (see above) which indicates that there are excitatory reflex pathways from peripheral orofacial nociceptors (*via* caudalis nociceptive neurones) to the alpha motoneurones in the

Figure 9. Increases in jaw muscle EMG activity reflexly induced by injection of the algesic chemical mustard oil into the rat TMJ region. **A** shows the time-course of the increased muscle activity (the EMG activity has been rectified and integrated). Note the biphasic character of the increase. **B** shows the site of mustard oil injection, and **C** shows EMG traces at representative time periods (From Yu et al. Effects of inflammatory irritant application to the rat temporomandibular joint on jaw and neck muscle activity. Pain 60:143–149, 1995.)

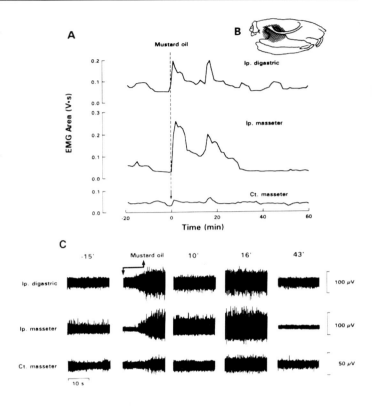

V motor nucleus supplying the jaw-opening and jaw-closing muscles. Co-contraction of these antagonistic muscles could provide a "splinting" effect that limits jaw movements in pathophysiological conditions affecting deep tissues such as TMJ and muscle. While these EMG patterns do not occur in awake humans when an algesic chemical (e.g. hypertonic saline) is infused into the jaw muscles, noxious orofacial stimulation can induce alterations in the normal alternating activity of the jaw-opening and jaw-closing muscles during mastication in humans as well as in animals. This includes enhancement of jaw-opening EMG activity during jaw-closing, and *vice versa*.

These and other findings appear inconsistent with many current and long-held concepts of the aetiologies underlying TMD pain, especially the so-called "vicious cycle" in which muscle hyperactivity leads to pain which leads to more muscle hyperactivity and so on. Heavy muscle exercise does appear to lead to microtrauma in muscles and connective tissue, usually followed by pain that peaks in about 24 hours, but it is unclear whether such processes characterise TMD pain. This so-called delayed onset muscle soreness occurs only after eccentric exercise, however (Chapter 8). Most elements of the vicious cycle hypothesis have not been experimentally tested or verified.

An alternative concept is the *pain adaptation model*, in which pain may result in agonist muscles becoming less active during a specific movement (e.g. the masseter muscle during jaw-closing) and antagonist muscles (e.g. anterior digastric) becoming more active in this movement, thereby limiting jaw mobility and possibly aiding healing.

Modulatory influences

In view of the multidimensional nature of pain, it is not surprising that pain can be modulated by a variety of pharmacologic agents and physical and psychological interventions. Several areas in the thalamus, reticular formation, limbic system, and cerebral cortex determine and regulate perceptual, emotional, autonomic, and neuroendocrine responses to noxious stimuli by utilising various excitatory and inhibitory neurochemicals. The modulatory effects differ from one person to another, which is consistent with the idea that pain is a highly personal experience that is susceptible to a variety of biological, pharmacological, psychological, genetic and environmental influences.

The intricate organisation of each subdivision of the V brainstem complex and the variety of inputs to each of them from peripheral tissues or from different parts of the brain provide a particularly important substrate for interactions between the various inputs. This modulation was an important element of the gate control theory of pain. Other modulation can also occur at thalamic and cortical levels and in the peripheral tissues themselves. The central modulatory processes release endogenous neurochemical substances, some of which underlie facilitatory influences on nociceptive transmission, while others exert primarily inhibitory influences that may involve presynaptic or postsynaptic regulatory mechanisms. These neurochemicals include, serotonin (5-HT), noradrenaline, GABA and opioids such as the endorphins and enkephalins. These neurochemical substrates are used by pathways that descend from structures elsewhere in the brain onto nociceptive pathways and modify incoming pain signals. These central pathways emanate from the periaqueductal gray matter, rostroventral medulla/nucleus raphe magnus, anterior pretectal nucleus, locus coeruleus and parabrachial area of the pons as well as the somatosensory and motor areas of the cerebral cortex, to name just a few. Electrical or chemical stimulation of these central sites activates descending pathways that project to the V brainstem complex and can inhibit V brainstem neuronal and related reflex and behavioural responses to noxious orofacial stimulation in experimental animals (Fig. 10). Stimulation of some of these pathways also relieves pain in human patients.

While these descending pathways exert their effects on nociceptive transmission by the release from their endings of neurochemicals such as 5-HT in subnucleus caudalis (Fig. 8), some chemicals (e.g. enkephalins, GABA) appear to be released from the endings of interneurones contained wholly within to the V brainstem complex (e.g. the substantia gelatinosa of subnucleus caudalis). The enkephalins are one of several opioid peptides that can act on specific opiate receptors in the CNS or peripheral tissues (e.g. mu, delta, kappa opiate receptors). The action of the narcotic analgesic morphine on opiate receptors in peripheral tissues was mentioned in a previous section but all three receptor subtypes are also widely distributed in the CNS. They are concentrated in several sites including the periaqueductal gray, amygdala, anterior cingulate cortex, and V subnucleus caudalis. All three opiate receptor subtypes have been implicated in the modulation of nociceptive processes: some exert facilitatory effects, others are inhibitory. For example, analgesia can be produced by the microinjection of certain opioids at these intra-cerebral sites. This appears to involve the activation of descending anti-nociceptive pathways that originate in these sites, and the descending inputs inhibit orofacial nociceptive transmission at the very first relay station, in subnucleus caudalis. Suppression of nociceptive transmission can also be induced by the application of opioids directly to subnucleus caudalis. This presumably acts on opiate receptors related to some of these descending inputs to the V brainstem complex or on opioid-containing neurones intrinsic to the subnucleus caudalis. These inhibitory

influences acting *via* the descending pathways or by actions within caudalis itself are thought to contribute to the analgesic efficacy of the narcotic opiate-related analgesics drugs (e.g. morphine and codeine).

The descending influences can also be activated by a variety of behavioural and environmental events and thereby modify pain. For example, increasing a patient's expectations that a drug will produce a powerful analgesic effect can result in a considerable increase in the drug's analgesic prop-

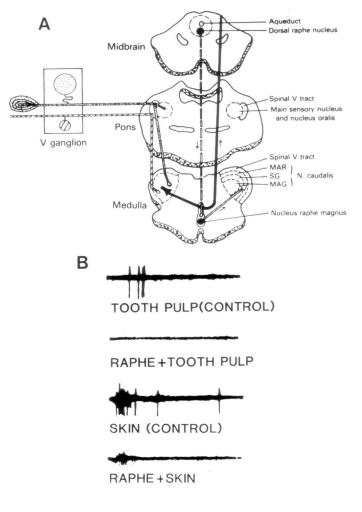

Figure 10. Ascending trigeminal nociceptive pathway and descending modulatory pathway that may suppress activity of neurones in nociceptive pathway. A. Nociceptive neurones in subnucleus caudalis that receive and relay information from small-diameter primary afferent fibres (*crosshatched pathway*) only (nociceptive-specific neurones), or from small-diameter afferent fibres and from both large-diameter primary afferent fibres (*stippled pathway*) (wide dynamic range neurones) predominate in the superficial (e.g. MAR) and deeper laminae of subnucleus caudalis. Responses of both types of neurones to noxious oral-facial stimuli can be suppressed by descending influences from dorsal raphe nucleus in periaqueductal gray and nucleus raphe magnus, as shown for the wide dynamic range neurone illustrated in B. Records here show that the neurone's responses to these noxious stimuli can be completely suppressed if tooth pulp or noxious skin stimuli that excite the neurone are interacted with electric stimuli delivered to the raphe system. Time duration of each record is 100 ms. SG: substantia gelatinosa; MAG: magnocellular lamina (Part A of figure from Dubner et al. 1978.)

erties, the so-called "placebo" effect (placebo is a Latin word meaning "I please"). This effect involves changes in the descending modulatory influences in pain, and may in part involve endogenous opioid processes. Cognitive processes associated with the context or environment in which a noxious stimulus is experienced, even a person's personality, psychological or emotional state, and previous life experiences, can also modify the descending influences. A good example is the anxious or dental-phobic patient who may experience more pain in the clinical setting than a relaxed patient who has previously experienced painless dental procedures.

Changes in the activity of the CNS processes underlying neuroendocrine function (e.g. hormone levels) and sleep can also influence the pain experience by modulating these descending pathways, and thus contribute to, for example, gender differences in pain and the modulation of pain by sleep. Nutritional factors can also influence pain expression, in part by influencing the function of some descending influences, and studies in animals have demonstrated phenotypic differences in pain sensitivity that may be due to genetic factors. It is also possible that pain sensitivity in humans may have heritable features.

In addition to the various descending influences noted above, nociceptive transmission is also subject to modulation by influences that are initiated by peripheral stimulation and involve the interneuronal circuitry existing with subnucleus caudalis (and the spinal dorsal horn). Some of these influences were envisaged in the large fibre-small fibre interactions proposed in the original gate control theory of pain. They include inputs from somatosensory afferents, as well as inputs into the CNS from visceral afferents such as those in the vagus nerve

carrying afferent input from arterial or cardiopulmonary baroreceptors into the CNS. Afferent modulatory effects can be used to some advantage clinically. Application to peripheral tissues of acupuncture and transcutaneous electrical nerve stimulation (TENS) may, for example, inhibit the responses of V brainstem nociceptive neurones evoked by noxious orofacial stimuli, and there are clinical reports of the effectiveness of these therapeutic procedures in reducing pain. Such stimuli are thought to act mainly by activating small-diameter somatosensory afferent inputs into the CNS, although nociceptive transmission can also be suppressed by non-noxious stimuli (e.g., vibratory or tactile) that excite large afferent nerve fibres. Small-fibre afferent inputs from various spatially-dispersed regions of the body inhibit neuronal nociceptive responses to other small-fibre afferent inputs: this is the so-called diffuse noxious inhibitory controls (DNIC) mechanism. In other words, pain in one part of the body can inhibit pain evoked from another part of the body. Such a mechanism may be related to findings in humans that pain perception can be decreased for example by applying noxious stimuli such as chemical irritants elsewhere in the body (so-called counter-irritation), and that noxious forearm ischaemia is very effective in reducing the intensity, unpleasantness and spatial referral of pulpal pain (see Fig. 7 in Chapter 5). It is not clear how much of the effectiveness of TENS and acupuncture can be explained by afferent inputs that bring about suppression of nociceptive transmission by segmental mechanisms, or by the afferent inputs exerting their suppressive effects through their activation of descending inhibitory influences from higher brain regions. The neurochemical basis for their suppressive effects also is unclear, although endogenous opiate-related mechanisms are at least partly involved.

Neuroplasticity and central sensitisation

The transmission of nociceptive signals is not only subject to suppressive influences from afferent stimulation, but can also be enhanced by alterations to the peripheral afferent inputs to the CNS that may result from inflammation or trauma of peripheral tissues and nerve fibres.

It was pointed out in a previous section that many caudalis NS and WDR neurones with a cutaneous receptive field also receive convergent afferent inputs from tissues that include tooth pulp, TMJ or masticatory muscle, which contributes to the spread and referral of pain that is typical of deep pain conditions involving these tissues. This extensive convergence of afferent inputs may also contribute to central neuronal changes that can be induced by inflammation or injury of peripheral tissues or nerve fibres. Chemicals released from the peripheral tissues or primary afferent nerve endings themselves by the injury or inflammation may enhance the excitability of peripheral nociceptors (i.e. peripheral sensitisation). This in turn may produce a barrage of nociceptive input into the CNS which can lead to prolonged functional alterations in subnucleus caudalis (and spinal dorsal horn) resulting in a state of increased excitability of caudalis neurones (Fig. 11). This is known as *"central sensitisation"*. For example, the nociceptive afferent activity caused by damage to or inflammation of tooth pulp, TMJ or muscle induces spontaneous activity, lowering of the activation threshold, receptive field expansion, and enhancement of responses of caudalis NS and WDR neurones that may also include a gradually augmenting response to a series of repeated noxious stimuli ("wind-up"). Central sensitisation is not restricted to subnucleus caudalis but also occurs in nociceptive neurons in subnucleus oralis and in higher brain regions such as the VPM thalamus, although caudalis is responsible for the expression of central sensitisation in these structures through its projections to both oralis and VPM thalamus.

An important concept stemming from these considerations is that the afferent inputs and brainstem circuitry are not "hardwired" but are "plastic". That is, the receptive field and response properties of the nociceptive neurones can be changed, at least in part, from the unmasking and increased efficacy of some of the extensive convergent afferent inputs to the nociceptive neurones that were noted above. The neurones' responses to these inputs are enhanced and their receptive fields are enlarged, resulting in a greater number of stronger inputs.

This neuroplasticity of the nociceptive neurones in the brainstem may, as noted earlier, be accompanied by prolonged increases in activity of both jaw-opening and jaw-closing muscles. The neuroplastic changes occurring in caudalis nociceptive neurones are relayed not only via ascending pathways to higher brain centres such as VPM but also onto the V motoneurones supplying these muscles via the connections of subnucleus caudalis with brainstem reflex centres such as the V motor nucleus. These prolonged increases in jaw-opening and jaw-closing activity may serve to limit jaw movement in pathophysiological conditions affecting the jaw, for example, when a masticatory muscle is injured or inflamed.

The neuroplastic changes that are reflected in an increased excitability in as-

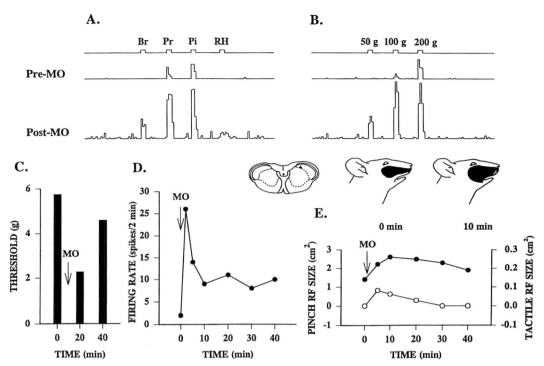

Figure 11. An example of a nociceptive-specific neurone recorded in the rat subnucleus caudalis and the changes in its spontaneous activity and mechanoreceptive field (RF) properties following mustard oil (MO) application to the right maxillary molar pulp. The top half (**A**) shows the neurone's responses to mechanical and thermal stimuli applied to the cutaneous receptive field. Upper trace is a marker of stimulation by brush (Br), pressure (Pr), pinch (Pi), and radiant heat (RH). Middle trace shows neuronal responses in control conditions (i.e., Pre-MO, before MO application). Lower trace shows neuronal responses to the same stimuli 20 min after MO application (i.e., Post-MO, after MO application). Top half (**B**) illustrates responses to graded mechanical stimuli (50 g, 100 g, 200 g); each stimulus given for 3 sec. Note that after MO application, this NS neuron became responsive to light tactile stimulation and radiant heating of its cutaneous receptive field, and strongly responsive to graded pinch stimuli. The bottom half shows the profound decrease in mechanical threshold at 20 min after MO application (**C**, arrow), the MO-induced burst of neuronal activity, and (**D**) the MO-induced expansion of the cutaneous pinch receptive field as well as the temporary appearance of a tactile receptive field (**E**, dots represent values of pinch receptive field size; circles represent values of tactile receptive field size). Inset figures illustrate histologically-confirmed recording site, and receptive field sizes before (0 min) and 10 min after MO application. (From Chiang et al, NMDA receptor mechanisms contribute to neuroplasticity induced in caudalis nociceptive neurons by tooth pulp stimulation. J. Neurophysiol. 80:2621–2631, 1998.)

cending and reflex nociceptive pathways and that underlie central sensitisation are produced by a cascade of events that starts with a noxious stimulus initiating a barrage of activity in nociceptive afferents that causes the release from their endings in the CNS of several chemical mediators, including glutamate and substance P (Fig. 12). These neurochemicals prolong neuronal depolarisation and increase the excitability of the nociceptive neurones via actions on glutamate (e.g. NMDA) and neu-

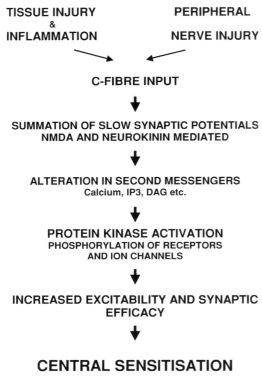

TISSUE INJURY
&
INFLAMMATION

PERIPHERAL

NERVE INJURY

C-FIBRE INPUT

SUMMATION OF SLOW SYNAPTIC POTENTIALS
NMDA AND NEUROKININ MEDIATED

ALTERATION IN SECOND MESSENGERS
Calcium, IP3, DAG etc.

PROTEIN KINASE ACTIVATION
PHOSPHORYLATION OF RECEPTORS
AND ION CHANNELS

INCREASED EXCITABILITY AND SYNAPTIC
EFFICACY

CENTRAL SENSITISATION

Figure 12. Events leading to the production of central sensitisation of central nociceptive neurones by peripheral injury or inflammation. (From Woolf, C., with permission.)

segmental and descending modulatory influences were outlined.

The net result of these neuroplastic changes is an increased central excitatory state that is dependent on peripheral nociceptive afferent input for its initiation, but may not be fully dependent on peripheral afferent drive for its maintenance. Central sensitisation can last for days or even weeks, and is thought to contribute to persistent pain and to the spontaneous pain and tenderness that characterise many clinical cases of injury or inflammation. Central sensitisation may enhance the effect of low-threshold mechanosensitive afferent inputs (which are not normally associated with pain) on nociceptive pathways in conditions associated with peripheral injury or inflammation, and thus could contribute to the allodynia that often is associated with pain conditions. It also can explain the hyperalgesia that is a feature of many persistent pain conditions, because it increases the response of central nociceptive neurones to A-delta and C-fibre nociceptive inputs. The increased receptive

rokinin receptors as well as other receptor classes. Activation of these receptors is particularly associated with removal of the voltage-dependent magnesium block of the NMDA receptor, the entry of calcium into the neurones, phosphorylation of the NMDA receptor, and a change in neuronal kinetics. Other ionotropic and metabotropic excitatory amino acid receptors as well as neurotrophins and kinases involved in the phosphorylation of receptors may also play a role. The central sensitisation may also involve disinhibition, which refers to a loss of some of central inhibitory processes that were mentioned earlier when

An understanding of how central sensitisation is initiated is central to the effective use of approaches such as pre-emptive analgesia in clinical management. For example, when surgery is likely to result in long-lasting postoperative pain (the best example being extraction of impacted third molar teeth), the administration of long acting local analgesia and anti-inflammatory drugs at the time of surgery may give better post-operative pain control even when the surgery is performed under general anaesthesia.

field size of the nociceptive neurones also appears to represent a central factor contributing to pain spread and referral, and the spontaneous activity of the neurones may contribute to spontaneous pain.

NMDA receptor antagonists have been shown to be effective in preventing the development of central sensitisation, e.g., their application to subnucleus caudalis can block the neuroplastic changes in caudalis nociceptive neurones and in the higher brain centres and reflex centres to which caudalis projects. However, because glutamate has widespread actions via NMDA receptors in the CNS, NMDA receptor antagonists may produce several side effects such as nausea and drowsiness. So while these considerations draw attention to the value of developing therapeutic approaches such as new analgesic drugs that target the chemical mediators in the CNS that develop and maintain central sensitisation, the challenge is to produce drugs that have effective pain-suppressing actions without the undesirable side effects.

Peripheral sensitisation also can contribute to pain spread, hyperalgesia and allodynia by increasing the excitability and decreasing the activation threshold of primary afferents. Thus, many pain conditions may involve a mixture of both peripheral and central sensitisation. For example, the pain and limitations in jaw movements that are characteristic of TMDs can be explained by the existence of peripheral and/or central sensitisation phenomena producing states of allodynia and hyperalgesia and pain spread or referral, as well as co-contraction of jaw-opening and jaw-closing muscles. The sensitivity of a "hot tooth" to thermal or mechanical stimuli applied to the inflamed tooth can also be explained by these mechanisms.

Injury to afferent nerve fibres themselves may also trigger a different set of mechanisms that result in central sensitisation. These include the initiation of abnormal impulses in the injured afferents, sprouting of the afferents into peripheral tissues (hyperinnervation) and the formation of neuromas (tangles of nerve endings), the development of functional contacts between sympathetic efferents and nociceptive afferents, changes in the phenotype of the afferent fibres, and structural reorganisation of the endings in the CNS of primary afferents due to central sprouting. Many of these changes associated with the afferent fibres and their central consequences, such as central sensitisation and changes (e.g. disinhibition) in segmental or descending influences, can persist for long periods and lead to the development of neuropathic pain conditions (see Clinical presentation of orofacial pain).

Many of the peripheral and central neural consequences of injury may also be the result of deafferentation, i.e., the partial or total loss of the afferent nerve supply from a particular body region. One extreme example is the denervation of a hand as a result of severe trauma to the wrist. Less extreme examples are the surgical or accidental transection of the inferior alveolar nerve, or the endodontic removal of an inflamed tooth pulp. Thus, the physiological consequences of deafferentation need to be taken into account when the aetiology of a number of orofacial pain states are considered. Deafferentation in the trigeminal innervation from endodontic therapy and tooth extraction is common. In addition, sensory alterations induced by neural trauma, compression or transection may initiate peripheral and central neural events leading in some cases to painful conditions such as V neuralgia, atypical facial pain, and burning mouth syndrome (see Clinical presentation of orofacial pain).

Table 4.

Spontaneous pain	• Pain intensity
	• Pain quality
	• Localisation
	• Time course
	• Modifying factors
Stimulus-evoked pain	• Thermal
	• Mechanical
	• Chemical
	• Electrical

Important points to examine in order to describe the orofacial pain complaint.

Assessment of orofacial pain

In light of the complexity of pain as a multi-dimensional and bio-psycho-social experience (Fig. 1), it is clear that it cannot be measured in physical units like weight in kilograms or height in centimetres. However, it is important to understand that there are several ways to assess pain and its effects systematically. The key to pain analysis is a standardised pain history and examination. Table 4 provides an overview of the subjective reports of pain. Later we will also consider adjunctive physiological and behavioural measures of orofacial pain.

Spontaneous pain

Pain intensity
Assessment of the intensity of the pain is the main step to gain an understanding of the pain complaint. The most used method is to ask the patient to place a mark on a 10-cm line with 0 labelled as "no pain" and 10 as "most imaginable pain". Although very simple, this visual analogue scale (VAS) can be considered the "gold standard" of pain assessment today. Numerous research reports have confirmed that it is a valid and sensitive technique for describing the intensity of pain. For some pain conditions, especially those that are persistent, the pain can best be described by VAS pain assessments of different aspects of the pain; for example, "how much pain right now", "how much pain during the last month" and "how much pain when it was worst". Sometimes it can also be useful to assess the unpleasantness of pain on a similar 0–10 VAS. There are many other related pain ratings scales, for example "0-1-2-3-4-5-6-7-8-9-10" (numerical) or "no – mild – moderate – severe – unbearable" (categorical) or combinations of various rating scales.

The pain scales used for children are different, and many different ones have been described. All pain scales have some limitations and their use may depend on the spe-

A major problem with clinical and experimental pain is the lack of a good vocabulary to describe its variable forms. Pain usually tends to be described in terms of the stimulus that might have caused it, e.g., "burning", "stabbing", "tearing". Pain language charts such as the McGill Pain Questionnaire (MPQ) have been developed to help to define more precisely what is being perceived. This problem was recognised by the English author Virginia Woolf who wrote: *"English, which can express the thoughts of Hamlet and the tragedy of Lear, has no words for the shiver and the headache .... The merest school girl, when she falls in love, has Shakespeare and Keats to speak for her, but let a sufferer try to explain a pain in his head to a doctor and language at once runs dry."*

cific purpose to assess the intensity of pain. In dental practice, the most important thing is to standardise and use the same scale with each individual patient in order to evaluate the efficacy of treatment or time course of the pain condition.

Pain quality

Another important parameter for the pain analysis is to obtain an understanding of the quality of pain. Just as taste can be sweet, sour, bitter, or salty (and umami), pain can have different characteristic qualities. For example, tension-type headache is described as "pressing" or "tightening" whereas migraine has a "throbbing" quality. Muscle pain is often described as "tense" and "taut" and toothaches are often "sharp" or "shooting". Trigeminal neuralgia is typically described as "stabbing" pain. It is clear that these words can assist in the differential diagnosis of pain, but also that the words are not unique or entirely specific to only one pain condition. The MPQ can be used to standardise verbal descriptions. This questionnaire is available in many different languages and takes advantage of the many verbal descriptors that people use to describe pain, i.e., the "language of pain". The MPQ also has the potential to be a multidimensional pain assessment tool since both the sensory-discriminative component and the affective part of pain can be calculated as indices depending on the words used to describe the pain.

Pain localisation

The localisation of pain is of course of immense importance but often it can be quite difficult for the patient to pinpoint its exact location. Some of the neurobiological reasons for this difficulty in locating pain particularly from deep craniofacial tissues have already been discussed under the terms of referral and spread of pain. In the clinic, it

is a good idea first to have the patient point to the painful area and then to ask the patient to draw the distribution of pain on an anatomical map (pain map). Since many patients (up to 70%) with pain in the orofacial region also complain about pain elsewhere on the body, a careful pain analysis should also include whole body pain maps. The head and face pain maps show distinct characteristics depending on whether or not the pain is coming from the neck muscles, jaw muscles, TMJ, teeth, or tension-type headache. For research purposes, such pain drawings can be further analysed by calculating the area and determining the centre point of the pain experienced by the patient.

Time course

The onset of pain and its duration will give important clues to the diagnosis. For example, was there a sudden onset (from trauma or dental treatment) or did pain gradually develop with no precipitating cause? Is the pain present every day or does the patient have any days without pain? Use of pain diaries can help to get a good overview of the painful condition. Fig. 13 shows a schematic representation of the time course of different types of pain.

There may also be major variations in the intensity of pain during the day. In some patients, orofacial pain is worst in the morning and lessens during the day, whereas the opposite can also occur. In the first situation, the dentist should consider, for example, sleep bruxism or rheumatoid arthritis as a contributing factor. It is also possible to see fluctuations during the week, during the month (e.g. menstrual cycle-related) and even during the year (e.g. worst pain during cold winters). There are many other possible time courses of pain but it is always essential to obtain an understanding of how it has

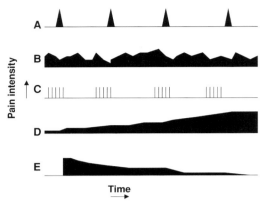

Figure 13. Illustration of theoretical time courses in different types of pain conditions in the orofacial region and head. In **A** the patient reports attacks of severe pain which are clearly separated by pain-free intervals. Pain of this type could point to a migraine, for example. In **B** there is continuous pain lasting for a prolonged period of time from which the patient never experiences complete relief, but there are some fluctuations in the general level of pain. This could be typical of myofascial pain or tension-type headaches. In **C** there are several bouts or attacks of strong pain, which are separated by pain-free intervals. The pain attacks (paroxysms) can then be absent for weeks or months and then return. This pattern is typical of V neuralgia. In **D** there is a slow, steady increase in pain over a longer period of time, which could be indicative of pain from malignant diseases. Finally, in **E** the pain suddenly appears and slowly diminishes. This could occur after an acute displacement of the articular disc of the TMJ followed by a natural remission.

developed over time. This information may not be available for the dentist who sees the patient for the first time. In that situation, the dentist will have to rely on the other information from the pain analysis and the dental examination of the orofacial structures, in order to exclude any acute pain condition due, for example, to pulpitis or an anteriorly-displaced disc in the TMJ.

Modifying factors

It is important to have a checklist to assess which orofacial functions are influenced by

pain and to what extent. Besides its time course (spontaneous remissions or exacerbations), pain can also be influenced by oral functions and in particular mastication. This is often the case in TMD pain patients, although some patients may actually gain relief from chewing. Yawning and wide opening of the mouth can be very painful for patients with TMJ problems. Pain may be associated with sleep problems, and stress and psychological factors (e.g. anger, depression) may also be clearly associated with pain. There has been a long debate on whether depression leads to pain or pain leads to depression, but it is often impossible and probably meaningless to try to establish a causal relationship.

Treatment is obviously meant to relieve the pain, but patients with persistent orofacial pain have often been subject to a number of treatments in the past without satisfactory results. In fact, they may even have worsened the pain, for example, in atypical odontalgia where extensive endodontic and extraction therapy normally does not solve the pain problem. The dentist should obtain information on the type of treatments provided, by whom (physician, physiotherapist, neurologist, psychologist, complementary medicine, etc.), and for how long, and in the case of pharmacological treatment what drug type and doses have been used. While it may be frustrating for the patient, the lack of an effect of a particular treatment can provide new information for the dentist about the underlying mechanisms; generally, however, these cases should be referred to pain centres and specialists.

■ Stimulus-evoked pain

Many orofacial pain conditions will have both a spontaneous component and also a stimulus-evoked component. This is strongly linked to the expressions hyperalgesia, hyperaesthesia and allodynia and the corresponding hypoalgesia and hypoaesthesia (see pain glossary). The underlying mechanism is the relationship between the intensity of a stimulus, the neural activity in the primary afferent fibre, the activity in the projection neurons and the perceived intensity of the stimulus (see also Primary afferent properties and peripheral sensitisation). These relationships are shown schematically in Fig. 14. In many pain conditions, the normal relationship between stimulus intensity and perceived intensity is shifted to the left.

It is also important to distinguish between pain evoked by different stimulus modalities (mechanical, thermal, chemical) or electrical stimuli, as outlined in the following sections.

Mechanical stimuli

Mechanical stimuli evoke a broad range of well-known sensations such as pressure, touch, vibration and tickle (Chapter 6). However, when you apply pressure to a normal muscle, pain is not be experienced until the pressure exceeds a certain magnitude, which is termed the pain threshold. This threshold is lower in a painful muscle (allodynia), and applying the pressure that is threshold for a normal muscle will evoke increased pain (hyperalgesia). These phenomena are usually demonstrable in patients with myofascial TMD problems and tension-type headache. However, mechanical allodynia can also be present around a tooth during chewing due to inflammation in the periodontal ligament. This can be revealed by the percussion test, i.e. tapping the tooth with a blunt dental instrument such as a mirror.

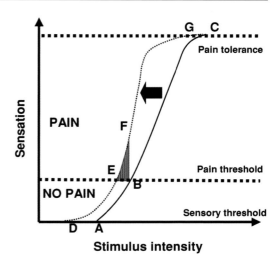

Figure 14. Schematic relationship between stimulus intensity (e.g., temperature or pressure) and the sensation evoked. ABC represents the normal relationship. A certain stimulus intensity is required in order to be detected by the subject (A: sensory threshold). As the stimulus intensity increases, there is an increased sensation (e.g. of warmth or pressure but not pain) until the pain threshold is reached (B). If the stimulus intensity continues to increase, there is an increased sensation of pain until the tolerance threshold is reached (C). In conditions with tissue injury pain and nervous system injury pain there is a shift of the stimulus-response curve to the left (arrow). DEG suggests decreased thresholds but also increased sensations at a given stimulus intensity, compared to ABC. DE represents hyperaesthesia, EF allodynia and FG hyperalgesia.

In the clinic you can test the mechanical sensitivity of muscles by standardised palpation and recording the graded responses (no pain – a little pain – moderate pain – strong pain) from the patient. Pressure algometers provide a quantitative value in physical units (e.g. kPa) of the pain threshold but are used mainly for research purposes. Touch sensations can simply be tested by a cotton swab or with special calibrated nylon filaments (von Frey hairs) applied to the facial skin or oral mucosa, which allows a quantitative assessment. Punctate sensations (pin-prick) can be tested by a blunt needle. Chair-side assessment will normally use the contralateral side (non-painful side) as a control and serves to determine whether or not there is a change in the mechanical sensitivity, but does not determine the magnitude of a change.

Thermal stimuli

Thermal sensations have been dealt with in Chapter 3; however, in painful states and in particular in some neuropathic pain states, there may be altered processing of thermal stimuli. This can be examined by applying cooled or heated metal objects to the painful area and using the contralateral non-painful side as a control. A more standardised technique is to use thermal elements with temperatures that are controlled more accurately, for example, aluminium bars kept in the refrigerator or in a heated water bath with a preset temperature. The magnitude of the subjective responses can then be graded on VAS or other verbal rating scales. Furthermore, maps of skin areas that respond differently to thermal stimuli in pain conditions affecting those areas can be compared with normal, non-painful skin areas. Finally, laboratory studies use radiant heat and skin temperature measurements to determine the thermal and pain thresholds to hot and cold stimuli. However, simple thermal stimulation procedures are used extensively to examine the vitality of the tooth pulp, e.g. the application of ice or warmed gutta percha to the tooth to determine whether there is hyperalgesia to cold or heat stimuli.

Chemical stimuli

The interaction between chemical stimuli and thermal sensation are considered in Chapter 2 in relation to taste and chemosensory function. However, chemical stimuli can also evoke pain. For example, sugar can exacerbate the pain of a toothache and can evoke pain from exposed dentine for a short period (Chapter 5), and so information from the patient on modification of pain by sweet and acid foods should also be taken into consideration.

Capsaicin (the burning ingredient in hot chilli peppers) and menthol (the cooling agent often used in chewing gum) bind to specific receptors (TRPV1) and are closely involved in nociceptive mechanisms. These algogenic chemicals are used in research laboratories to investigate primary and secondary hyperalgesia, and in clinical studies as pain-provoking stimuli to determine the responsiveness of the patient.

Electrical stimuli

Electrical stimulation of nerves does not elicit a natural sensation but rather a sudden, unpleasant jolting sensation. This is the result of bypassing the peripheral endings and directly stimulating peripheral nerve fibres. Depending on the stimulus intensity, it is likely that a mixed set of afferent fibres will be activated that range from non-nociceptive mechanosensitive fibres to high-threshold A-delta and C-fibres. The sensation will vary depending on the stimulus intensity, stimulus configuration (electrical pulse durations and frequency) and characteristics of the stimulating electrode. In Dentistry, electrical stimuli are commonly used to test the vitality of the tooth pulp (Chapter 5) and the predominant sensation is pain, although there may be a narrow range of stimulus intensities which elicit a non-painful sensation. It must be remembered that stronger electrical stimuli applied to the crown of a tooth to test pulp vitality can spread and activate afferent fibres from the periodontal ligament and gingiva, which may provide false positive responses.

■ Adjunctive measures of orofacial pain

Since pain is more than a simple sensation, some biological markers and associated physiological and behavioural responses can also be used as additional measures of the processing and consequences of pain. In some circumstances, these may be useful in the differential diagnosis of orofacial pain.

Electromyography (EMG) is a neurophysiological technique that measures the electrical signals (action potentials) from skeletal muscle fibres when they contract (Chapter 7). EMG has been used in research laboratories to determine the consequences of nociceptive inputs and processing of pain on muscle activity. However, EMG and the as-

Microneurography is far too complicated to be used in routine examinations of orofacial pain patients. Experimentally, a somewhat similar technique can be used during orthognathic surgery of the mandible when there is a significant risk of damaging the inferior alveolar nerve. In this technique, a needle electrode is inserted to record the electrical changes evoked in the mandibular nerve near the foramen ovale when the mental nerve is stimulated with repeated electric stimuli. As long as the nerve remains intact, the stimulus will continue to evoke action potentials. If it is damaged, the nature and size of the nerve electrical recordings will change.

sociated techniques that measure bite force and jaw movements are not a routine part of the orofacial pain analysis in the dental office, and their value in orofacial pain diagnosis remains controversial.

Many attempts have also been made to determine whether *trigeminal reflexes* can be used as objective measures or correlates of orofacial pain. This is mainly based on the finding that there is a correlation between the amplitude of the reflex response and the intensity of the stimulus, for example, the jaw-opening reflex in animals and the nociceptive limb withdrawal reflex in man. It has also been reported that orofacial pain can influence trigeminal reflex activity, e.g. experimental muscle pain enhances the monosynaptic jaw-stretch reflex and shortens the duration of the silent period in the masseter muscle evoked by electrical stimulation of orofacial tissues (e.g. Fig. 4 and 6 in Chapter 8). These findings indicate a connection between trigeminal reflex circuits and nociceptive pathways, but the use of trigeminal reflex recordings for assessment of orofacial pain is not warranted since the necessary sensitivity, specificity or prognostic value of this approach has not been established. Recordings of trigeminal reflexes may, however, be indicated if lesions (e.g. stroke or degenerative diseases in the brainstem) of the reflex pathways are suspected and need to be ruled out.

Microneurography has been used to study the responses of periodontal receptors (Chapter 6) and also in pain research. This technically-demanding method has contributed greatly to the understanding of nociceptive processing. With this technique, the activity of single peripheral nerve fibres can be recorded while as the subject reports his/her subjective responses at the same time. Several different classes of C-fibres have been identified with this technique, for example, fibres responding with different sensitivities to thermal, mechanical and chemical stimuli.

Imaging tests such as radiological examination or computerised tomograms (CT) scans provide excellent information on bony structures, and magnetic resonance imaging (MRI) gives valuable information on soft tissues, i.e., these investigations can help to reveal tissue injury and provide an explanation for a painful condition. However, they do not provide direct measures of pain, and gross changes have been seen, for example, in the form or shape of the condyle without associated pain. Thus, there is no simple or direct relationship between the amount of tissue injury and the magnitude of pain. The dentist should therefore carefully consider when and why radiographs or other imaging studies should be used to identify a possible structural cause of pain. A rule of thumb is that a diagnostic test should make a difference in the diagnosis and treatment plan in order to be justified. Generally, there will be indications for an imaging test of e.g., the TMJ in relation to trauma or suspicion of systemic joint disorders (rheumatoid arthritis), ankylosis, tumours, before surgical intervention, and in special cases where documentation and follow-up or reassurance of anxious patients is warranted. Finally, it must be noted that structural changes in the CNS at the cellular level associated with chronic pain are not detectable by the current imaging techniques.

Functional MRI (fMRI), electroencephalography (EEG) and *magnetoelectroencephalography* (MEG) can be used in the research laboratory to assess changes in the activity of the cortex and other regions in the CNS that are related to the processing of pain. *Positron emission tomography* (PET) is another sophisticated technique, which shows rather crudely the patterns of neuronal activity of the living human brain while it is pro-

cessing painful stimuli. Such studies have taught researchers a lot about the complexity of the brain in the processing of pain and which regions and circuits are involved in the sensory-discriminative and affective-motivational components of pain. PET images have also illustrated the networks in the brain related to placebo responses and hypnosis, thereby coupling the physiology of pain to its psychology. At the moment, however, the clinical utility of these brain-imaging techniques is limited and it is not possible to use a PET or fMRI scan to establish, for example, that "this patient has a neuropathic pain condition due to deafferentation of the upper second left molar and there is a significant emotional disturbance associated with the pain condition".

Autonomic parameters such as heart rate, blood pressure, sweat secretion, temperature, dilation of the pupil and many other physiological measures related to the function of the autonomic system are also coupled to pain. Measurement of these signs can be useful when severe autonomic dysfunction is part of the pain complaint (e.g. complex regional pain syndromes) but are rarely used in relation to orofacial pain conditions. The general problem with measures of autonomic function in relation to pain is that they are not specific to pain but may also change during other emotional reactions (anger, fear, aggression) and, furthermore, they normally tend to habituate which means that the responses become smaller over time.

Psychological and behavioural tests are important for diagnosis and management. In several examination systems (e.g., the so-called Research Diagnostic Criteria for TMD), there are checklists of dysfunctional behaviour, e.g., how much has pain interfered with the patient's ability to work and to engage in social activities. Furthermore, various symptom checklists can be used to obtain a measure of depression and somatisation scores.

The patient's treatment-seeking pattern is also important to establish since you may use quite different management approaches for the patient who has seen several other dentists or pain specialists before coming to you, or if you are the first dentist to see the patient. Other behavioural measures like the facial expression of the patient can also be valuable. Interestingly, it has been shown that there is good relationship between pain and certain facial expressions, which can be coded and quantified. Tightening of the eyes, lowering of the eyebrows (frowning), and tense lips are often associated with pain and may especially be helpful in evaluating the level of pain in children or in patients with impaired language. The type and dose of medication already used by the patient for relief of pain is also important to consider; however, one should be cautious using this as a direct measure of pain behaviour since successful treatment can be associated with either an increased or a decreased consumption of analgesics.

Nerve blocks by administration of local anaesthetics (e.g. lidocaine or bupivacaine) can be valuable in the pain analysis if the source of pain remains obscure. The painful area (e.g. tooth, jaw muscle or TMJ) or the relevant nerve can be injected and the pain intensity monitored on a VAS before and after the injection. A robust decrease ($> 50\%$) in pain would suggest that nociceptive input from that particular region contributes to the spontaneous pain, although placebo responses and pain referred from another site should also be considered. Preferably, a double-blind technique (i.e., both the dentist and patient not knowing if an active or inactive solution is being injected) should be used to avoid bias and expectancy effects. This technique is very powerful and can be

recommended for differential diagnosis even if the sensitivity and specificity of the test not has been clearly described in relation to orofacial pain.

Blood tests should be carried out primarily to rule out systemic diseases (e.g. rheuma factor in rheumatoid arthritis) or leukocytosis in acute infections, but will not help in the diagnosis of most orofacial pain complaints. However, elevated erythrocyte sedimentation rates are indicative of temporal arteritis, and folate, vitamin B-12 and iron deficiencies should be checked in patients with a presumed burning mouth syndrome. Biological markers of nociceptive activity and pain are not yet available, although patients with widespread muscle pain such as fibromyalgia may have increased plasma levels of 5-HT and prostaglandins (PGE_2), and synovial fluid samples from patients with TMJ osteoarthritis may have increased levels of 5-HT, PGE_2, cytokines and neuropeptides such as substance P and CGRP. More research is needed before assessment of these substances can be recommended for dental practice.

In summary, dentists should be able to assess orofacial pain complaints in a standardised manner and know which parameters are important in the clinic. They also need regular updates of their knowledge on the usefulness and limitations of current and future developments of adjunctive measures of pain, as this field is changing quickly. There is no single measure of pain which will encapsulate the entire bio-psycho-social aspect of pain, but a number of useful clinical and laboratory techniques have been outlined.

Clinical presentation of orofacial pain

In the following section some of the most common, and a few rarer, orofacial pain conditions are briefly described. These are listed according to the proposed mechanism-based classification of pain (Table 2). The intention is not to give a complete overview of all the different orofacial pain conditions but rather to provide neurobiological descriptions of some examples of clinical pain. More detailed information is available in specific textbooks on orofacial pain.

Transient orofacial pain

This type of pain can be elicited from virtually any orofacial structure during many dental procedures, for example, by probing a dental cavity or dentine-exposed surface, measuring gingival pocket depths, placing orthodontic appliances, drilling or scaling the teeth, inserting a needle, etc. The biological explanation for the reason that many people find it unpleasant and painful to go for a routine dental examination is because the orofacial tissues are densely innervated by free endings of nociceptive afferents that are easily stimulated during dental procedures, the primary somatosensory cortex specifically related to the orofacial region is very large, and because of the special psychological meaning and importance that this region has to people. The dentist can often anticipate this transient type of pain and tailor appropriate pain control to each individual patient and situation.

Pain from tissue injury

Inflammation is a natural consequence of tissue injury arising from e.g., mechanical or thermal trauma, viral or bacterial infections or cancer lesions. It can influence the excitability of nociceptive afferent endings in the peripheral tissues (peripheral sensitisation) and thereby enhance the pain of the injury, and CNS changes (e.g. central sensitisation) may also contribute to the pain (see basic neurobiology of orofacial pain section). In

trauma, there will normally be injury to more than one type of tissue, and the clinical manifestation will depend on which tissues are involved. Deep pain has characteristics that are quite distinct from those of superficial types of pain in terms of its quality (aching, cramping *versus* sharp, burning) and localizability (diffuse *versus* localised). Inflammation of a muscle (myositis) will cause swelling, loss of function and pain in much the same way as inflammation of the oral mucosa (mucositis), but the clinical manifestations may differ depending on the physical properties and functions of the involved tissue. For example, inflammation in the tooth pulp (pulpitis) will be different from gingival inflammation (gingivitis) due to the relative rigidity of dentine and enamel.

The most common types of pain in dental practice are *toothaches* (odontalgias) associated usually with reversible or irreversible pulpitis (Chapter 5). Pulpitis may start as an increased response to hot or cold stimuli and later pain may be spontaneous but exacerbated by heat and cold stimuli. Toothaches usually have a "sharp" or "dull" quality and sometimes a "throbbing" component. The intensity of the pain is described by many patients as extremely severe, in particularly in the acute stages. There can be bouts of pain attacks lasting minutes to hours. The tissue damage is highly localised, but the pain may spread and be referred to the ipsilateral face and jaw. The clinical examination should include a meticulous examination for dental caries and defective restorations and eventually radiography, in addition to a careful dental history (caries, trauma, dental treatment). Sensory testing with electrical and thermal stimuli will also be of benefit: the rule of thumb is that application of thermal stimuli to a tooth with irreversible pulpitis will produce a longer-lasting pain whereas cold or heat stimuli applied on a tooth with reversible pulpitis will evoke a sharp and more intense pain than on a normal tooth. Other common odontalgias include *periapical periodontitis*, which can be the consequence of irreversible pulpitis. Acute periapical periodontitis is associated with severe pain that is difficult to locate to a single tooth; there also may be both mechanical and thermal hyperalgesia. In the chronic stage, the pain is usually moderate, and mechanical hyperalgesia will commonly be present. Other more special cases of toothaches can be cracked or partially fractured teeth, barodontalgia (tooth pain triggered by changes in barometric pressure in the external environment), and referred pain from remote and other craniofacial structures.

Another frequent painful inflammatory condition is *pericoronitis*, which is related to accumulation of food debris and oral microflora around a partially-erupted third molar. *Gingivitis* and *periodontitis* are also very common inflammatory conditions which are associated with tissue injury but rarely produce symptoms of pain, although acute painful exacerbations can occur. Tissue injury pain is also encountered following oral surgery procedures and tooth extractions.

Maxillary sinusitis causes cheek pain and tenderness of the zygomatic arch and teeth, due to inflammation of the lining of the maxillary sinus that often occurs in relation to nasal colds. It may sometimes be confused with odontalgias due to referral or projection of pain to the teeth in the maxilla but history and clinical examination in addition to radiographs and provocation by bending the head will help to diagnose this pain problem.

Pain due to lesions of the oral mucosa can have numerous causes, for example, infections (e.g. herpetic stomatitis, candidiasis, acute necrotizing gingivostomatitis), immune system disorders (erosive lichen planus, aphthous stomatitis), traumatic and iatrogenic injuries, neoplasia, nutritional and metabolic diseases. Usually, such painful conditions will be associated with the other signs of inflammation such as reddening and swelling or direct signs of tissue injury.

Inflammatory conditions in the jaw muscles (myositis) or TMJ (synovitis and capsulitis) can occur after mechanical trauma, for example, from a blow to the face or from infection as a complication to third molar surgery or systemic infections. Localised inflammatory reactions (osteoarthritis) or systemic arthritis (rheumatoid arthritis; psoriatic arthritis) may be present in the TMJ and are often associated with quite severe tissue destruction.

In summary, there are many and varied painful conditions in the orofacial region that are associated with tissue injury; however, the underlying mechanisms of the pain most likely involve similar neurobiological events such as peripheral and central sensitisation.

Nervous system injury pain

The third major category according to the mechanism-based classification is pain arising from nervous system injury. In the orofacial region, one of the most unpleasant conditions is *trigeminal neuralgia*. Neuralgia simply means pain in the distribution of a nerve, and often it has a paroxysmal character (bursts of attacks). This is a rather rare condition but important to differentiate from the odontalgias because the management is very different. Trigeminal neuralgia is sudden, unilateral, severe, brief, stabbing, recurrent pain usually in the distribution of the maxillary or mandibular branches of the trigeminal nerve, and much less commonly in the ophthalmic division. The pain is sharp with electric shock-like stabs felt in the skin or buccal mucosa and is often triggered by light mechanical contact on a specific location known as the trigger point. The pain attacks are short (lasting only seconds) but can occur repetitively (minutes apart) and are then followed by a refractory period (Fig. 13C). Between the attacks, the patient is largely asymptomatic and there are no clear changes in somatosensory sensitivity. The aetiology and pathogenesis of trigeminal neuralgia are poorly understood, but it can occasionally be secondary to benign or malignant brain tumours, multiple sclerosis or facial trauma.

Other types of neuralgias have been described in relation to the facial nerve (geniculate neuralgia), intermedius nerve, glossopharyngeal nerve, hypoglossal nerve, vagal nerve, and occipital nerve. Furthermore, there are some extremely rare conditions which involve nervous tissues like Tolosa-Hunt syndrome, Raeder syndrome and short-lasting, unilateral neuralgiform pain with conjunctival injection and tearing (SUNCT). *Post-herpetic neuralgia* can also affect the trigeminal nerve (usually the ophthalmic branch) and is a complication of acute herpes zoster infection. Damage of the large nerve fibres with loss of myelination is thought to be involved in the pathology.

Simple extraction of a tooth and even endodontic treatment causes peripheral nerve injury and deafferentation, which may sometimes have peripheral and central neural consequences (see Basic neurobiology of orofacial pain). Despite the numerous surgical procedures and extractions of teeth performed every day in dental practice, there are rather few patients who complain about persistent nerve injury pain. This may be because the orofacial tissues are highly vascularised which facilitates regeneration but also because the injured nerves are usually quite small as a reason why so few patients complain of persistant orofacial pain compared

with those in the extremities. While pain certainly can appear when a peripheral branch of the trigeminal nerve is injured, for example during major surgery on the jaws, hypoaesthesia and numbness are more common.

Idiopathic types of orofacial pain

TMD is a collective term which covers a number of painful conditions in musculo-skeletal tissues (e.g. jaw muscles, tendons, TMJ) which may be accompanied by limitations of jaw movements and clicking or grating noises in the TMJ. The mechanisms of pain in these conditions are not completely understood but may involve some of the same events as discussed in the previous sections, including both peripheral and central sensitisation. It is useful to distinguish between three major categories of TMDs, namely, myofascial pain; disc displacements with or without reduction; and arthralgia, osteoarthrosis and osteoarthritis in the TMJ. There can be problems in the musculo-skeletal system other than those listed above, such as dislocation of the condyle, ankylosis etc., but these conditions are rare.

Myofascial TMD pain simply means that the patient complains of jaw muscle pain and that there are increased responses to palpation of these muscles (mechanical hyperalgesia). There is also often referral of pain to other craniofacial tissues on the ipsilateral side. Its aetiology is unknown, but female gender, depression and the presence of multiple other pain conditions are significant risk factors. Some of the other risk factors that have been suggested are grinding or clenching of the teeth, and certain types of malocclusion such as cross-bite. It is fair to say that dentists in the past have focused on the occlusal aspects; however, extensive research has shown that occlusion generally has little to do with the cause of myofascial TMD.

Displacement of the disc in the TMJ with reduction is associated with clicks during jaw movements when the disc returns to its normal position, whereas disc displacement without reduction means that the disc is permanently displaced, often in the mediolateral direction of the condyle, and constitutes a mechanical hindrance to mouth opening which therefore will be limited (<35 mm between the incisors).

Arthralgia is defined as pain in the joints, and TMJ arthralgia is characterised by local pain on palpation of the TMJ. Osteoarthrosis is considered a degenerative disorder in which the surface of the condyle is worn and there are coarse grating sounds (crepitation) from the TMJ but without pain. Osteoarthritis in the TMJ has already been briefly considered under tissue injury pain, and inflammatory reactions play a major role for the destruction and for the presence of pain.

Due to the diversity of TMD pain conditions, it can often be difficult to pinpoint one single causative factor. Generally, they are today viewed as multifactorial problems with some anatomical, neuromuscular and neurobiological and psychosocial factors, which can act as predisposing, precipitating or aggravating factors in an individual patient.

Atypical odontalgia is a very troublesome condition for both the patient and the dentist because this type of pain can initially be difficult to distinguish from conventional odontalgias with pain localised to the tooth or to the site where the tooth used to be. Hence, the patient may receive excessive and unnecessary dental treatment with multiple root canal treatments and extractions without any change in their pain. *Atypical facial pain* can be both unilateral and bilateral and can have both intermittent or continuous time courses often with a throbbing quality of the pain. These two pain conditions are difficult to treat successfully, and indeed some dentists consider atypical odontalgia and facial pain to be predominantly psychological in origin because of the associated emotional signs, stress and depression and because of the lack of recognisable tissue injury. It has also been proposed that they could represent neuropathic pain conditions arising from deafferentation and long-term neuroplastic changes of the type described in the previous sections. In these cases, it is important for the dentist to stop all further dental interventions unless there are clear signs of tissue pathology, and to refer the patient to a pain specialist.

Finally, *burning mouth syndrome* is a relatively common orofacial pain condition especially in middle-aged and elderly women, particularly after menopause. It is characterised by a burning, smarting pain on the tongue, lips and hard palate. Visual inspection of the oral mucosa does not reveal signs of inflammation and the condition is quite refractory to dental treatment.

Headaches

Some pain conditions do not fall easily into the proposed mechanism-based classification. Examples of these include the primary headaches such as migraines, cluster headaches and other trigeminal autonomic cephalgias. These headaches are sometimes referred to as neurovascular headaches. The pathophysiology of *migraines* is not completely clear but is thought to involve an interaction between neurovascular inputs, myofascial nociceptive inputs and supraspinal effects. Both peripheral and central sensitisation and neurogenic inflammation could also contribute to the pain. Some types of headache may also have a strong genetic predisposition. The pain in migraines with aura (classical migraine, with visual, sensory or speech problems) or without aura (common migraine) are most often unilateral, moderate to severe in intensity, and have a pulsating quality that is aggravated by physical activity. Migraines come in attacks lasting up to 3 days and the patients often report nausea, vomiting, and increased sensitivity to sounds and light. There are several variants of migraine and the dentist must ensure that these patients are examined by a neurologist or pain specialist.

Cluster headache is, as the name suggests, a pain condition which occurs in series of attacks, which usually are extremely painful and associated with autonomic reactions such as tears in the eye, blocked nose, oedema of the eyelid and facial sweating. This is one of the rare pain conditions which primarily occurs in men. The dentist should exert great care not to mistake this pain condition for an acute pulpitis or apical periodontitis and start unnecessary dental treatment. *Paroxysmal hemicrania* has many of the same characteristics as cluster headache but pain attacks are shorter, more frequent and occur mainly in females and are unique in responding to indomethacin medication. *Carotidynia* is described as a dull aching, sometime throbbing pain near the upper portion of the carotid arteries, with referred pain to the teeth, face and head on the same side. *Temporal arteritis* is associated with a unilateral or bilateral headache with mainly continuous or throbbing pain associated with muscle pain in the temporal region: biopsies and blood tests may help to establish the diagnosis.

Dentists can expect to see many patients with *tension-type headaches* which, in contrast to the migraines, are extremely frequent. Some studies have reported that up to 80% of the population may experience this type of headache at least once in their life. The tension-type headaches can be divided into infrequent (<12 days per year), frequent (>12 and <180 days per year) or chronic (>180 days per year). The pain is described as a pressing or tightening pain of mild to moderate pain intensity, bilateral, and not aggravated by physical activity. Both peripheral and central sensitisation of muscular inputs are thought to be involved.

In addition, headaches can be due to numerous other reasons such as head and neck trauma, cranial or cervical vascular disorders, substance abuse, infections, and psychiatric disorders.

Other aspects of orofacial pain

Pain can be referred to the orofacial region, and in particular to the teeth, from distant sources such as the heart (during angina), neurovascular disorders (migraine), maxillary sinuses, nasal mucosa and ears. The dentist needs to be aware of these patterns of pain referral, which are thought to be explained by central convergence of afferent inputs from various cranial and cervical nerves onto common projection neurons in the subnucleus caudalis (see Brainstem nociceptive transmission).

Finally, it needs to be mentioned that in very rare cases, *psychiatric disturbances* (hallucination, hysteria, hypochondrias) and somatisation problems may be the main reason for the pain. A careful dental, medical and psychosocial history in addition to uncharacteristic and non-specific results in the pain analysis may suggest this diagnosis, and these patients must be referred to pain specialists, clinical psychologists or psychiatrists for further evaluation and management.

■ Pain therapy

The dentist needs a good understanding of the neurobiology and psychosocial aspects of pain in order to treat and manage clinical pain. The transient type of pain can often be effectively prevented by administration of local anaesthetics. For example, inflammatory pain can usually be treated effectively and sometimes virtually prevented by the appropriate use of anti-inflammatory agents such as NSAIDs (see below). However, neuropathic pain and idiopathic pain conditions are much less amenable to therapy, and can normally be managed but not cured. A natural goal is to obtain the best possible pain relief with the least invasive means. If the cause of pain can be identified (for example dental caries or bacterial infection around an impacted lower third molar), the cause should obviously be treated. This is fortunately the case for most patients with acute orofacial pain but not always for the

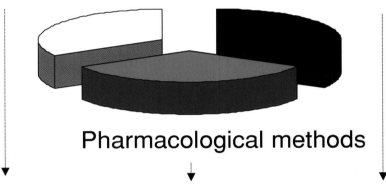

Psychological methods   Physical methods

Pharmacological methods

Information	Local anaesthetics	Stretch therapy
Counseling	Non-opioid analgesics	Jaw exercises
Education	Salicylates	Massage
Stress management	Acetaminophen	Ultrasound
Biofeedback	Nonsteroidal anti-inflammatory	Soft laser
Relaxation	Steroids	Heat / cold
Hypnosis	Opioids	TENS
Cognitive-behavioural	Anxiolytics and sedatives	Acupuncture
Psychotherapy	Antiepileptics – anticonvulsants	Oral splints
	Antidepressants	
	Muscle relaxants	
	NMDA receptor antagonists	
	Serotonin agonists	

Figure 15. Overview of pain therapy modified from Schmidt, RF: Fundamentals of Sensory Physiology, Springer-Verlag, 1986. In most orofacial pain conditions, physical, pharmacological and psychological methods can be combined to control or manage the pain. The selection of the specific methods will depend on the underlying mechanisms of pain and individual psychosocial features, i.e., pain therapy needs to be tailored to the needs of each person.

persistent types. If there is no longer any sign of tissue pathology, then symptomatic treatment will be necessary. It can be useful to view pain management as a "combined package" with different modalities (Fig. 15). These modalities can be combined in numerous ways tailored to the individual patient to interact with the nociceptive processing and pain at different levels of the neuroaxis.

If we consider the nociceptive trigeminal pathways (Fig. 4), then it is logical to consider combining approaches that target both peripheral mechanisms and central processes to control or manage painful conditions.

■ Peripheral targets

A typical way for the dentist to manage many types of pain is the administration of *local anaesthetics* (e.g. lidocaine/lignocaine, bupivacaine, mepivacaine, articaine), either through transmucosal or transdermal injections, or topical application. Injections can be performed as nerve blocks (e.g. at the inferior alveolar nerve, mental nerve, infra-orbital nerve) or as submucosal infiltrations where the finer nerve branches are blocked. Local anaesthetics bind to the interior of the axonal membrane and prevent depolarisation and thus propagation of action potentials. Usually there is some preservation of the touch sensation (since local anaesthetics preferentially block small-diameter affer-

> Lidocaine is sometimes also given systemically by anaesthesiologists to relieve certain types of pain, e.g. post-herpetic neuralgia.

ents), and the patient should be informed about this. The efficacy of local anaesthetics varies depending on their chemical and physical properties, particularly their pKa, and on the condition of the peripheral tissues (e.g. the presence of inflammatory conditions may be associated with the release of chemical substances, particularly H^+, that can counteract the local anaesthetic effect). The analgesia usually begins within a few minutes, and lasts 1–4 hours and even more depending on the local anaesthetic used. This is adequate for most dental procedures, including oral surgery. Longer-lasting local anaesthetics can be used to reduce post-operative tissue-injury pain and central sensitisation.

Prior to injections, topical anaesthetics can be applied (e.g. benzocaine, EMLA® paste) to reduce the transient pain evoked by the penetration of the needle. A number of special techniques are also used for local anaesthetic injection. For example, intraligamentous injection can block a single tooth and is useful both for very focal pain control and for differential diagnosis of odontalgias in order to identify the painful tooth. As more knowledge is gained from the peripheral aspects of nociception and the upregulation of receptor types, further refinement and more effective local anaesthetics are likely.

Salicylates (e.g. aspirin) have been used for more than 100 years as analgesic, antipyretic, anti-inflammatory and anti-rheumatic drugs. They act principally in peripheral tissues where they prevent the synthesis of prostaglandins. They are normally considered safe and effective drugs for mild to moderate intensities of tissue injury pain and headaches. Care needs to be taken with their use in patients with certain medical problems, for example, anticoagulant medication, because of their well-known effect on platelet activity. Some patients are allergic to salicylates.

Nonsteroidal anti-inflammatory drugs (NSAIDs) (e.g. ibuprofen, naproxen, keterolac) prevent the formation of prostaglandins from arachidonic acid through blockage of the enzyme cyclo-oxygenase. Their efficacy in tissue-injury types of pain and in particular post-operative pain has been thoroughly documented and NSAIDs are amongst the most commonly used drugs in dental practice. Great care needs to be taken with their use in particular in situations requiring sustained administration and in medically-comprised patients because of their gastrointestinal side-effects. Recently, a selective cyclo-oxygenase-2 inhibitor has been marketed which is claimed to reduce side-effects; however, the evidence on this point is incomplete, and a conservative approach to their use is recommended. Interestingly, the NSAIDs may also have CNS effects.

Acetaminophen is another class of aspirin-like analgesics where the effect is believed to involve peripheral actions (e.g. weak inhibition of prostaglandin synthesis) but central effects are also likely. It is particular useful as an alternative to NSAIDs and salicylates in patients with gastrointestinal problems. The aspirin-like drugs have been combined with weak opioids like codeine, but the additive effects are only marginal.

Adrenocortical steroids and their chemical derivatives (e.g., dexamethasone, methylprednisolone, betamethasone) have a variety of biological effects but can also be used for short periods as potent anti-inflammatory agents to manage acute, intense inflammatory conditions (e.g. intra-articular injection in TMJ osteoarthritis, or intramuscular injection in myositis).

A number of *physical methods* have also been used to target peripheral pain mechanisms in dental practice. For example thermal stimulation (heat, cold), massage and stretching of painful muscles are believed to have an effect on blood circulation and local tissue repair processes, and by slowing nociceptive transmission from the injured site. Nevertheless, these effects can be difficult to separate from central effects; that is, activation of descending inhibitory systems, release of analgesic substances like endorphins and enkephalins, and cognitive-behavioural aspects could also play a part. It is also not clear to what extent and why acupuncture and TENS are effective in the management of for example persistent TMD types of pain, but a central modulatory component seems likely.

Occlusal splints have for many years been the most important part of TMD management and often also tension-type headaches. Insertion of a splint in the upper or lower jaw will alter the peripheral sensory inputs from, e.g., periodontal receptors, mechano-sensitive receptors in the jaw muscles, oral mucosa and facial skin, but the consequences of this for trigeminal sensory and motor function are not clear. There is little scientific support for any neurophysiological mechanism that might underlie the efficacy of occlusal splints, and indeed more recent studies have cast doubt on whether occlusal splints are any more effective than placebo splints (i.e. splints designed not to interfere with the occlusion). It has also been suggested that occlusal splints have a strong effect on the cognitive-behavioural dimension of pain, e.g. by increasing awareness of oral habits and facilitation of relaxation, and the splint may in fact best be compared with a non-harmful "occlusal crutch".

Central targets

The analgesic effect of *opioid* drugs (e.g. morphine, fentanyl) has been known for a long time and they remain amongst the most potent analgesics available today. They exert their analgesic effect through actions on several specific receptor types (mu, delta, kappa) located throughout the CNS; however, recent studies have also indicated the presence of opioid receptors in peripheral tissues. The efficacy of opioids has been clearly demonstrated on both tissue-injury types of pain and nervous system injury types of pain. Their main disadvantages are the risk of respiratory depression, sedation and the development of dependency and abuse. Opioids are required only in selected cases in dental practice, e.g. for post-surgical pain management or very intense and persistent orofacial pain problems, and their use should normally be restricted to pain specialists.

Antiepileptic drugs, i.e., anticonvulsants, (e.g. carbamazepine, oxcarbazepine, phenytoin) can be used for management of trigeminal neuralgia. The presumed site of action is a stabilising effect on sodium channels which prevents high-frequency neuronal discharges in the CNS. More recently, antiepileptic drugs like gabapentin have been introduced and shown to be effective in the management of post-herpetic neuralgia and diabetic polyneuropathy, but the evidence of their efficacy in most orofacial pain conditions is not impressive.

Anxiolytics and sedatives (e.g. diazepam, lorazepam) can be useful in very nervous or dental-phobic patients since anxiety and stress can increase the perception of pain. There is also some evidence that short-term trials of benzodiazepines can be useful in more persistent types of TMD pain, and it has been suggested that they may also be effective in burning mouth syndrome. However, there is little scientific evidence to support their general use in the management of orofacial pain conditions.

Dentists should be aware of the analgesic effect of *antidepressants*, in particular the tricyclic antidepressants (e.g. amitriptyline, imipramine). This analgesic effect is not directly related to their anti-depressive effect but could be due to their multiple site of actions, e.g. blockage of the re-uptake of noradrenaline and serotonin, in addition to antagonistic effects on NMDA receptors. They are now the first drug of choice in many neuropathic pain conditions and can also be tried in persistent types of musculoskeletal pain, e.g. tension-type headache and persistent TMD pain. Care needs to be taken in their use, since tricyclic antidepressants are contraindicated in certain clinical conditions, e.g. in patients with heart problems and glaucoma, and their prescription and monitoring of plasma concentrations should preferably be done by pain specialists. Interestingly, tricyclic antidepressants have recently been shown to possess local anaesthetic-like effects. It should also be remembered that a finite number of dental patients

The drugs that have come to be known as *"muscle relaxants"* are misleadingly named, as they do not act directly on skeletal muscles. Rather, they exert their effects on circuits in the central nervous system that ultimately control muscle activity. These drugs should not be confused with drugs that relax muscles directly, such as curare-like drugs which block neuromuscular transmission, and dantrolene which prevents excitation-contraction coupling in skeletal muscle fibres by blocking the release of Ca^{2+} from the sarcoplasmic reticulum.

will be taking these drugs for the treatment of their depression.

The NMDA receptor has been widely implicated in the neuroplastic neuronal changes which could underlie persistent orofacial pain (see Brainstem nociceptive transmission) but so far clinical trials with *NMDA receptor antagonists* (e.g. ketamine, dextromethorphane) have shown only modest analgesic effects and their clinical use is compromised by side-effects such as sedation and hallucinations. Since NMDA receptors are present not only within the CNS, but also in the periphery (see Primary afferent properties and peripheral sensitisation), it might be possible in the future to administer NMDA receptor antagonists locally, but this will await further studies.

Muscle relaxants with central actions (e.g carisoprodol, cyclobenzaprine, tolperisone hydrochloride) have frequently been prescribed for tension-type headache and myofascial TMD due to the assumption that muscle spasms are a central part of their pathophysiology. This assumption has now been challenged, however, muscle relaxants appear to be moderately effective in these conditions, perhaps due to other effects such as blocking sodium channels or antidepressant-like actions.

Vascular headaches such as migraines respond to *serotonin-receptor agonists* (e.g. $5HT_{1B/1D}$) which may counteract neurogenic inflammation by constriction of dilated cranial extracerebral blood vessels, reduction of neuropeptide release from peripheral nerve endings around cranial blood vessels and central inhibition of impulse transmission in subnucleus caudalis. These drugs (e.g. sumatriptan) should normally be prescribed by a neurologist or other pain specialists.

Finally, *psychological and behavioural* therapy should be considered. In the simplest case, this may consist of providing the patient with simple information about the procedures, reasons for the pain problem, prognosis and reassurance. Distraction or directing the attention away from transient types of pain (e.g. by music, movies) is easily implemented in dental practice. Hypnosis may also be a relevant treatment option both for acute pain control and for management of persistent orofacial pain conditions in patients who respond to this approach.

It has been shown that self-care instructions and monitoring can provide at least as good pain relief as the usual dental approaches (e.g. occlusal splints) to TMD pain patients, and that in more severely affected patients, the inclusion of comprehensive care provided by a clinical psychologist will provide a significant advantage compared with the usual dental treatment. While psychotherapy and extensive cognitive-behavioural therapy normally fall outside the scope of dental practice, it nevertheless appears important to tailor the treatment to each individual patient. Various degrees of psychological intervention should not be considered as treatments of last resort, but rather used concurrently with pharmacological or physical treatments. Further research is needed to define the advantages of combinations of psychological-behavioural management and other treatment modalities.

In summary, there is a wide range of techniques and methods to control and manage orofacial pain, with which the dentist must be familiar. The specific choice will depend on the individual patient and the experience and expertise of the dentist. Dentists must be able to predict procedural pain and to arrange the necessary methods for pain control. For orofacial pain patients, it is important for the dentist to provide them with a tentative diagnosis and to establish realistic treatment goals.

Conclusions

In this chapter we have described the definition and classification of orofacial pain from a contemporary perspective. The underlying neurobiological mechanisms of orofacial pain have been presented, with emphasis on the normal nociceptive transmission process and alterations in this process that are characterised by peripheral and central sensitisation and neuroplastic changes. Although these basic mechanisms play a vital role in our understanding of the clinical manifestation of orofacial pain, it is equally important to consider the psychosocial or psychophysiological dimensions of pain when orofacial pain is assessed, and not least when intervention is required.

Finally, this chapter has some broad guidelines for management of various orofacial pain conditions. These guidelines are likely to differ between different countries and dental schools, and will require constant revision and updating.

Glossary

- Allodynia: Pain due to a stimulus which does not normally provoke pain, i.e. lowered threshold.
- Analgesia: Absence of pain in response to stimulation which would normally be painful.
- Anaesthesia dolorosa: Pain in an area or region which is anaesthetic.
- Causalgia: A syndrome of sustained burning pain, allodynia, and hyperpathia after a traumatic nerve lesion, often combined with vasomotor and sudomotor dysfunction and later trophic changes.
- Central pain: Pain initiated or caused by a primary lesion in or dysfunction of the central nervous system.

- Central sensitisation/hyperexcitability: The increased excitability of nociceptive neurones in the central nervous system that can be induced by a nociceptive afferent barrage into the central nervous system following tissue injury.
- Dysaesthesia: An unpleasant abnormal sensation, which may be either spontaneous or evoked.
- Hyperalgesia: An increased response to a stimulus which is normally painful, i.e., increased pain response.
- Hyperaesthesia: Increased sensitivity to stimulation, excluding the special senses.
- Hyperpathia: A painful syndrome characterised by an abnormally painful reaction to a stimulus, especially a repetitive stimulus, as well as an increased threshold.
- Hypoalgesia: Diminished pain in response to a normally painful stimulus, i.e., raised threshold to activation.
- Hypoaesthesia: Decreased sensitivity to stimulation, excluding the special senses.
- Neuralgia: Pain in the distribution of a nerve or nerves.
- Neuritis: Inflammation of a nerve or nerves.
- Neuroplastic changes: The changes in the properties of primary afferents and neurones in the central nervous system that may occur following tissue injury and during development and maturation of the nervous system. They reflect a dynamic state of the morphological, biochemical and physiological properties of the afferents and neurones.
- Neurogenic pain: Pain initiated or caused by a primary lesion, dysfunction, or transitory perturbation in the peripheral or central nervous system.
- Neuropathic pain: Pain initiated or caused by a primary lesion or dysfunction in the nervous system.

- Neuropathy: A disturbance of function or pathological change in a nerve: in one nerve, mononeuropathy; in several nerves, mononeuropathy multiplex; if diffuse and bilateral, polyneuropathy.
- Nociceptor: A receptor preferentially sensitive to a noxious stimulus or to a stimulus that would become noxious if prolonged.
- Noxious stimulus: A stimulus that damages normal tissues.
- Pain threshold: The least experience of evoked pain which a subject can recognize.
- Pain tolerance level: The greatest level of pain which a subject is prepared to tolerate.
- Paraesthesia: An abnormal sensation, whether spontaneous or evoked.
- Peripheral sensitisation: The increased excitability of nociceptors following peripheral tissue injury or repeated noxious stimulation.
- Referred pain: Pain felt outside the region of primary lesion
- Projected pain: Pain due to disturbances along the course of a nerve fibre or its central connections which is felt as shooting pain in the peripheral distribution of that nerve.

■ Selected references

Dionne R, Phero JC, Becker DE (eds). Management of pain and anxiety in the dental office. WB Saunders 2002.

Dubner R, Sessle BJ, Storey AT (eds). The Neural Basis of Oral and Facial Function. New York: Plenum Press 1978; 483 pp.

Lund JP, Lavigne GJ, Dubner R, Sessle BJ. Orofacial pain. From basic sciences to clinical management. Quintessence 2001.

Merskey H, Bogduk N (eds). Classification of chronic pain, 2. ed. IASP Press 1994.

Okeson JP. Management of temporomandibular disorders and occlusion, 5. ed. Mosby 2003.

Ren K, Dubner R. Central nervous system plasticity and persistent pain. J Orofac Pain 1999;13:155–163.

Sessle BJ. Acute and chronic craniofacial pain: brainstem mechanisms of nociceptive transmission and neuroplasticity, and their clinical correlates. Crit Rev Oral Biol Med 2000;11:57–91.

Sessle BJ. The neural basis of temporomandibular joint and masticatory muscle pain. J Orofac Pain 1999;13:238–245.

Svensson P, Graven-Nielsen T. Craniofacial muscle pain: Review of mechanisms and clinical manifestations. J Orofac Pain 2001;15:117–145.

Tooth pulp

James W. Hu

Goals:
- To describe the structure and functions of the human tooth pulp.
- To understand the peripheral and central neural mechanisms involved in toothache.
- To describe clinical examples of changes in the tooth pulp under physiological and pathophysiological conditions.

Key words:
Toothache; nerve; receptor; dentine; inflammation; hydrodynamics; pulpitis.

■ Introduction

Teeth and pain have always been intimately related and pain has always been important for the dental profession. The first recorded history of dental practice is in ancient Egypt about 2600 BC, and the diagnosis and management of toothaches have been integral components of dental practice since Dentistry became a recognized profession in the late 19th century. The Danish story-teller Hans Christian Andersen suffered frequently from toothaches and described his experience in this way: "My teeth cause me tremendous pain: the nerves are really fine keys on which the indiscernible pressure of the air plays, and so there is a concert in the teeth, now piano, now crescendo, all tunes of pain caused by changes of climate".

Even today, toothache remain one of the most common reasons for people to seek dental treatment. Under normal physiological conditions, intact and healthy teeth will not give rise to any painful sensations even when stimulated with cold or hot. However, if damage occurs to the hard tissues, the tooth may become exquisitely sensitive to natural stimuli as Hans Christian Andersen has so eloquently described. It is essential for the dentist to understand the complexity of the structure and function of the tooth pulp in order to diagnose and manage this situation. However, the tooth pulp has functions other than simply signalling tissue damage. It is intimately related to the function of dentine, supplying its nutrients and promoting its repair. For this reason, the tooth pulp and dentine are often referred to as the dentine-pulp complex. Knowledge of the functions of the tooth pulp is therefore also critical in everyday dentistry when one is drilling or cutting enamel and dentine and during other operative procedures. Think, for example, what happens to the tooth pulp when the tooth is deliberately moved by orthodontic forces or is accidentally avulsed.

This chapter provides a detailed description of the physiological aspects of the human tooth pulp.

Tooth structure

The tooth is a mineralised hard tissue composed of enamel, cementum, dentine and pulp, which is supported by periodontal tissues (Fig. 1A). Enamel is the most highly mineralised and therefore the hardest tissue in the body. Cementum is a specialised connective tissue which resembles bone, except that cementum is avascular and does not undergo resorption and remodelling. Dentine is also a mineralised and avascular connective tissue with approximately one million dentinal tubules per tooth, each of which is filled with a process from an odontoblast cell, and may contain nerve terminals. Finally, the pulp is a highly vascular and richly-innervated connective tissue forming the soft core of the tooth. The connective tissue in the pulp consists of fibres (mainly colla-

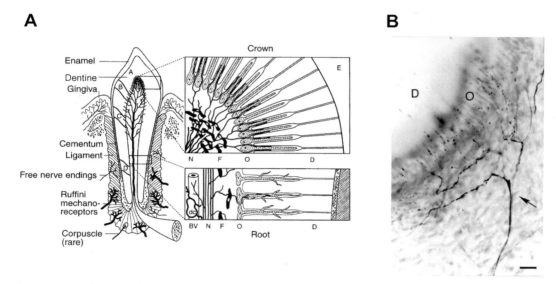

Figure 1. (A) Schematic of a mature erupted tooth and its dentinal, pulpal, and periodontal innervation. In the dentinal zones labelled A-D, more than 40% of the dentinal tubules are innervated at the tip of the pulp horn (zone A) and decreasing percentages of innervated dentinal tubules in zones B (4–8%), C (0.2–1%) and D (0.02–0.2%). The higher magnification panels show differences in intradentinal nerve (N) incidence, pulpal fibroblasts (F), odontoblasts (O), dentine (D), and enamel (E) for the crown and root. Odontoblasts form a barrier that separates the subodontoblast plexus from the rest of the pulp. Perivascular dendritic cells (dc) and blood vessel (BV) innervation are shown in the root diagram (lower left panel). The innervation of periodontal tissues is mainly concentrated in the root region where the maximal torque occurs as the result of forces acting on the crown, and by specialized low-threshold direction-sensitive mechanoreceptors, such as Ruffini endings, and pain-sensitive free nerve endings. (B) A single dental A-delta fibre labelled immunochemically with CGRP shows multiple branches from its parent axon (about 4 μM diameter). Some the fine nerve terminals entering the dentine tubules are shown as black streaks; however, this is limited to the base of the dentinal tubule near the odontoblast layer. Modified and reprinted from Byers, 1984, 1994 with permission.

gen), cells (odontoblasts, fibroblasts, undifferentiated mesenchymal cells as well as mast cells in inflamed pulps), and a matrix (proteoglycans and fibronectin), further details of which can be found in textbooks of dental histology.

Extensive axon branching is a very important anatomical characteristic of dental nerve fibres that is highly correlated to their unique physiological properties. Various levels of axon branching have physiological and potential clinical implications. Fig. 1B shows that branching of a 4 μm thick "parent" axon at the subodontoblast plexus level enables a relatively small number of dental afferent fibres to innervate a very large number of dentinal tubules. Near the apex of the tooth, the alveolar nerve branches to innervate every accessory apical canal. Finally, the extensive branching of axons within the alveolar nerves results in each dental afferent neuron innervating multiple teeth. This contributes to the poor localisation of toothache, neurogenic inflammation and reinnervation of reimplanted teeth. Because of the extensive axon branching, injury of dental nerve fibres may result in consequences that are less serious than those that occur when cutaneous sensory afferent fibres are injured, such as local areas of paraesthesia. The extensive axon branching may contribute to the unusual ability of dental afferent fibres to regenerate and to reinnervate the dentinal tissues.

In contrast to other connective tissues in the body, the tooth pulp is encapsulated and protected by hard tissue walls. Hence, the tooth pulp has a very low compliance because the surrounding dentine prevents any significant volume changes if the pressure within the pulp chamber changes. This means that the equilibrium between the various factors that affect blood flow and the circulation of tissue fluid in the tooth pulp is critical to the health of the tooth pulp, as described later.

The tooth pulp also contains a large number of free nerve endings. Each tooth may be innervated with up to 1000 afferent (sensory) neurones originating from the maxillary or mandibular division of the trigeminal (V) nerve. Afferent fibres innervating the teeth comprise less than 0.1% of the 500,000 trigeminal neurones, but each nerve fibre branches, tapers and arborizes extensively (Fig. 1B), especially in the coronal part of the tooth, contributing to the formation of the so-called subodontoblastic plexus. Some of these very fine free nerve endings also enter the dentinal tubule but extend only about one-third of the distance (<100 μm) from the subodontoblastic plexus to the outer surface of the dentine. This is important to remember when one is trying to understand the basis for the sensitivity of exposed dentine, e.g. at the dentinoenamel junction (see later).

■ Blood flow

Unlike dentine, the tooth pulp is amply supplied with arterioles, venules and lymph vessels. Small arteries or arterioles enter the tooth pulp *via* the main apical foramen and accessory foramina. Together with the nerve supply, they pass axially in the root pulp towards the coronal pulp. Arterio-venous (AV) anastomoses are shunts between arterioles and venules: these are a common feature in the pulpal circulation, and enable blood to bypass the capillary beds. Under normal conditions, the capillary bed is empty and the AV shunts permit regional control of pulpal blood flow by shunting of blood directly from arterioles to venules. Capillary loops pass between the odontoblasts towards the predentine, but the capillaries do not enter into the dentinal tubules. Around 90% of pulpal capillaries are found in this subodontoblastic zone and this is the major site of nutrient and gas exchange within the subodontoblastic plexus. The capillaries drain into venules that merge to form the central pulpal venules which run parallel to the arterioles and nerve bundles. In a healthy tooth pulp, blood occupies about 5% of the total volume. The tooth pulp has a high blood flow around 40–50 ml/min per 100 g of tissue, which is comparable with the most active tissues in the body, such as the brain or liver.

The blood flow in the tooth pulp is controlled by the autonomic nervous system, primarily by sympathetic efferent nerve fibres. Furthermore, activity in nociceptive afferents can also influence pulpal blood flow by the release of vasodilatatory substances The blood flow and transcapillary pressure determine the rate of formation of interstitial fluid and thereby affect the intrapulpal pressure. Due to the rigid dentine walls, small increases in volume produce major changes in pressure. Experimental studies in animals have shown that increases in pulpal temperature by laser radiation cause increases in blood flow and extravasation. Extravasation is the leakage of plasma proteins from venules to the interstitial space, and is a feature of inflammation. In the pulp, extravasation increases intrapulpal pressure. Several pro-inflammatory neuropeptides such as calcitonin gene-related peptide (CGRP), substance P and vasoactive intestinal polypeptide (VIP) are released near blood vessels and have vasodilatatory effects, whereas vasoconstriction is under the influence of nor-adrenaline, mainly via α_1 and to a lesser degree by α_2 adrenoreceptors, as well as neuropeptide Y and its receptors on the vascular smooth muscles. Inflammation of the tooth pulp induced either by bacterial or mechanical trauma will therefore have consequences on local blood flow regulation and can lead to increases in pressure in the pulp chamber. The increased intra-pulpal pressure may then compromise the blood flow, leading to tissue hypoxia and eventually to tissue necrosis. It should also be emphasized that administration of local anaesthetics containing the vasoconstrictor nor-adrenaline will impede blood flow for hours, which may leave the tooth pulp more vulnerable, for example, during tooth preparation.

Dentine-pulp permeability barrier

Tight junctions between odontoblasts and the connective tissue in the pulp constitute a selectively-permeable barrier which regulates the movement of interstitial fluids and solutes (including nutrients) between the tooth pulp and the dentinal tubules (Fig. 1). In intact teeth, the barrier is permeable to water and small ions but impermeable to larger metallic ions. This barrier constituted by the odontoblasts creates a localized "micro-environment" within the dentinal tubules that facilitates dentine matrix deposition and subsequent mineralisation. Dentinal tubules also provide routes for the passage of substances, including bacteria, to and from the pulp. Dentinal tubules extend the full thickness of dentine and taper from the pulp outwards; hence, there is a higher moisture concentration in deep cavity preparations that can affect the bonding strength of resin to this part of the cavity wall.

Several factors can affect dentine permeability: these include the patency and thickness of the tubules, the dentine area involved, the concentration gradient between pulp and dentine tubule fluid, dentinal fluid flow and the permeability of the odontoblast barrier. Increased intravascular volume (e.g. due to arteriolar dilation or venous constriction) or increased interstitial fluid volume (e.g. due to increased capillary permeability or lymphatic blockage and consequent intradental pressure increase) will tend to increase the volume of the pulp. However, since the tooth pulp is contained in a low-compliance chamber, the volume changes may result in dentinal fluid movements which are very important for activation of the neural endings that evoke pain (see later, Mechanisms of dental sensation/hydrodynamic theory), as well as increases in pulp chamber pressure which may be a factor in initiating tissue necrosis.

Role of odontoblasts

In addition to the roles mentioned above, odontoblasts regulate dentine matrix production, repair and calcification (for details, see dental histology textbooks). Odontoblasts are derived from neural crest cells, but are not excitable cells in the classical sense (like nerve cells). However, like all other cells, they have a membrane potential determined by the intracellular and extracellular ion concentrations generated by membrane transporters. Despite the fact that free nerve endings (unmyelinated fibres) are found preferentially in dentinal tubules in close relation with the odontoblast processes, odontoblasts do not function as sensory receptors and they lack gap junctions and presynaptic structures to pass signals directly to the free nerve endings in the subodontoblastic plexus.

The release of neuropeptides and neurotrophic factors, such as CGRP and NGF, has profound long-term effects on the structure and sensitivity of the tooth. Both chronic inflammation and frequent stimulation of periodontal tissues (for example due to bruxism) may lead to increased pulpal blood flow and calcium metabolism, which in turn may stimulate increased dentine production (*via* formation of reparative dentine) and hence reduce the size of the pulp cavity. These morphological changes may render the tooth pulp less sensitive and the tooth more brittle. Although lacking direct synaptic connections, odontoblasts and nerve endings can have profound functional interactions via chemical transmission. Since odontoblasts change shape after mechanical stimulation or disturbance which induces fluid movements in the dentinal tubules, it is tempting to suggest that odontoblasts could act as mechanical transducers. For example, the fluid movement-induced distortion of odontoblastic cell shape may cause them to release ATP which could then activate $P2X_3$ receptors on the nerve endings (see later: Peripheral receptor mechanisms).

Nerve supply

In the tooth pulp, nerve action potentials are conducted along small-diameter (A-delta or C) primary afferents of the V nerve. The mandibular division (V_3) innervates the lower dental arch, and the maxillary division

(V_2) innervates the upper dental arch. The tooth pulp is innervated not only by sensory V afferent nerve fibres but also by post-ganglionic sympathetic efferent axons. The latter cause the pulp vessels to constrict by releasing noradrenaline. Their cell bodies are located in the superior cervical ganglion, from which axons pass to the tooth pulp with the branches of the V nerve along the blood vessels. Unlike the skin or other oro-facial tissues, vasodilation in the tooth pulp does not seem to be controlled directly by parasympathetic cholinergic efferent fibres. Rather, vasodilation is controlled by changes in sympathetic tone and the local release of neurogenic substances and neuropeptides from sensory afferents as well as the transmitter substance nitric oxide (NO) which is a short-lived gas molecule produced in the endothelial cell lining of the blood vessels.

Several neurochemicals have been found in nerve endings (e.g. ATP, glutamate, substance P, CGRP, VIP, NGF) and in immunocompetent cells in the tooth pulp (e.g. histamine, 5-HT, prostaglandins, bradykinin, opioids). These neurochemicals have been implicated in the responses of the pulp afferent fibres to noxious stimulation, injury and inflammation, as well as being involved in processes related to regeneration and repair. It is therefore important to realize that the pulp innervation is in a dynamic state in which many factors (e.g. injury, the ageing process, and the drilling of dentine during dental restorative procedures) can affect the release of neurochemicals and thereby alter the blood flow in the tooth pulp.

◼ Peripheral receptor mechanisms

Most of our present understanding of sensory receptors in tooth pulp afferents is based on *in vitro* and anatomical studies.

Some aspects of receptor physiology have not yet been linked to the nerve terminals within the intradental tissues *in vivo*.

Sensory receptors are located in the peripheral terminals of afferent nerve fibres and are able to detect environmental change (stimulus). Like synaptic receptors in the central nervous system, sensory receptors are divided into two major classes: ionotropic and metabotropic receptors (Table 1). Ionotropic receptors gate ion channels directly, i.e. activation by ligands leads to ion exchanges *via* the receptor pore subunits. This results in membrane potential changes in excitatory cells such as neurons. Metabotropic receptors gate ion channels indirectly; i.e., they are activated by ligands to turn on the intracellular G-protein coupled signal pathway, in order to produce their physiological effects. The ligands can be endogenous chemicals similar to neurotransmitters; however, a physical stimulus, such as heat, cold or mechanical distortion may activate directly some receptors without any ligand involvement.

Each nerve fibre as well as its terminals where the transduction occurs may contain multiple receptor types. The existence of one or more particular receptor type on a nerve fibre will usually determine its response properties, e.g. the appropriate receptors will cause one sensory nerve to be a mechano-nociceptor and another to be a polymodal nociceptor (Chapter 4).

We will discuss three ionotropic receptors that are associated with the dentine-pulp complex and may be involved with the sensory transduction process. This involves membrane potential changes due to ion exchanges within a receptor pore composed of different subunit proteins.

Purinergic ATP-sensitive P2X$_3$ receptors
In vitro studies have shown that both ATP and mechanical force can excite single rat

Table 1. Representative receptor types occurring in the tooth pulp and dentine and their functional significance.

	Receptor Type	Ligand or Activator	Anatomical Evidence	Physiological Evidence	Sensation in Human
Ionotropic	P2X$_3$	Mechanical ATP	Co-expressed with CGRP		Pain
	TRPV1	Capsaicin, H$^+$ (low pH) Heat (threshold =45°)	8% for pulp but 20% for small diameter skin afferent fibres	Activated by capsaicin applied to pulp, and heat	(Dull) pain
	TRPV2	Mechanical Heat (threshold >50°)	20% pulp and co-expressed with CGRP		
	ASIC	H$^+$	33% and co-expressed with CGRP		Pain
	"Sodium"	Na$^+$	Wide-range sensations		
Metabotropic	BK1, BK2	Bradykinin	Exist	Inflammatory mediator and sensitisation of afferent	Pain
	NK1	Substance-P	Exist		
	NK-2	Neurokinin A			
	NK-3	NKB			
	TrkA	Nerve Growth Factor	Exist		
Opioid – μ	Endorphin, Enkephalin		Exist		Attenuating pain
	CGRP	CGRP	Exist	Vasodilator	
	PGE2	PGE2	Exist	Inflammatory mediator and sensitisation of afferent	

molar tooth pulp cells. In human teeth, purinergic ATP-sensitive P2X$_3$ receptors have been found in nerve terminals closely associated with the odontoblast processes. Both myelinated and unmyelinated P2X$_3$ receptor-positive afferent fibres have been identified near the subodontoblastic plexus. This location makes these ATP-sensitive receptors prime candidates for mediating sharp pain from the dentine, although their possible involvement in also mediating dull pain from the tooth pulp cannot be ruled out.

It has been suggested that these receptors could contribute to the sensation of pulpal pain if drilling, mechanical stimulation or air-blasting of the exposed dentine or tooth pulp could induce the release of ATP either by cell lysis or through direct mechanical distortion arising from intradental fluid movements. The ATP could then excite the nerve fibres in the dentinal tubules by binding to $P2X_3$ receptors. However, there is at present no experimental evidence that mechanical distortion induces ATP release from odontoblasts.

TRPV1 receptors

In vitro studies have provided evidence that transient receptor potential vanilloid 1 receptors (TRPV1, also named as vanilloid receptor 1, VR1) are polymodal and can be activated by capsaicin (a pungent extract from hot chilli peppers which is used experimentally to activate nociceptors), low pH (protons) and noxious heat ($>45\,°C$). Capsaicin can activate C-fibres, but not A-delta fibres in the tooth pulp. Immunochemical studies suggest that only about 8% of sensory afferent fibres in the tooth pulp have TRPV1 receptors, and these are probably small to medium size A-delta and C fibres. Only 20% of TRPV1 neurones in the tooth pulp co-express CGRP, an important marker for nociceptors in the tooth pulp, whereas other TRPV1-expressed neurones from the V nerve (e.g. skin and deep tissues) show much higher proportions of CGRP co-expression. These TRPV1-linked receptors are thought to be responsible for mediating dull pain from the tooth pulp, e.g. due to electrical stimulation with a pulp tester, intense noxious heat, or inflammation.

TRPV2 receptors

Histological studies show that TRPV2 (or VR1-L) receptor-positive afferents from the tooth pulp have much larger cell bodies on average than the corresponding TRPV2 receptor-positive afferents from the skin, which suggests that these afferent fibres from the tooth pulp resemble mechanically sensitive A-beta and A-delta fibres. Twenty-six percent of V skin afferent fibres show posi-

tive TRPV2 immunoreactivity compared with 37% of afferent fibres from the tooth. These TRPV2 positive afferents from the tooth pulp also co-express CGRP immunoreactivity. In cutaneous nociceptors, TRPV2 receptors are associated with type I A-delta mechano-nociceptors that have a high thermal threshold ($>50\,°C$) and are mostly sensitive to noxious mechanical stimulation.

Other receptors

One-third of sensory afferent neurones in the tooth pulp express the acid-sensing ion channel (ASIC) receptor protein immunoreactivity, and 36% of them also co-express CGRP. During inflammation in the tooth pulp, the tissues become acidic, and the ASIC receptor may contribute to the detection of protons, e.g., in inflammation. Sodium channel receptors are of course also present in all afferent fibres including those from tooth pulps and contribute to nerve conduction and possible sensory transduction: local anaesthetic drugs blocks sodium channel receptors to stop nerve conduction. Opioid receptors (mu (µ) receptor subtype) have also been demonstrated in human pulp tissues. Animal experiments have shown that morphine blocks the activation of A-delta intradental afferent fibres by mustard oil, which raises the possibility that at least part of the opioid analgesic effect may occur peripherally, i.e., in the tooth pulp, in addition to the well-known analgesic effects which occur centrally (Chapter 4).

Other intradental cells also have metabotropic receptors whose action may modulate the excitability of other ionotropic receptors (such as sodium channels) during transduction. Indeed, several metabotropic receptor ligands such as bradykinin, histamine, and prostaglandin (E2 subtype) are algogenic and can evoke action potentials in animal single-fibre recording experiments (Fig. 3C) and pain sensation when applied to exposed human pulp (but not to exposed dentine, see below).

Mechanisms of dental sensation

Our understanding of the peripheral mechanisms of dental sensation is based upon electrophysiological recordings from single nerve fibres from the pulp in a small number of human studies and a large number of animal studies (Figs. 2, 4, 5, Table 2).

Toothaches may arise from the tooth pulp and/or dentine. Because of the unique nature of the sensitivity of dentine, it has been a great challenge to understand how pain is transduced in teeth. Dentine is porous and a

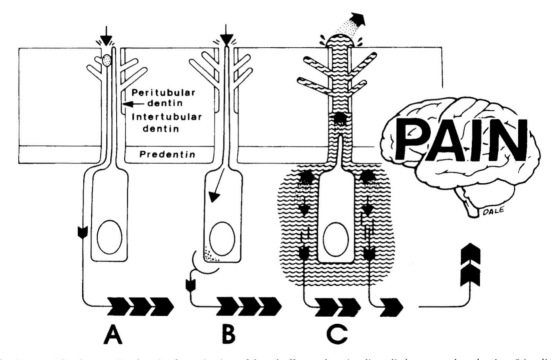

Figure 2. The three major theories for activation of dental afferents by stimuli applied to enamel or dentine. Stimuli are indicated by arrowheads. The so-called *neural theory* (**A**) attributes activation to excitation of the nerve endings within the dentinal tubules, leading to action potentials that are conducted along the parent primary afferent nerve fibres in the pulp into the dental nerve branches and then to the brain. The *odontoblastic transduction theory* (**B**) proposes that the stimuli initially excite the odontoblast process or body, the membrane of which may come into close apposition with that of the nerve endings in the pulp or in the dentinal tubule. The odontoblast then transmits the excitation to the associated nerve endings. However, lack of evidence for either synapses or neurotransmission between odontoblast and dentinal nerve opposes this theory. The *hydrodynamic theory* (**C**) proposes that the stimuli cause displacement of the fluid within the dentinal tubules. Stimuli such as drilling of dentine, probing and air-drying of exposed dentine, mechanical irritation of pulp, and application of hyperosmotic solutions promote liquid displacement within the dentinal tubules. The displacement occurs in either an outward or an inward direction. This mechanical disturbance is thought to activate (*via* fluid movements and/or ion transport) mechanoreceptors in the nerve endings in the dentine (most likely within the dentinal tubules) or pulp (unlikely). This theory has the most experimental support. Modified and reprinted with permission from Ten Cate (1998: Oral Histology: Development, Structure and Function. Ed. 5. St Louis: Mosby).

good thermal and electrical insulator, which gives it unique physical properties and neural responses. For example, a small temperature change at the neck of a tooth causes pain (the enamel is absent at the cemento-enamel junction and dentine is often exposed because of wear from tooth-brushing), whereas a comparable temperature change in the skin will only evoke a minute sensation of warmth or cooling. Algogenic compounds such as KCl, bradykinin or histamine cause pain when applied to abraded skin, but do not elicit toothache when applied to dentine in shallow cavity preparations. However, hyperosmotic solutions of innocuous compounds such as sucrose can evoke pain when applied to exposed dentine.

The unique anatomical structure of the tooth has led to three major theories being proposed to explain how stimulation of dentine by various means leads ultimately to the sensation of pain (Fig. 2).

- The *Neural Theory* proposes that transduction is mediated by free nerve endings within the dentinal tubules, i.e., pain is generated from nerve endings in the same way that it is in other parts of the body. The key problem with this theory is the distance between the site of stimulation and the nerve endings which are activated.

- The *Odontoblast Theory* suggests that the stimulus is transduced by the odontoblastic processes in the dentinal tubules and is then transferred to the nerve endings within the dentine-pulp complex. However, there is no evidence for electrical or chemical synapses between odontoblasts and nerve endings.

- The *Hydrodynamic Theory* proposed by Brännström is based on the idea that stimulation of the dentine causes the fluid in the dentinal tubules to move (i.e., its hydrodynamic action). This fluid movement excites mechanosensitive receptors on the nerve endings in the subodontoblastic plexus. Fig. 4 shows an experimental set-up in which this hydrodynamic phenomenon and its neural correlations was recently tested. This theory accounts for most of the observations related to the transduction of various stimuli into pain in the dentine.

■ A-beta and A-delta nerve fibres in dentine

The conduction velocities of the fastest-conducting intradental nerve fibres are within the A-beta range. These fibres are sensitive to vibration of the tooth and may have purely mechanoreceptive functions. However, the properties of these intradental mechanoreceptors are clearly different from those of periodontal receptors (Chapter 6): their lack of direction sensitivity, their vibration tuning profiles (they follow up to 250 Hz vibration), their responses to increasing force of mechanical stimuli, and their relatively restricted intra-dentinal receptive field. It is clear that they lie within the tooth because intra-pulpal local anaesthesia blocks their activity without blocking periodontal receptor activity.

The conduction velocity of some pulpal afferents may be different along the section of nerve that lies inside the tooth (i.e., in the A-delta range of $2.5–40$ ms^{-1}) compared with the section that is outside it (e.g., A-beta speeds of $40–80$ ms^{-1} when in the trunk of the inferior alveolar nerve). This suggests that the diameter of some pulpal nerve fibres is less within the pulp than in the parent myelinated axons (shown schematically in Fig. 1A and in Fig. 1B). As stated earlier, CGRP is an important marker for

A: SINGLE AFFERENT FIBRE RECORDING SET−UP IN DOG

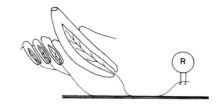

B: AFFERENT FIBRE SIZES

C: RESPONSE PROPERTIES

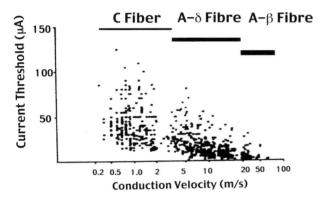

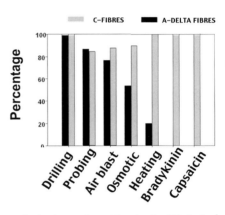

Figure 3. Properties of single dental afferent fibres recorded from anaesthetized experimental animals. (A) A single strand of nerve bundle was dissected from a cut nerve to give a very small number of afferent fibres. The conduction velocity was determined and various stimuli applied in order to show the response properties of the sensory receptor in the pulp (e.g., Fig. 5B). The threshold of electrical stimulation of the pulp was negatively correlated with the conduction velocity of the 3 groups of afferent fibres, i.e., fast-conducting A-beta fibres had the lowest threshold, whereas slowly conducting C fibres had the highest threshold. (B) The distribution of responses found in Aβ, Aδ and C fibres is a good index of the relative proportion of each type of afferent fibre. (C) The proportions of single fibres that responded to various forms of mechanical and chemical stimulation. Data from both dog and cat experiments are combined in this figure. Modified and reprinted from Narhi and Hirvonen, 1987 and Narhi et al, 1992, Byers and Narhi, 1998 with permission.

these intradentinal afferents and usually associated with cutaneous nociceptors (Fig. 1B). This group of fibres might mediate the so-called "pre-pain" sensation that is perceived when a near-threshold electrical stimulus is applied to a human tooth. Studies using single-fibre recording techniques have found that intradental A-delta and A-beta fibres respond to dentinal stimu-

lation in a similar way, indicating that both fibre groups are involved with dentine sensitivity and suggesting that they might belong to the same functional group. A-fibres respond to probing and drilling of dentine, air-drying of exposed dentine, mechanical irritation of pulp, and to application of hyperosmotic solutions of fluids such as sucrose (Figs. 2, 4). These stimuli can cause a

Figure 4. Measurement of hydrodynamic action and its neural response. A shows the *in vitro* experimental set-up devised for this purpose by Andrew and Matthews. The tip of the crown of a dog's canine tooth was been ground down to expose the dentinal tubules and the surface was etched with phosphoric acid. This surface was then sealed with a cap which was connected to a capillary filled with milk in Ringer solution so that minute fluid movements of the fluid column could be observed through a microscope. The nerve connected to the tooth was carefully dissected to preserve its viability and a single nerve strand was isolated for electrophysiological recording. This was stimulated with the electrical stimulator (R/S) to determine its conduction velocity. Heat, pressure or cold stimuli could be applied to the tooth through the cap on its crown. Examples of results obtained with this set-up are shown in B and C. In B, the number of action potentials evoked in a 5-second interval is plotted against the velocity of movement of the fluid in the capillary (indicating the movement of fluid in the dentinal tubules) when either positive or negative pressure was applied to the exposed dentinal surface This shows that the A-delta fibre (conduction velocity is 28.7 $m \cdot s^{-1}$) generated more action potentials when the fluid moved out of the tubules in this instance. The fluid flow velocity, pressure and the action potential response is shown in C. Changing the pressure applied to the cap (lower trace) induced fluid flow in the capillary, indicating outward fluid movement in the dentinal tubules (middle trace). This triggered action potentials (vertical lines in top trace) only when relatively high negative pressure was applied, which would presumably have been felt as pain in an intact animal (or human). However, pressure changes and movement of fluid in the dentinal tubules in the opposite direction did not activate this nerve fibre, and would presumably not have been accompanied by the sensation of pain. Modified and reprinted from Andrew and Matthews, 2000 with permission.

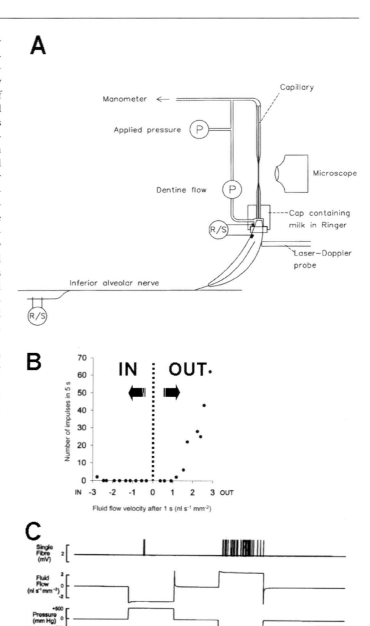

minute amount of fluid to move outward in the dentinal tubules (hydrodynamically), thus causing transduction at the nerve terminal and evoking action potentials (Fig. 4), possibly by structural/membrane distortion of a mechanoreceptor. As noted above, ATP-sensitive $P2X_3$ receptors may be the neural correlates for this hydrodynamic action.

The sensitivity of these myelinated nerve fibres depends on whether the dentinal tubules at the dentine surface are open or blocked. An etched, open dentinal surface greatly enhances their sensitivity, whereas a layer of varnish, potassium oxalate or potassium nitrate crystals or high fluoride concentrations (the active ingredients in some toothpastes) are believed to "plug" the opening of the dentinal tubules and prevents fluid movement, thus rendering these fibres less sensitive. Removal of intra-dental fluid will totally disable the A-fibre sensitivity. These findings are in accordance with the idea that A-fibres are activated by a hydrodynamic mechanism. Some A-delta fibres are insensitive to hydrodynamic stimuli; however, the terminals of these afferent fibres are most likely distributed in the pulp rather than near the odontoblasts.

As noted previously, several chemicals are released from the peripheral tissues or primary afferent nerve endings by tissue injury or inflammation, and these substances can increase the excitability of peripheral nociceptors, resulting in nociceptor or peripheral sensitisation (Fig. 5, see Chapter 4). Peripheral sensitisation may also develop in pulpal afferents following e.g. a crack in the dentine, leakage from a filling, or local pulpal inflammation, resulting in a decrease in the activation threshold and an increase in their excitability and expansion of their receptive fields. More severe intradental inflammation may involve central sensitisation (see later).

C-fibres in the tooth pulp

In a normal healthy tooth, only rather intense stimuli which affect the pulp tissues will activate intradental C-fibres (conduction velocity <2.5 ms^{-1}; summarized in Table 2). These fibres are polymodal, meaning that they can be activated by several different types of stimuli such as algogenic chemicals, intense heating or cooling of the tooth crown and mechanical stimulation, e.g. during drilling in deep cavities. Their activation threshold is usually high which may be explained in part by the insulating properties of enamel and dentine. Nevertheless, the response profiles to heat imply TRPV1 or TRPV2 receptor involvement in the activation of intradental C-fibres. Intense cold stimuli evoke dull pain; however, the receptor type that mediates this is unknown. Mechanical stimulation of pulp tissue or application of bradykinin, histamine, or capsaicin to the exposed pulp are also effective stimuli for activation of pulpal C-fibres; however "hydrodynamic" stimulation of the dentine of a normal tooth is insufficient to activate these C-fibres (Fig. 3C). In C-fibre terminals, neuropeptides, especially the vasodilators substance P and CGRP, are co-released with neurotransmitters such as glutamate or serotonin, and modulate blood flow within the pulp.

Neurogenic inflammation

Chapter 4 describes how activation of nociceptors may lead to the release of the vasodilator CGRP from sensory nerve terminals and cause increases in the local blood flow, resulting in neurogenic inflammation. Inflammation can also be triggered by invasion of microorganisms, for example, through cracks in the enamel and/or exposed den-

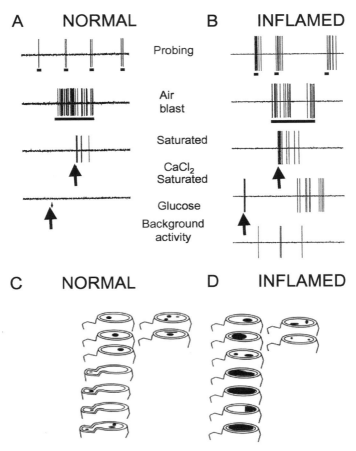

Figure 5. Examples of responses of single intradental A-delta afferent fibres arising in the tooth pulp to probing, air-drying, and hyper-osmotic solutions applied to exposed dentine. These data were obtained in an experimental set-up such as that shown in Fig. 3A. The vertical lines in A, B are action potentials in single afferent nerve fibres. The records shown in A show the response obtained from healthy dog teeth. The records in B were obtained from dog's teeth in which inflammation was induced by drilling a cavity in the cervical dentine one week earlier. In healthy teeth (**A**), the response of a single afferent fibre was always brief and occurred only during the stimulus, whereas the response of the inflamed teeth (**B**) was stronger but and not closely time-locked to the stimulus. There were also additional responses to the hyper-osmotic stimulus and background activity. C and D show the receptive fields (RFs) of single pulp nerve fibres in normal and inflamed dog incisor teeth that were located by probing the dentine. Note that the RFs are much larger in these inflamed teeth (**D**) than in the healthy normal teeth (**C**). A is reprinted from Narhi et al, 1996. B shows data modified from Narhi et al, 1994, C is reprinted with permission from Byers and Narhi (1999) with permission.

tinal tubules. Dental cracks or injury lead to extensive sprouting of intradental nerves into the exposed area as shown by CGRP immunoreactivity studies, which may con-

tribute to hypersensitivity of the tooth pulp. Inflammation also leads to the release of a wide range of endogenous substances from pulpal tissues including the nerve terminals.

Table 2. Sensory Afferent Fibres of Normal Teeth.

	A-β Fibre	A-δ Fibre	A-δ Fibre (Insensitive to hydrodynamic stimulation)	C fibre
Location	Dentine	Dentine	Pulp	Pulp
Function	Tactile sensitivity and pain	Tactile sensitivity and pain	Pain	Pain
Reflex Effect	Vascular effects, Jaw opening in animals.	Vascular effects, Jaw opening in animals.	(Jaw Immobilisation)	(Jaw Immobilisation)
Pain Quality	Sharp, well-localized dentinal pain	Sharp, well-localized dentinal pain	Unclear	Poorly-localized, dull pain
Hydrodynamic Reactivity	Yes	Yes	No	No
Response to Noxious Heat	Transient Response	Transient Response	Yes	Yes
Peptide Expression	CGRP	CGRP	CGRP	CGRP Substance-P
Receptor Expression	$P2X_3$ TRPV2	$P2X_3$ TRPV2	TRPV1 TRPV2	TRPV1 TRPV2

Note: The information contained in this table only applies to dentine-pulp complex.

Immunocompetent cells such as macrophages and mast cells release cytokines and histamine. Pulpal tissues also promote the synthesis of prostaglandins and bradykinin. Nerve terminals release neuropeptides such as pro-inflammatory NGF, vasodilator CGRP or substance P; hence, this form of inflammation is termed "neurogenic". These inflammatory mediators activate nerve terminals (*via* metabotropic receptors). Many mediators or neurotransmitters are algogenic, pain-producing substances, e.g. bradykinin and prostaglandins. Some, such as NGF which not is directly associated with a painful sensation, are pro-inflammatory substances. Vasodilators promote extravasation and cause oedema that raises intradental pressure in the non-compliant pulp chamber and may eventually result in pulpal necrosis. Both CGRP and substance P contribute to the vasodilation, but this extravasation of interstial fluid is mediated mainly by substance P. Another important marker of inflammation is the low (acidic) pH resulting from cell breakdown, which can activate ASIC and TRPV1 receptors.

Like other cutaneous and deep afferent nerves, pulpal afferents usually branch many times before and after entering the apices of several teeth. This contributes in several ways to the well-known difficulty in locating a painful tooth. It obviously provides an anatomical explanation for the sensation, but also may be the substrate for the induction of neurogenic inflammation in adjacent, possibly healthy teeth. The activation of nociceptors in an inflamed pulp can cause neuroactive substances such as CGRP or substance P to be released from the terminals of the branches that innervate the pulps of nearby healthy teeth, thereby increasing their sensitivity.

Increased intradental temperatures (>42 °C) may lead to increased blood flow. This increase is neurogenic because it can be blocked by the application of local anaesthetics or by denervating these teeth. At even higher intradental temperatures (>48 °C), plasma protein extravasation occurs. This can be blocked by pre-treating the animal with repeated systemic doses of capsaicin, which reduces C-fibre function, but not by blocking sympathetic activity. These changes can also be explained by the mechanisms of neurogenic inflammation. The severe consequences of increased temperatures in the tooth pulp must be kept in mind when operative procedures are performed on a tooth. Thus, water-cooling of rotating instruments is absolutely essential.

■ Central neural mechanisms

Brainstem organisation

The neurones in the V brainstem complex are somatotopically arranged with the oral and perioral structures represented in the dorsomedial aspect in each component of the V brainstem complex. In the subnucleus caudalis, this inverted, medially-facing pattern of representation of the face and mouth also has a second superimposed ring-like representation pattern in its antereocaudal aspect, i.e., the receptive fields of the perioral region are found in the rostral part of the subnucleus, and receptive fields of the more lateral regions of the face are more caudal. This second somatotopic pattern in the subnucleus caudalis has been referred to as an "onion-skin" pattern of organisation. The clinical significance of this onion-skin or-

ganisation is that pain may be referred from one tooth to another area not necessarily limited to its own quadrant, i.e., pain can spread vertically to teeth of the neighbouring ipsilateral division of V (e.g. Fig. 7).

Most evidence indicates that the subnucleus caudalis is the principal, but not the exclusive brainstem relay site for V nociceptive information. Intradental afferent axons branch within the descending V spinal tract and make synaptic contacts in the V brainstem complex (Chapter 4). While the central terminals of the nociceptive afferents from the skin of the face are distributed mainly in the most caudal subnucleus caudalis, the intradental afferents (at least the A-delta fibres which contain CGRP) are found in the rostral as well as the caudal subnuclei (oralis, interpolaris, and caudalis). Lesions of the subnucleus caudalis in experimental animals and surgical transection of the V spinal tract at the rostral pole of subnucleus caudalis in humans in patients with trigeminal neuralgia (see Chapter 4) reduce the behavioural, muscle reflex and autonomic responses to orofacial noxious stimuli. These lesions have some effect on thermal perception, but have little or no effect on tactile sensibility or intra-oral pain conditions such as toothache: this, indicates the involvement of more rostral nuclei such as the subnucleus oralis in these conditions.

Electrical stimulation of the tooth pulp activates both nociceptive and non-nociceptive neurones in both subnucleus caudalis and oralis. Many of these pulp-sensitive neurones can be activated by many inputs from other tissues. The majority of these nociceptive neurones (wide dynamic range and nociceptive-specific neurones) can be activated by more than one tooth and many other noxious inputs. This phenomenon is termed convergence, i.e. of multiple inputs onto the same neurone. The poor localisation of toothache and the frequent occurrence of pain referral in the orofacial area are likely to be related to these convergence patterns from tooth pulp afferents onto the central nociceptive neurones.

In subnucleus oralis, the dental A-delta afferents make strong synaptic contacts with low-threshold mechanoreceptive (LTM) neurones (i.e., they are activated at stable latency by low-threshold electrical pulpal stimulation). Another important feature of these oralis LTM neurones is the high occurrence of convergence from both pulpal and periodontal inputs. This convergence also qualifies these neurones as pre-motor interneurones in orofacial reflex pathways that may involve jaw-opening reflexes (in animals) and mastication. Furthermore, the extensive convergence of afferent inputs also implies the integration of the sensory and motor interaction between teeth, periodontium and jaw muscles (see Chapter 6, 7).

The jaw-opening reflex in animals (but not humans) can be evoked both by low-threshold mechanical stimuli such as tapping the tooth (innocuous), and by noxious stimuli such as air-blast onto the exposed pulpal tissues. Although noxious stimulation can evoke a jaw-opening reflex in experimental animals, the electrical pulp-induced jaw-opening reflex is not a reliable measure of orofacial nociception due to the potential activation of other low-threshold afferents from the skin, gingival or mucosal tissues (Chapters 4 and 6).

Electrical stimulation of the tooth pulp evokes responses in the subnucleus caudalis nociceptive neurones that are more variable in latency and response than those in subnucleus oralis neurones, suggesting the involvement of multiple synapses or slowly-conducting afferent fibres (A-delta or C-fibres). These differences are further shown in the response patterns evoked by noxious heat ($>50\,°C$) stimulation of cat canine teeth for the pulpal-activated subnucleus oralis and subnucleus caudalis neurones. Only subnucleus caudalis nociceptive neurones show a consistent response to repeated noxious heat (Fig. 6), whereas the pulp-driven oralis LTM neurones fail to respond consistently. Different receptor types of the A and C fibres (possibly of the heat-sensitive TRPV1 receptor type) terminate in the subnucleus caudalis neurones that mediate both hydrodynamically-induced dentinal pain and the inflammation-induced widespread pain of pulpitis (see below), whereas only hydrodynamically-induced dentinal pain of the ATP-sensitive/mechanosensitive type (of A-delta fibres) activates the subnucleus oralis neurones that mediate dentinal pain.

Central neuronal reaction to injury and inflammation

Central sensitisation-induced neuroplastic changes can be observed in the nociceptive neurones receiving dental convergent afferent inputs (Chapter 4). For example, Fig. 11 of the Chapter 4 shows that the properties of a subnucleus caudalis nociceptive-specific neurone change after damage or inflammation of a tooth pulp. Following the application of mustard oil (which stimulates small fibres and induces inflammation) to the anaesthetized rat maxillary molar pulp, the responses of the central nociceptive neurone to these inputs are greatly enhanced. These neuronal properties are reflected in an increased likelihood of spontaneous activity, expansion of the mechanoreceptive field, lowering of the activation threshold, and increased responses to suprathreshold stimuli.

The enhancement of responses arising from central sensitisation can occur in nociceptive-specific and wide dynamic range neurones in caudalis and can be considered

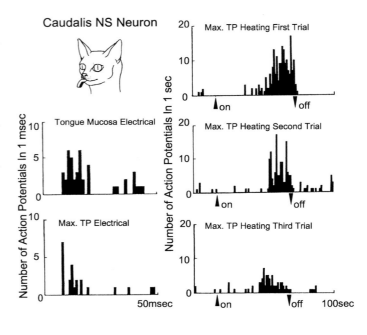

Figure 6. Responses of a nociceptive-specific neurone in the cat trigeminal system. The mechanoreceptive field of this neurone in nucleus caudalis is indicated by the black area on the tongue. This neurone responded to electrical stimulation of the maxillary tooth pulp TP (bottom left panel) and tongue (middle left panel). The frequency of the action potentials that were evoked during a 50 ms period are shown. The right-hand panels show the responses of the same neurone to three consecutive bouts of noxious heat stimulation of the maxillary canine tooth (>55 °C for 60 s). This stimulus evoked a response only when the temperature of the core of the pulp reached a certain range: this explains the long delay between the onset of the stimulus and the onset of the response. Similar stimuli failed to evoke reliable discharges in subnucleus oralis LTM neurones (data not shown). Reprinted from Hu and Sessle, 1984 with permission.

as a model for irreversible pulpitis. The increased spontaneous activity may contribute to spontaneous pain, and the expansion of receptive fields may contribute to the spread and referral of pain. The dramatic reduction in activation threshold may result in allodynia, and the increased response to suprathreshold stimulation may contribute to the hyperalgesia found in irreversible pulpitis. These pulpal inflammatory-related neuroplastic changes are C-fibre and NMDA receptor mechanism-dependent and long lasting (Chapter 4). These alterations have also been observed in nociceptive neurones of the subnucleus oralis as well as in the thalamus, i.e., at higher levels of nociceptive processing. The changes in both oralis and thalamus are, however, critically dependent upon the processing within the subnucleus caudalis. One reason for the dependency of the subnucleus oralis nociceptive neurones

on noxious processing in the subnucleus caudalis is that C-fibre afferents terminate only in the subnucleus caudalis where the central sensitisation process is being initially processed.

Neuroplasticity is believed to be an important process in the transition of acute to chronic pain following other types of nerve injury, such as injury to the inferior alveolar nerve. Irreversible pulpitis is associated with allodynia, hyperalgesia and pain spread or referral (Fig. 7), and is often considered one of the most severe pain conditions a person may experience. Neuropathic pain conditions also result from neuroplastic changes associated with peripheral nerve injury, although such problems rarely occur following injury to the nerves innervating teeth. Indeed, neither endodontic root-canal treatment nor extraction of teeth usually produces severe or longer-lasting adverse effects, despite the fact that both procedures involve peripheral nerve injury (deafferentation). There are relatively few case reports of "phantom" toothache, which is toothache that is perceived to originate in a previously-extracted or endodontically treated tooth. In animal studies, pulpectomy produces sensory disturbance in the mechanosensitivity of low-threshold mechanoreceptive neurones in the subnucleus oralis and main sensory nucleus, but generally fails to produce extensive or persistent neuroplastic changes in the nociceptive neurones in the subnucleus caudalis. Fortunately for the dentist, these results imply that these frequently used dental procedures have only modest consequences for the neural pathways. Nevertheless, the findings of neuroplastic changes open a window for understanding, for example, atypical odontalgia and facial pain when the normal healing and regenerative capacity is compromised in some patients.

During tooth shedding from deciduous to permanent dentition, the remarkable regenerative capacity of the tooth pulp afferents does not lead to sensory disturbances. In contrast, neuropathic pain may develop following mandibular third molar extraction or surgery if there is injury either to the inferior alveolar nerve which is composed of mixed dental and cutaneous sensory afferent fibres, or to the lingual nerve. The incidence of such nerve injuries appear to be in range of $<5\%$ for acute dysaesthesia and $<0.5\%$ for development of chronic neuropathic pain conditions. Neuroplastic changes associated with neuropathic pain conditions such as behavioural expression of allodynia and hyperalgesia and neuronal neuroplastic changes have been observed in a rat model of injury to the inferior alveolar nerve: hence, this model may help to design better treatments in the unfortunate situation of iatrogenic nerve damage in dentistry.

Clinical correlates

Toothache

The most conspicuous clinical manifestation of tooth pulp physiology (or more accurately, pathophysiology) is, of course, toothache. Observation and reports from human subjects during clinical and experimental procedures indicate that toothache is perceived in only a limited number of forms. Electrical pulses generated by a pulp tester at an intensity very close to the threshold of pain can induce a non-painful sensation called "pre-pain". This pre-pain sensation or paraesthesia may be due to the recruitment of a few nociceptive afferent fibres, but not enough to give rise to normal pain sensation. In contrast, drilling, probing and hyperosmotic stimulation of exposed dentine, and thermal stimulation of the tooth all seem to evoke only pain, i.e., without any sensation of touch, heat or cold. It is interesting that high-energy lasers which are used to remove caries and for cavity preparation appear to cause less pain and discomfort than traditional dental drills, which suggest that mechanical stimuli may play a significant role in the discomfort experienced by patients undergoing conventional restorative procedures. Carious lesions in enamel or dentine may lead to pulpitis which may be either reversible or irreversible, and which may progress to necrosis of the pulp.

The rule of thumb is that:

- in conditions with a reversible pulpitis, application of either heat or cold to the tooth produces a short-lasting sharp and intense pain;
- when the pulpitis is irreversible, either heat or cold produces a long-lasting pain; and
- when the pulp is necrotic, no stimuli evoke any sensation from the tooth pulp.

In general, the pain associated with pulpitis is dull and may radiate to wide areas of the face and jaw, indicating central sensitisation. Mechanical stimulation of exposed dentine of an otherwise healthy tooth induces a sharp, piercing and relatively well-localized pain. Intense heating or cooling evokes dull pain. The quality and intensity of different toothache types may reflect functional differences in intradental nerve and central neural pathways.

It must be kept in mind that peripheral sensitisation can also contribute to hyperalgesia and allodynia by increasing the excitability and decreasing the activation threshold of primary afferents. Thus, many pain conditions may involve a mixture of peripheral and central sensitisation. In clinical practice, tapping a tooth can reveal its clinical condition. An inflamed tooth pulp becomes hypersensitive, which is an indication of mechanical allodynia, whereas tapping on a normal tooth (which activates mechanical receptors in the periodontal ligament) will not provoke pain.

Following a careful dental history (caries, trauma, dental treatment), the clinical examination should include a careful examination for dental caries and defective restorations, and include radiography. Sensory testing with electrical and thermal stimuli will aid in diagnosis since application of hot or cold stimuli to a tooth with reversible pulpitis will evoke a sharper and more intense pain than it will from a normal tooth. On the other hand, cold or heat stimuli applied on a tooth with irreversible pulpitis will produce longer-lasting pain, indicating the involvement of central mechanisms.

Modulation of toothache

Modulation of toothache can take place at three levels, namely, at the peripheral, brainstem and supra-trigeminal levels. Exogenously-administered drugs can also act at these three levels. At the peripheral level, the tooth pulp is a confined structure and pulpitis can limit drug delivery due to a compromised blood supply. Provided that they can reach the pulp, opioid analgesics that modulate central pathways can also act through the opioid receptors on tooth pulp afferents. If the toothache is associated with only minor and focal inflammatory changes, i.e., no widespread inflammation corresponding to an overt pulpitis, NSAIDs can suppress local inflammation, thus reducing the pain sensation. In addition, NSAIDs may also have central suppressive effects on brainstem nociceptive neuronal activity to produce analgesia through their action in reducing the activity of the elevated levels of COX-2 enzyme activities that occur in second-order neurones as the result of inflammatory pain. Chapter 4 points out that a number of mechanisms act at the brainstem level to modulate incoming nociceptor signals: these include segmental inhibition, descending modulation from the raphe system (e.g. the periaqueductal gray and nucleus raphe magnus) and diffuse noxious inhibitory control (DNIC). Fig. 7 illustrates an experiment that demonstrates this DNIC process. A tourniquet was applied to the arm of two patients who had widespread pain in the oro-facial area (shown by the shading) which was the result of irreversible pulpitis. The occlusion of the circulation of the arm for several minutes induced moderate levels of pain in the arm, which then led to a shrinking of the area from which the pain was perceived to the single inflamed tooth. Acupuncture to control dental pain may act in a similar way.

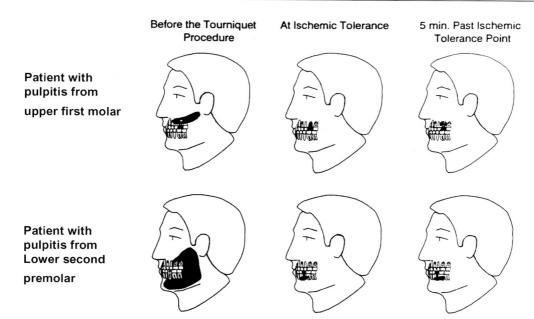

Figure 7. The effect of remote pain on the distribution of pain arising from a single inflamed tooth in two patients. The figurines on the left show patterns of spread of pain that are commonly encountered. However, this distribution changed when a tourniquet was inflated on the left forearm to restrict blood flow and induce ischaemic arm pain lasting for two to three hours. The painful area then shrunk to the single responsible tooth. This is an example of DNIC (described in more detail in Chapter 4). The distribution of pain in the face of the patient shown in the lower row of figurines fits the so-called "onion-ring" distribution of orofacial pain. Reprinted from Sigurdsson and Maixner, Pain 1994;57:265–275 with permission.

Degeneration, regeneration and age-related changes

Humans are "diphyodonts," that is, they have only two sets of teeth throughout their lives: i.e., the deciduous and the permanent teeth. The process of replacement of the deciduous teeth with permanent teeth involves resorption and shedding of deciduous teeth: this inevitably results in injury of their nerves and inflammation. When the permanent teeth erupt, they are re-innervated from the alveolar nerves. However, children rarely suffer any longer-lasting pain or sensory disturbances from this naturally-occurring nerve injury process, which is another indication that not all nerve injuries result in pain. Permanent teeth are significantly more densely innervated than primary teeth. When a deciduous tooth is replaced by a permanent tooth, the latter becomes innervated by the same nerves that formerly supplied the deciduous tooth. How the additional permanent (molar) teeth are then innervated when they erupt is an interesting puzzle.

The deciduous to permanent tooth succession triggers neuroplastic changes in subnucleus oralis LTM neurones: the proportion of neurones with convergence of both pulpal and periodontal inputs is lower in kittens with deciduous teeth than it is in the adult cat. Peripheral injury/inflammation may lead to extensive changes both at the periphery (such as sprouting of C-fibres that express CGRP) as well as in the brainstem (reorganisation in subnucleus oralis).

Dental nerves apparently possess the ability to regenerate and to re-innervate tooth pulps. This is intriguing because the tooth is the only tissue other than skin and bone which is regularly auto-transplanted (e.g. after avulsion). These reimplanted teeth may be re-innervated and became vital again, which does not occur spontaneously in severed digits or limbs that are surgically reattached: instead, meticulous reconnection of nerves is required to restore sensory (and motor) function. There are two possible explanations for this phenomenon. Either the tooth contains a high concentration of neurotrophic factors such as nerve growth factors that induce reinnervation of the tooth by the parent dental nerve (i.e., superior or inferior alveolar nerve), or the dental nerve is continuously producing branches of growing axons to innervate the tooth pulp. (Note that successful tooth reimplantation is also critically dependent upon the preservation of cementum and periodontal ligament cells.)

Teeth also become re-innervated after their nerves are sectioned. When teeth are denervated in experimental animals, the dental nerves always find their way back to the denervated tooth *via* alternative nerves, such as upper cervical nerve roots. However, the reinnervation does produce some abnormalities, such as reduction of nerve density within the dentinal tubules.

In aging, secondary or reparative dentine is formed, which gradually shrinks the volume of the tooth pulp chamber and root canals. It also reduces the neuropeptide concentrations of dental innervation. In general, aging reduces the sensitivity as well as the trophic influence of dental nerves: these physiological changes may lead to cracks and chips, but rarely to the loss of teeth.

■ Summary

This chapter has reviewed the fundamental physiology of the tooth pulp. Since the tooth pulp chamber is a low-compliant environment, microcirculation as well as odontoblasts and other specialized cells play a role to maintain normal function. Toothache is the most critical function of the pulp and serves as an important warning signal for underlying pathology, such as inflammation. There are two types of toothaches: one originates from dentine and the other from pulp. Dentine pain is the result of its unusual structure: heat, cold and hyper-osmotic substances can cause dentine pain when the dentinal tubules are exposed because they induce fluid movement within the dentinal tubules which then activates sensory receptors in the subodontoblastic nerve plexus (hydrodynamic action). However, common pain-causing substances such as bradykinin and histamine do not elicit pain when applied to the dentine. Pulpal pain is usually the result of inflammation within the pulp which may lead ultimately to irreversible pulpitis or necrosis.

■ Selected references

Andrew D and Matthews B. Displacement of the contents of dentinal tubules and sensory transduction in intradental nerves of the cat. J Physiol 2000;529:791–802.

Brännström M. The hydrodynamic theory of dentinal pain: sensation in preparations, caries, and the dentinal crack syndrome. J Endod 1986;12:453–457.

Byers MR and Narhi MV. Dental injury models: experimental tools for understanding neuroinflammatory interactions and polymodal nociceptor functions. Crit Rev Oral Biol Med 1999;10:4–39.

Chiang CY, Park SJ, Kwan CL, Hu JW and Sessle BJ. NMDA receptor mechanisms contribute to the trigeminal nociceptive neuronal plasticity induced by mustard oil application to the rat molar tooth pulp. J Neurophysiol 1998;80:2621–2631.

Hilbrand C, Fried K, Tuisku F and Johansson CS. Teeth and tooth nerves. Prog in Neurobiol 1995;45:165–222.

Hu JW and Sessle BJ. Comparison of response of cutaneous nociceptive and non-nociceptive brainstem neurones in trigeminal subnucleus caudalis (medullary dorsal horn) and subnucleus oralis to natural and electrical stimulation of the tooth pulp. J Neurophysiol 1984;52:39–53.

Sessle BJ. Acute and chronic craniofacial pain: brainstem mechanisms of nociceptive transmission and Neuroplasticity, and their clinical correlates. Crit Rev Oral Biol Med 2000;11:57–91.

Narhi M, Yamamoto H, Ngassapa D and Hirvonen T. The neurophysiological basis and the role of inflammatory reactions in dentine hypersensitivity. Arch Oral Biol 1994;39Suppl:23S–30S.

Mechanosensation

Mats Trulsson and Greg K. Essick

Goals:
- To describe the different types and functions of mechanoreceptors in the human orofacial region.
- To understand the role of mechanoreceptors as both exteroceptors and proprioceptors in signalling information from the orofacial region.
- To describe similarities between the human orofacial region and hand in terms of sensory innervation, functional behaviour, and underlying motor control.
- To understand clinical examples of how orofacial mechanoreceptors enable patients to adapt to contemporary dental treatments that replace lost natural teeth.

Key words:
Mechanoreceptors; face; mouth; teeth; trigeminal; tactile sensibility; cutaneous sensibility; oral mucosa; sensory-motor control; mastication.

Introduction

Mastication, speech and facial expression are among the most complex motor behaviours that humans perform. To enable fluent speech, the precise manipulation of food particles between the teeth, and the delivery of an expressively whistled tune requires that the activity of tens to hundreds of muscles is accurately coordinated and sequenced. Forces of hundreds of Newtons in magnitude are generated and exerted by the jaw in directions appropriate for crushing the toughest of foods, yet at the same time the immediately adjacent soft tissues are kept clear of the occlusal surfaces of the teeth. To accomplish these feats, the brain must constantly access, process, and take into account information from the jaw, tongue, lips, and cheeks as well as information about the location and physical properties of food substances in the mouth. Specialized receptors in the orofacial tissues provide this information. They are classified as mechanoreceptors to distinguish them from other types of receptors in the orofacial region that respond best to other modalities of stimulation (e.g., thermoreceptors, chemoreceptors and nociceptors). These receptors are arranged to respond preferentially to the mechanical strains that occur in the tissues during function. It is the mechanoreceptors that provide information about substances in the mouth, necessary for guiding formation, manipulation and cleavage of the food bolus during chewing. Because these receptors are sensitive to deformation of the tissues, they additionally serve a proprioceptive role in the specification of the positions and movements of the masticatory structures during function.

The practice of clinical dentistry provides ample opportunity to witness the importance of orofacial mechanoreceptors to the motor control of the face and mouth. Local (dental) anaesthesia of sensory nerves to the jaw, lips and tongue results not only in impairment of sensation, including the elimination of painful sensations from nociceptors in the tooth pulp, but also in impairment of motor activities, particularly those requiring precise control of the orofacial musculature. Speech is difficult to articulate without error, and facial expression becomes awkward in the absence of sensory feedback of the consequences of subtle degrees of facial muscle activation. Saliva escapes the mouth (drooling) as lip continence fails from the lack of sensory monitoring. Upon attempts to chew, the lips, tongue and cheeks are poorly discriminated from food substances: as a result, errors in motor control occur and these soft tissues are damaged, particularly in children. Although the motor impairments resolve with the return of sensory function, they can persist for long periods of time in patients who experience trigeminal nerve injuries and permanent sensory impairment from, e.g., orthognathic surgery and accidental fracture of the mandible.

As a consequence of the dense and diverse supply of mechanoreceptors for motor control and of the development of the forebrain in man, orofacial receptors also serve a vital role in perception. No other area of the body is served by a more extensively developed somatosensory system, resulting in perceptions of tactile events that are unsurpassed in detail. Foods differing slightly in texture and physical properties are more easily discriminated even than by the highly-sensitive fingertips and result in rich tactile experi-ences of crunchiness, crispiness, and fattiness. Fine grit that is readily appreciated upon occlusion of the teeth is not detected by other means of oral or digital examination. The texture and "mouth-feel" of food combine with its flavour (taste and smell) to determine our culinary enjoyment. Remarkably, information from mechanoreceptors alone has been shown to result in taste perception. Providing that the mechanoreceptive innervation remains functionally intact, taste experiences can occur on tongue areas that have lost the ability to transmit gustatory information. For example, patients with injuries of the lingual nerve often report an improvement in the taste of foods after surgical repair of the nerve. Careful laboratory testing, however, reveals that only the tactile (mechanoreceptive) afferents in the lingual nerve usually regenerate.

■ Cutaneous and mucosal mechanoreceptors

It may not immediately occur to you, but the functions of the trigeminal sensory and motor systems are very analogous to those of the hand, particularly in relation to the precise manipulation of objects. This is reflected in the exceptional innervation density of the perioral tissues and the hand, and the large areas of sensory and motor cortex that process the sensory information and control the motor activities of these two vital areas of the body. Hence, while the primary focus of this chapter is on mechanoreception in and around the mouth, the properties of mechanoreceptors in the hand will also be summarised as there is a larger body of experimental data from the hand mainly because it is technically easier to gather such data from the upper limb.

Cutaneous mechanoreceptors in the human hand

Historical perspective and methods to study mechanosensation

The functional properties of cutaneous mechanoreceptors in man were first characterized 35 years ago in the glabrous (non-hairy) skin of the hand. Subsequent studies of other areas of the human body, including the orofacial region, employed similar recording techniques and approaches in classifying mechanoreceptors. In these studies, a thin wire electrode was inserted without anaesthesia through the skin into the median nerve at the upper arm or wrist. This technique, known as microneurography, enables the action potentials of individual sensory axons to be observed and recorded. After the electrode is placed to record the activity of only one axon, the area of skin on the palm or ventral surface of the digit that it innervates is identified and characterised. This area is known as the receptive field for that sensory axon. The mechanoreceptors in the skin of the hand were found to be innervated by fast-conducting, large-diameter, myelinated Aβ axons, and to respond vigorously to subtle mechanical deformation applied to their receptive fields.

> The amount of force required to evoke an action potential or to change an Aβ-fibre axon's ongoing discharge defines its threshold. This is determined experimentally by prodding the receptive field with fine nylon filaments (so-called von Frey hairs or Semmes-Weinstein aesthesiometers). The filaments differ in diameter and thus the amount of force applied when they buckle. The same instruments are used clinically to measure thresholds for touch perception, which is often impaired in patients after injury to the trigeminal nerve. Based on their sensitivity to very low forces, often less than 0.001 N (i.e., equivalent to a weight of 0.1 gram), the Aβ-fibre axons are classified as low-threshold mechanoreceptors to distinguish them from high-threshold mechanoreceptors and mechanonociceptors that signal information about pressure and impending or actual trauma to the skin, respectively. The term mechanoreceptor is used exclusively in this chapter to refer to those that exhibit low thresholds.

Classification of mechanoreceptors

Four functionally distinct types of mechanoreceptors were described for the glabrous skin of the human hand in the early studies. In concordance with previous experiments conducted on animals, these four types can be distinguished by the following properties: (i) by the rate at which their discharge activity adapts to sustained supra-threshold forces, and (ii) by the size and borders of their receptive fields (Fig. 1). Two types adapt quickly ("Fast-Adapting", or FA I and FA II) to sustained skin deformation, i.e., they respond only to the onset, and sometimes the removal, of a stimulus. The other two types adapt slowly (Slowly-Adapting, or SA I and SA II). In addition to being dynamically sensitive to the application of the stimuli, the SA mechanoreceptors signal the magnitude of sustained skin deformation.

The type I mechanoreceptors have small receptive fields, typically 2–8 mm in diameter on the finger tips, with well-defined borders. These properties and the high densities of these receptors on the finger tips

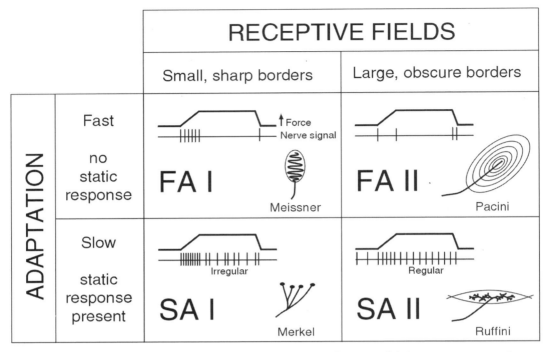

Figure 1. Classification of cutaneous mechanoreceptors based on the adaptation of their responses to a step increase in force and on their receptive field properties. Graphs illustrate a typical train of impulses (lower trace) to indenting forces applied to the receptive field (upper trace) for each receptor type. All receptors respond to the onset of the stimulus, but only the slowly adapting ones continue to respond to its sustained presence (static response). The structure of the nerve terminal ending of each receptor type is also schematically shown. (Modified from Johansson RS, Vallbo ÅB: Trends in Neuroscience 6:27–32, 1983).

(about 200 receptors/cm^2) make type I mechanoreceptors particularly well-suited for encoding highly detailed spatial information, e.g., for extracting information about the fine form and texture of objects that are touched and manipulated with the finger tips. In contrast, the type II mechanoreceptors are fewer in number and have receptive fields that are larger with less well-defined borders. Typically, their receptive fields cover a whole finger or much of the palm when defined by taps with a pencil. The very sensitive FA type II mechanoreceptors are easily excited by high-frequency mechanical oscillations produced by a tuning fork held on the skin. The SA type II mechanoreceptors

readily respond to lateral skin stretch produced by stimuli both near and at a distance from the area in the receptive field that is most sensitive to mechanical stimulation. These observations indicate that the different types of mechanoreceptors extract information about different aspects of mechanical deformation of the skin. The information extracted is determined by the manner in which each receptor terminates in the tissues.

Modes of termination in the skin

It is thought that each of the four different types of mechanoreceptors terminate in morphologically-specific nerve endings: FA I are Meissner corpuscles; SA I are Merkel cells; FA II are single Pacinian corpuscles; and SA II are single Ruffini endings. These four types of specialized nerve endings are illustrated schematically in Fig. 1. The Meissner corpuscles (FA I) are located in the papillary ridges of the dermis. Each consists of a series of cross laminations interleaved with nerve endings to form a column. Several FA I nerve fibres may terminate in the column. Collagen fibres between the laminae connect the corpuscle to the basement membrane of the epithelium. The Merkel cell neurite complexes (SA I) are located at the bases of the epidermal ridges and consist of modified epithelial cells associated with disk-like expansions of nerve fibre terminals. The modified epithelial cells are strongly connected to the surrounding epithelium. The Pacinian corpuscles (FA II) are the largest receptor ending, some reaching 1 mm in length, and are found in the deeper layers of the skin as well as in the subcutaneous tissues. Each consists of concentric layers of Schwann's cell lamellae surrounding one single nerve fibre terminal. The Ruffini endings (SA II) are located in the dermis and consist of long spindle-shaped capsules. The nerve terminals are intermingled with collagen fibrils that pass longitudinally through the corpuscle and anchor the receptor in surrounding collagen at its poles. These specialized nerve endings determine the manner in which mechanical energy from tissue deformation is transformed to graded receptor potentials (electrical energy), which in turn determine the discharge of the axons. In contrast to the different specialized nerve endings, the myelinated sensory axons carrying the signals from the endings into the central nervous system are thought to be identical.

In addition to mechanoreceptors supplying the glabrous skin of the human hand, mechanoreceptors in the hairy skin of the hand and arm have been studied, initially in the radial nerve and more recently in the lateral antebrachial cutaneous nerve. Studies of the hairy skin of the hand and forearm, as well as studies of the hairy skin of the leg, have found a fifth type of mechanoreceptor that responds to movement of individual hairs. These hair follicle receptors are typically rapidly adapting and sensitive to different directions of hair movement.

Low-threshold C-fibre mechanoreceptors
Collectively, the different types of low-threshold mechanoreceptors described above for glabrous and hairy skin relay precise information about the timing, location, and magnitude of mechanical events. More recently, yet another class of low-threshold mechanoreceptors has been described in the hairy skin of the arm and leg but is not found in the glabrous skin of the hand. The sensory afferent axons from these receptors are noticeably different from those of the mechanoreceptors discussed above, being small-diameter, slowly-conducting, unmyelinated C-fibres. These do not provide precise information about the timing of mechanical events. In fact, because their action potentials travel so slowly (about $1 \text{ m} \cdot \text{s}^{-1}$), they often reach the brain after the removal of the stimulus to which the receptors are responding. An interesting feature of these tactile C-fibre mechanoreceptors is their high sensitivity to light, low-force, mechanical stimuli that move slowly across the receptive fields – just like when a mother strokes the hand carefully across the cheek of her baby. Although the role of these mechanoreceptors is unclear, there is mounting evidence to suggest that they are associated with the socially-relevant and affective attributes of touch, evoking sensations of pleasantness and comfort. These mechanoreceptors have been identified in the

human face in recordings from the supra-orbital nerve, and appear to be particularly prevalent in the forehead.

Cutaneous and mucosal mechanoreceptors in the human face and mouth

Types of afferents

The facial skin and oral mucosa is innervated by sensory nerve axons in the trigeminal nerve which are grouped together into bundles or fascicles. Morphological studies of the terminals of these axons reveal both free nerve endings and a variety of specialized nerve endings: Meissner corpuscles, Merkel cells, Ruffini endings and hair follicle receptors. The hair follicle receptors in the hairy skin of the face are considered functionally equivalent to the Meissner corpuscles in the vermilion of the lip and the oral mucosa. Pacinian corpuscles are rare or lacking in most areas of the face and mouth, the ventral side of the tongue being a noted exception.

Densities of innervation and perceptual correlates

Recordings have been made both from multi-unit nerve fascicles (which are simultaneous recordings from hundreds of axons or nerve fibres within a nerve bundle) and single axons in different branches of the human trigeminal nerve, including the inferior alveolar (lower teeth) and mental (chin) nerves, the infraorbital (upper lip and mid-face) and supraorbital (forehead) nerves, and the lingual (tongue) nerve. Recordings from whole nerve fascicles indicate that the innervation territories of individual fascicles (known as fascicle fields) vary considerably. However, some regions of the orofacial complex appear to be included in most of the fascicle fields of a nerve. For example, most fascicle fields in the infraorbital nerve encompass a part of the upper lip vermilion and the corner of the mouth (Fig. 2A, top). For the lingual nerve, all fascicle fields include the tip of the tongue (not shown in Fig. 2). Given the concentration of axons from different fascicles, it can be concluded that the vermilion and the tip of the tongue are areas with particularly high densities of mechanoreceptive innervation.

Recordings from single trigeminal axons, like those from the human hand and arm, reveal that the mechanoreceptive innervation of orofacial soft tissues comprises receptors with both rapidly and slowly

The dense tactile innervation of the orofacial region is reflected in the huge size of the trigeminal nerve and its large representation in the primary somatosensory cortex of the brain. Roughly half of the primary somatosensory cortex processes information from the oral, facial and pharyngeal regions. Moreover, the large volume of cortex dedicated to the tongue and lips is rivalled only by that dedicated to the finger tips. The large cortical representation explains our heightened awareness of the face and mouth, and why, amongst other things, patients so readily detect (and complain about) rough areas on the surfaces of their teeth and scratches on prostheses. It has also been shown that human subjects perceive the size of small objects examined with the tongue to be larger than they do when they explore them with their fingers.

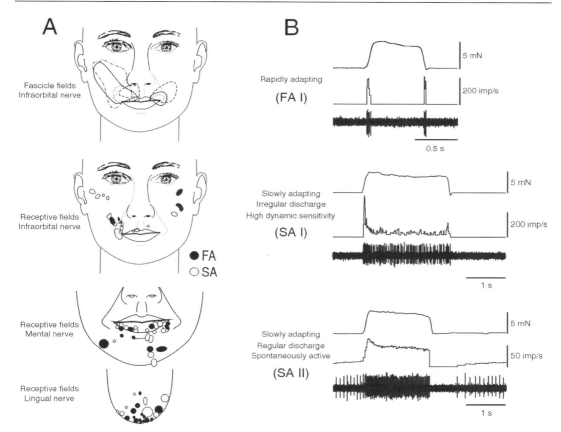

Figure 2. A, Innervation territories of nerve fascicles (top) and receptive fields of single mechanoreceptive afferents (below) identified in records from the infraorbital, mental and lingual nerves. **B,** Example of recordings from the three different types of tactile receptors in the orofacial region. The three types show response properties similar to those of tactile receptors in the human hand, i.e., FA I, SA I and SAII, and differ most notably in the adaptation of their responses to sustained application of force to the receptive field. For each panel the upper trace is the applied force in mN, the middle trace is the instantaneous frequency response in impulses per second and the lower trace is the electrical afferent nerve recording. (Modified from Johansson RS, Trulsson M, Olsson KA, Westberg K-G: Exp Brain Res 72:204–208, 1988 and Trulsson M, Essick GK: J Neurophysiol 77:737–748, 1997).

adapting response properties (Fig. 2B). Like the hairy skin of the hand, most mechanoreceptors in the facial skin and the vermilion are slowly adapting (SA) with small and well-defined receptive fields (Fig. 2A, middle). Slowly-adapting mechanoreceptors also seem to predominate in the buccal mucosa. In contrast, most mechanoreceptors terminating superficially in the tongue have

extremely small and well-defined receptive fields and adapt quickly (FA) to maintained tissue deformation (Fig. 2A, bottom). The sensory innervation of the face and cheeks resembles that of the hairy skin of the hand and arm; whereas the sensory innervation of the tongue tip resembles that of the fingertips. These differences in sensory innervation are well-suited for the functional specialization of the different areas. The tongue-tip and fingertips serve to manipulate and explore objects in the mouth and by the hand, respectively. In contrast, mechanoreceptors supplying the skin of the face and back side of the hand serve to signal facial and finger movements. Functional movements of the face and fingers produce complex time-varying patterns of skin stretch that stimulate these mechanoreceptors.

The high density of mechanoreceptors with small and well-defined receptive fields at the tip of the tongue and the lips is reflected in the high spatial resolution acuity of these areas. Testing of two-point discrimination suggests that the area of highest tactile acuity of the body is the tip of the tongue, followed by the lips and the tip of

Subjects who differ in lingual tactile acuity also differ in taste sensitivity to the bitter substance 6-*n*-propylthiouracil (PROP), a chemical substance routinely used in studies to classify subjects as to taster status (see Chapter 2). Subjects who are supertasters (i.e., who perceive PROP to be very bitter) also tend to be "superfeelers" and exhibit the highest lingual spatial acuity. In contrast, subjects who are non-tasters (perceive PROP to be mildly bitter or tasteless) tend to exhibit the lowest spatial acuity. Mounting evidence suggests that these differences in the sensory innervation of the tongue underlie, in part, differences in food preferences, such as preference for sweet versus non-sweet foods, and in related lifestyle choices and health risks.

the fingers (Fig. 3A). Two points of contact are felt as two points when separated by as little as 1 mm on the tip of the tongue, and 2–3 mm on the lips and finger tips.

Recent studies of lingual tactile acuity have sought to take into account the role of the tongue in manipulative and explorative activities. Subjects were instructed to use the tongue to examine and identify letters of the alphabet that were embossed on Teflon strips. The height of the smallest letter that could be identified was taken as an index of tactile acuity, with recognition of smaller heights indicating greater tactile acuity of the subject's tongue. It was found that normal subjects differ almost three-fold in their lingual spatial acuities (threshold letter heights range from 2.5 mm to 6.8 mm) and that acuity is inversely related to the density of fungiform papillae (the mushroom-shaped papillae) on the anterior tongue.

Functional properties of individual afferents and perceptual correlates

In general, the mechanoreceptors that supply the human facial skin, lips and oral mucosa have properties similar to mechanoreceptors that supply the human hand, i.e., three of the four types of mechanoreceptors described in glabrous skin (FA I, SA I and SA II afferents; Fig. 2B) and hair follicle receptors. Slowly-adapting mechanoreceptors with a high dynamic sensitivity (i.e., they respond vigorously to the onset of the mechanical stimulus) and an irregular discharge during maintained tissue deformation resemble the SA I receptors in the glabrous and hairy skin of the human hand (Fig. 2B, middle). Another group of slowly adapting mechanoreceptors characterized by a regular discharge rate and spontaneous activity is similar to SA II units (Fig. 2B, bottom). An important feature of SA II units is their exquisite sensitivity to lateral skin stretch, even

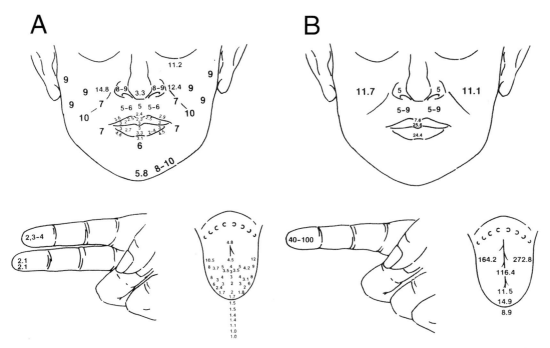

● **Figure 3.** A, Spatial variations in the two-point discrimination threshold obtained from different published studies. Each number represents the mean threshold in millimeters obtained from one study (numbers outside the tongue represent additional studies of the tongue tip). Two distinct points of contact are not felt at separations below the threshold. The tip of the tongue is the most tactually acute area of the body with a threshold of 1 mm. B, Spatial variations in tactile detection thresholds. Each number represents the mean threshold in milligrams weight obtained from one study. The threshold is the minimum force at which contact with a filament stimulus can be felt. The perinasal skin is the most tactually sensitive area of the body with thresholds as low as 5 mg-wgt. (Modified from Rath EM, Essick GK: J Oral Maxillofac Surg 48:1181–1190, 1990. Copyright © 1990. Reprinted with permission of American Association of Oral and Maxillofacial Surgeons.)

when this is applied far from the zone of maximal sensitivity within the receptive fields. Rapidly-adapting mechanoreceptors in the orofacial region resemble those of the FA I units in the glabrous skin of the hand (Fig. 2B, top). Importantly, no mechanoreceptors encountered in human recording experiments have showed response properties similar to those of Pacinian-corpuscle afferents (FA II), which concurs with psychophysical findings from humans and with neurophysiological and morphological findings from other species. That is, the orofacial

region, unlike the hand, is notably insensitive to high frequency vibrations and mechanical transients, the stimuli to which FA II mechanoreceptors are most sensitive.

With the exception of sensitivity to high-frequency mechanical events, the tactile sensitivity of the orofacial tissues is as high, or higher, than other areas of the body. This can be attributed to both high innervation densities of mechanoreceptors and high mechanical compliance (i.e., ability to be deformed) of the tissues. A high innervation density favours the likelihood that an area will be innervated by some of the more sensitive afferents. In this regard, individual mechanoreceptors of each type differ greatly in their sensitivity to mechanical stimuli (thresholds vary 10-fold or more). The high compliance of most orofacial soft tissues assures that even low forces produce deformation and strain of the specialized nerve endings of the mechanoreceptors. The exquisite sensitivity of the orofacial region to touch is exemplified by the delicate perinasal skin. Filament-like stimuli that deliver only 5–9 mg-weight are detected when applied to this area (Fig. 3B). For comparison, the minimal mechanical stimuli that can be detected on the finger tip are 40–100 mg-weight.

Mechanoreceptive signals during orofacial motor activities

Speech gestures
The nerve-recording experiments and findings described above indicate that mechano-

Precise measurement of tactile sensitivity on the facial skin cannot be easily made for some individuals for a rather unusual reason. In the absence of trigeminal nerve injury, the threshold force for perception is actually less than that which can be delivered by the commercially available instruments for clinical neurosensory testing (i.e., graded nylon filaments or Semmes-Weinstein aesthesiometers). This is because these instruments were designed for testing sensitivity on the skin of the hand, arm, and leg, and these areas are notably less sensitive than the perioral tissues.

receptors in the orofacial region serve as *exteroceptors*, signalling information to the brain about environmental stimuli that are brought into contact with the body. Recordings have also been made from the infra-orbital nerve during natural orofacial behaviours such as speech gestures, chewing, licking, and swallowing and from the lingual nerve during simple tongue movements. These showed that mechanoreceptors supplying the face, lips, and buccal mucosa discharge vigorously not only when the tissue is touched, but also in response to deformations of the tissue that occur during voluntary lip and jaw movements (e.g., during contact between the lips or the generation of air pressures for speech sounds). The precise nature of the responses indicates that these mechanoreceptors also serve as proprioceptors, signalling detailed information about the consequences of muscle activation on the soft tissues. This is demonstrated in Figs. 4A and B which show examples of afferent responses recorded from the infraorbital nerve when a subject was asked to enunciate ['a:pA], the Swedish word for monkey. The multi-unit activity from nerve fascicles that innervate the corner of the mouth responded in a tri-phasic manner (see middle trace of Fig. 4A). These three phases correspond to (1) mouth opening, (2) lip closure (arrow) and (3) the build-up of intraoral air pressure and lip-opening movement for the [p]-release sound. For comparison, Figure 4B exemplifies the response of a single mechanoreceptor in the buccal mucosa that responded only to the second phase, i.e., lip closure. These and similar data indicate that the complex multi-unit activity observed from the nerve fascicles during speech originates from signals in individual skin and mucosal afferents that respond preferentially to unique and different phases of multi-phasic speech gestures (see also Chapter 10 on speech).

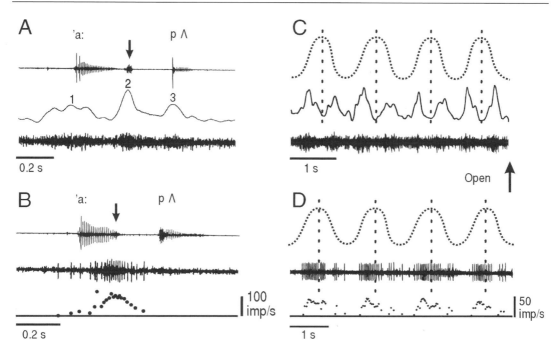

Figure 4. Afferent activity during speech gestures and chewing movements recorded from the infraorbital nerve. A and B illustrate multi-unit and single-unit activity evoked when the subject said ['a:pʌ], respectively. A, Audio signal, rectified and filtered nerve signal and microelectrode record represented in top, middle and bottom traces, respectively. B, Slowly adapting afferent with receptive field located in the buccal mucosa about 1 cm lateral to the corner of the mouth. Audio signal, microelectrode record, and instantaneous discharge frequency represented in top, middle and bottom traces, respectively. Arrowheads in A and B indicate a moment of rapid lip movements resulting in "pop-puff" sounds in the audio record. C and D, Multi-unit and single-unit activity during chewing movements, respectively. C, Top trace is of chewing movement; middle trace and bottom trace as in A. D, Same slowly adapting afferent as in B. Top trace as in C; middle trace and bottom trace as in B. (From Johansson RS, Trulsson M, Olsson KA, Abbs JH: Exp Brain Res 72:209–214, 1988).

The capacity of mechanoreceptors to signal proprioceptive information about movement and deformation of the facial tissue during function is particularly important for the control of the facial muscles (i.e., those muscles innervated by the facial nerve). In contrast to most skeletal muscles including the jaw-closing muscles and the tongue, histological and physiological studies have shown that the facial muscles lack receptors that are traditionally considered proprioceptors (see Chapter 8), i.e., they have no muscle spindles, Golgi tendon organs, or joint receptors. However, since the muscles insert directly into the soft tissues of the face, their contractions deform the skin in very specific patterns during function. Fig. 4 shows that the strains induced in the tissues during speech, for example, evoke rich and time-varying patterns of mechanoreceptor activity that can be interpreted in a meaningful way by the central nervous system.

Chewing movements

The facial skin is also deformed by jaw movements that are brought about by the masticatory muscles during chewing. These deformations are equally effective in stimulating the mechanoreceptors as those deformation produced by contraction of the facial muscles. Figs. 4C and D show recordings from the infraorbital nerve in a subject performing chewing movements. The multi-unit signal in Fig. 4C exhibits two peaks of discharge activity during each cycle of vertical jaw movement, one during jaw opening and another during closing. For comparison, Fig. 4D exemplifies the responses of a single slowly-adapting mechanoreceptor in the oral mucosa during chewing. This afferent responded most vigorously during jaw opening. Other afferents (not shown) responded most vigorously during jaw-closing movements. These and similar data indicate that the mechanoreceptive afferents supplying the face and buccal mucosa signal information about jaw movements, and that different mechanoreceptors in different locations respond preferentially to different movements. These signals are likely to be important in the control of mastication (see Chapter 8).

Tongue movements

Many mechanoreceptors in the human lingual nerve differ from those in the infraorbital nerve. In contrast to the mechanoreceptors innervating the facial skin and buccal mucosa, the afferents that terminate superficially in the tongue do not respond to tongue movements unless the receptive field of the afferent is brought into contact with other intra-oral structures or objects in the mouth. As an example, the fast adapting afferent in Fig. 5A responded each time the subject moved the tongue so that the receptive field on its tip contacted the lower incisor. However, afferents situated deeply in the tongue muscles (probably the terminal endings of muscle spindle afferents) encode

information about voluntary tongue movements in the absence of direct contact with the receptive field (Fig. 5B).

Clinical considerations: Facial muscle actions in retaining full dentures

The complexity of the discharge from mechanoreceptors supplying the oral and lingual mucosa and those situated deeply in the tongue suggest that they provide information on the exact position and amount of

In addition to their role in the retention of full removable dentures, mechanoreceptors in the oral mucosa must also provide tactile sensibility for the prosthetic teeth. In the absence of natural teeth, periodontal mechanoreceptors which normally serve this function are not present. Patients who are well-adapted to wearing dentures exhibit better retention and higher dental tactile sensitivity than patients with poor adaptation. For example, these patients can detect the presence of thinner foil interferences between the upper and lower prosthetic teeth than patients with poor adaptation and poor retention. It is unclear whether better tactile sensitivity of some denture-wearers is a cause or an effect of the improved retention. Nevertheless, good adaptation to full dentures requires sensory and motor training with the prostheses. Good retention probably facilitates the learning of tactile cues from the prosthetic teeth to replace those previously provided by periodontal mechanoreceptors.

food in the mouth: this information is important for guiding manipulation and formation of the food bolus during chewing. The afferents in the face, lips and buccal mucosa also discharge vigorously in a highly systematic manner to deformation of the tissues that occur during orofacial movements, thereby providing proprioceptive information to motor control circuitry in the brain.

The observation that similar strains also occur in soft tissues when an object contacts and moves across the skin or mucosa is relevant to clinical dentistry. The signals from the mechanoreceptors activated in this way have an important role in the retention of full removable dentures that are supported only by the oral mucosa. The retention of a newly fabricated removable denture is dependent on physical factors, that is, a close fit between the prosthesis and the underlying mucosa. With time, however, the fit deteriorates as the tissues remodel. This makes the role of the facial muscles progressively more important in the retention of the prostheses during function. Which facial muscles need to be contracted and by how much is determined by the mechanoreceptors whose discharge indicates movements of the denture bases. The importance of this mechanism is

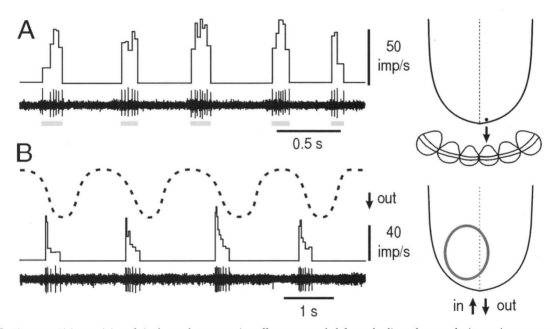

Figure 5. Firing activity of single mechanoreceptive afferents recorded from the lingual nerve during active tongue movements. **A,** Data from a rapidly adapting, superficially located receptor that exhibited a small receptive field (small dot) on the tip of the tongue. A burst of impulses (marked by the gray bars) was elicited each time the subject moved the tongue so that the receptive field was brought into contact with the lower incisor tooth. Top trace, instantaneous discharge frequency; bottom trace, nerve recording. **B,** Data from a slowly adapting, deeply located receptor that responded each time the subject protruded the tongue. Upper tracing indicates the outwards and inwards movements of the tongue. Care was taken to assure that the receptive field (large oval drawn on anterior tongue) did not contact oral structures during the active tongue movements. Middle and lower tracings as in **A.** (From Trulsson M, Essick GK: J Neurophysiol 77:737–748, 1997).

underscored by the effect of topical anaesthesia of the oral mucosa on denture retention: It has been estimated that as much as two-thirds of the retention is lost when the mucosa underlying a full lower denture is anaesthetized. Muscular retention, which depends on the mechanoreceptors in the oral mucosa, is particularly important to patients for whom the stability of the denture base is not optimal, e.g., patients whose lower alveolar ridge is greatly resorbed.

Periodontal mechanoreceptors

The periodontal ligament attaches the roots of the teeth to the alveolar bone. Although viewed most often as a mechanism for supporting the teeth, the periodontal ligament is also an important sensory organ that is richly supplied with low-threshold mechanoreceptors. About 300 mechanoreceptive afferents are thought to supply the ligament of each tooth in humans. These provide information about tooth loads that is essential for the fine motor control of the jaw during function. They also are the receptors for the conscious perception of tactile sensations that one experiences when forces are applied to natural teeth.

Structure and innervation

Sensory nerve fibres invade the apex and lateral foramina of the tooth sockets in the alveolus and terminate in the periodontal ligament. Although free nerve endings and a variety of more complex endings have been described, recent studies demonstrate a consistent occurrence of Ruffini-like endings in close relation to the ligament's collagen fibres in animals (Fig. 6). Similar endings are present in the periodontal ligament of humans. Like the low-threshold mechanoreceptors in the skin and oral mucosa, the Ruffini-like endings in the periodontal ligament send their signals into the central nervous system along fast-conducting, large-diameter, myelinated Aβ axons. Unlike the Ruffini endings in the skin, the Ruffini-like endings in the periodontal ligament are not encapsulated. They also vary in complexity from large-branched endings with finger-line extensions in contact with collagen fibres to small, simpler endings. The variation in the complexity of their morphology suggests a diversity in function. Even though other receptor endings, such as Meissner's corpuscles, are not prevalent in the periodontal ligament, variations in the Ruffini-like ending suggest that the information transmitted by the periodontal mechanoreceptors is more varied and richer in content than would otherwise be the case.

Most of the cell bodies of the nerve fibres that innervate the periodontal mechanoreceptors are located in the trigeminal ganglion, with a lesser number in the trigeminal mesencephalic nucleus. Interestingly, the two groups of periodontal mechanoreceptors supply different, albeit overlapping, areas in the periodontal ligament (Fig. 7). The ganglion afferents are distributed throughout the ligament from the marginal gingiva to the root apex, with the highest concentration around the middle of the root. The mesencephalic nucleus afferents, on the other hand, are concentrated near the apex of the tooth. The two groups of afferents terminate centrally at different sites in the brain stem, suggesting that their inputs serve different, although currently undefined, functional roles. Different jaw actions produce loads on the teeth that differ in magnitude, direction and duration. Thus, it is likely that different jaw functions stimulate the two groups of afferents differently.

Figure 6. Nerve endings in rat periodontal ligament: (1) Complex Ruffini-like endings with ensheathed axons; (2) Simple Ruffini-like endings with ensheathed axons; (3) Simple Ruffini-like endings with free, small, myelinated axons; (4) Free unmyelinated axons. Receptors in loose connective tissue around capillaries (CAP): (5) Simple Ruffini-like endings with free, small, myelinated axons; (6) Free unmyelinated axons (From Byers MR: J comp Neurol 231:500–518, 1985. Copyright © 1985. Reprinted by permission of Wiley-Liss, a division of John Wiley & Sons, Inc.)

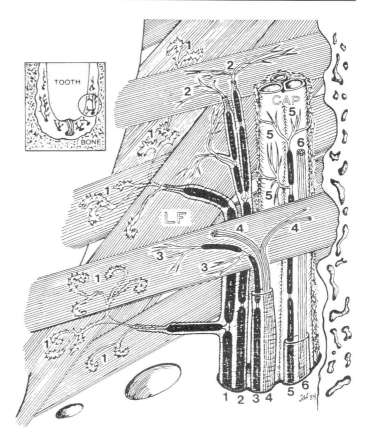

Stimulation of periodontal mechanoreceptors

During biting and chewing on food, the teeth are subjected to complex time-varying patterns of forces. When a force is applied to a tooth, the tooth moves slightly in its socket. Clinically, this is sometimes observed as *fremitus*, the slight movement that can be felt by the finger on a tooth upon its contact with the opposing teeth. This movement induces stresses and strains in the periodontal ligament. Depolarising receptor potentials and action potentials are generated in response to the tension created in the collagen fibres, probably through compression of nerve terminals sandwiched between the collagen fibres. The output from an individual periodontal mechanoreceptor depends on both the sensitivity of the receptor and the effectiveness of the tooth movement in producing strain in its Ruffini-like ending.

A large number of mechanical factors determine the effectiveness of the movement in producing strain, including the size and shape of the tooth, the point of rotation (fulcrum) of the tooth, the point of application of the force, and the presence of adjacent teeth with proximal contacts. The effect of this on the receptors then depends on the precise location of the Ruffini-like ending

179

Figure 7. Site of termination of nerve fibres with cell bodies in the trigeminal ganglion (TG) and trigeminal mesencephalic nucleus (MS) in the periodontal ligament of a cat canine tooth. To the right is shown the relative density of the innervation. The diagram is based on counting clusters of silver grains in four autoradiographic sections at each ligament level for each tooth (From Byers MR, Dong WK: J comp Neurol 279:117–127, 1989. Copyright © 1985. Reprinted by permission of Wiley-Liss, a division of John Wiley & Sons, Inc.)

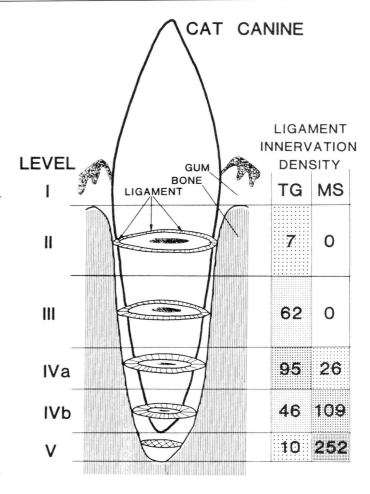

about the root(s), the receptor's orientation with respect to the surrounding collagen fibres and the visco-elastic properties of the periodontal ligament. As a consequence of these mechanical factors, different mechanoreceptors supplying the same tooth are not equally sensitive to force applied in different directions to the crown. Each receptor is optimally stimulated by forces applied in directions that most effectively strain its Ruffinilike ending.

■ Findings from animal studies

Adaptation to tooth loads

Recordings from periodontal mechanoreceptors in animals have revealed both slowly- and rapidly-adapting responses like those from mechanoreceptors in the human skin. The vast majority of the receptors was classified as slowly-adapting whereas a small minority was rapidly-adapting. Both classes were sensitive to the direction, magnitude and rate at which controlled experimental forces were applied to the crowns of the teeth. While some periodontal receptors could be designated as very rapidly adapting and other as very slowly adapting, many appeared to be both rapidly and slowly adapting depending on the conditions under which they were studied. The inability to classify these receptors equivocally implied that distinct subgroups of rapidly and slowly adapting mechanoreceptors might not exist in the periodontal ligament.

Further animal studies of receptors using different magnitudes and directions of force applied to the crowns of the teeth has helped resolve this question. When weaker forces were applied to receptors that appeared to adapt slowly to higher forces, some behaved like rapidly-adapting receptors. That is, they responded only to the onset of application of the stimulus, but did not continue to discharge when the stimulus probe was held against the crown of the tooth. This observation raised the interesting possibility that, unlike cutaneous mechanoreceptors, all periodontal mechanoreceptors are slowly-adapting, and that rapidly-adapting responses result from sub-optimal stimulation of the receptors. Indeed, those receptors initially classified as slowly-adapting were found to have lower response thresholds than those classified as rapidly adapting. Greater forces to the teeth were required to evoke responses in rapidly adapting receptors, indicating that mechanical conditions were not optimal for their stimulation. Similar observations were made in an experiment in which it was shown that periodontal mechanoreceptors terminate primarily between the fulcrum and the apex of the tooth. Those receptors closer to the fulcrum exhibited rapidly-adapting responses, whereas those nearer the apex exhibited slowly-adapting responses. However, in this experiment forces were applied perpendicular to the long axis of the teeth, which produces weaker strain, and thus less stimulation, of receptors near the fulcrum.

It was concluded from these animal studies that all periodontal mechanoreceptors are probably slowly adapting and possess the capacity to discharge continuously during sustained tooth loads, provided that the force is strong enough and applied in an appropriate direction. This finding agrees nicely with the consistent occurrence of Ruffini-like endings in the periodontal ligament and their similarity to the Ruffini endings of slowly adapting type II (SAII) mechanoreceptors in the human skin. Even in the earliest studies, a resemblance in response properties between the periodontal mechanoreceptors and the SA II mechanoreceptors found in the skin was noticed, namely, the presence of spontaneous activity, a steady discharge response to steady loads, relatively weak responses to the onset of stimuli, and directional selectivity in the effectiveness of loads (see Fig. 1 and 2). All of the available evidence suggests that re-

Periodontal mechanoreceptors enable patients to readily detect when new restorations are high in occlusion. However, in most if not all cases, increased fremitus cannot be detected clinically. The dentist must rely on articulating paper (film or tape) and Mylar shim stock, as well as the patient's comments, to adjust the occlusion. In contrast to restorative dentistry, increased fremitus can be detected after orthodontic treatment, but it decreases to normal with time.

sponses recorded from fast-conducting, Aβ-fibre periodontal mechanoreceptors originate in Ruffini-like endings in the periodontal ligament.

Receptor function after nerve injury and orthodontic forces

Injury to the sensory branches of the trigeminal nerve in humans commonly occurs after accidental trauma to the face and after maxillofacial surgical procedures such as orthognathic surgery. Animal experiments have shown that, like other damaged sensory axons, periodontal mechanoreceptive afferents regenerate following damage, with responses returning as early as 6 weeks after injury. However, the response characteristics of the regenerating sensory axons differ from those of undamaged axons. The mechanoreceptors respond to fewer directions of loading and are less sensitive to the magnitude of force and its rate of application to the crowns of the teeth. With time, the response characteristics tend to normalize, but even after long periods of recovery the response properties of the regenerated afferents do not always return to normal.

Interestingly, the same changes in response properties are observed in periodontal receptors after orthodontic treatment. Receptor sensitivity becomes progressively impaired over the period of time during which orthodontic forces are applied to the periodontium. After the tooth is moved into its new desired position and the tissues are allowed to heal, the response properties of the mechanoreceptors approach normal. However, the receptors continue to respond to fewer directions of force than normal and with fewer action potentials upon loading. It has been suggested that the altered receptor characteristics result from disorganization of the ligament's collagen matrix and direct injury to the nerve terminals. Consistent with this view, histological studies of the innervation of the periodontal ligament demonstrate that nerve injury does occur as a result of orthodontic forces and may be permanent.

The clinical significance of the altered response properties of the periodontal mechanoreceptors after nerve injury and orthodontic tooth movement is unknown. Alterations in jaw function and oral motor behaviours often accompany these events. However, they are usually attributed to impairment in sensory function of the cutaneous and mucosal receptors in the case of nerve injury and to the altered mechanics of chewing in the case of orthodontic treatment. It is likely that the brain learns to reinterpret the altered patterns of discharge from the periodontal mechanoreceptors in much the same way it must after dental treatments (including prosthodontics, orthodontics and oral surgery) that alter the occlusion and thus the way forces are distributed to the teeth. The impact of the altered response properties on the tactile sensibility of the teeth has not been determined.

■ Findings from human studies

Temporal aspects of loading teeth

The technique of microneurography has been used to study the functional properties of the periodontal mechanoreceptors in human subjects (Fig. 8A). Controlled forces were applied to small nylon cubes cemented to the incisal edges or occlusal surfaces on individual teeth. The neural discharge was recorded in response to forces applied in four directions in the horizontal plane (lingual, facial, mesial, distal) and in the two axial directions (up and down; Fig. 8B). Recordings from the inferior alveolar nerve revealed that human periodontal mechanoreceptors discharge continuously during sus-

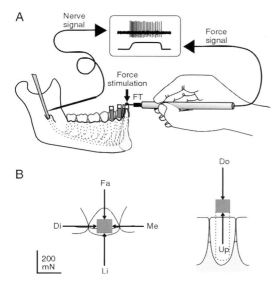

A, Nerve signal, Force signal, Force stimulation, FT

B, Do, Fa, Di, Me, Up, 200 mN, Li

Figure 8. A, Recording from periodontal mechanoreceptors in the inferior alveolar nerve in man. Forces are applied to the central incisor by the use of a hand-held probe equipped with force transducers (FT) for continuous force measurement. Note the small nylon sphere at the end of the probe and the nylon cubes attached to the teeth. B A tooth is shown in the horizontal plane (left) and in a vertical plane (right). Each of the six directions of stimulation are represented by the arrows: Fa, Me, Li, Di, Do and Up refer to facial, mesial, lingual, distal, downward and upward, respectively. The forces were applied to each of the five free faces on the nylon cube cemented to the tooth just above its edge. The probe slipped off the cube if the force was not applied perpendicular to the faces, assuring that data was collected only in the desired direction of force application. The upward force (Up) was applied with a nylon loop (not shown). (From Trulsson M, Johansson RS: Prog Neurobiol 49:267–284, 1996)

mechanoreceptors (about 70%) are active spontaneously and discharge regularly in response to forces applied to the teeth (Fig. 9A). The highly-regular, metronome-like discharge of the periodontal and SAII mechanoreceptors is striking and indicates that each afferent terminates in a single site at which mechanical strain is converted to neural discharge.

Coding of the spatial aspects of loads applied to teeth and functional considerations

Periodontal mechanoreceptors are normally broadly tuned to the direction of tooth loading (Figs. 9A and B): That is, the afferents typically respond to forces applied to the receptor-bearing tooth in two to four of the six test directions. Due to the broad directional tuning, an individual periodontal mechanoreceptor provides ambiguous information about the direction of a force applied to the tooth. However, analyses based on vector calculations show that information about the precise direction of force is represented reliably in the activity from small populations of periodontal mechanoreceptors.

The use of vector calculations to identify differences in the periodontal mechanoreceptors that supply the anterior and posterior teeth is illustrated in Fig. 9B and C. Based on the receptors' response to forces applied in each of six test directions, its single "preferred direction" was calculated by vector summation (thick arrow in Fig. 9B). The vectors in Fig. 9C represent the preferred directions for the population of periodontal mechanoreceptors that have been studied in the human mandible. Each cluster of arrows represents the vectors calculated for all of the mechanoreceptors that were examined in all teeth of that type (anterior teeth, first premolars, the second premolars and the first molars). The number of

tained loading of the teeth. However, consistent with the animal studies described above, it was found that the receptors' slowly adapting nature might not be recognized if the stimuli are limited to directions of application that activate the receptors poorly. Like slowly adapting type II (SA II) mechanoreceptors in the skin, most human periodontal

vectors shows the number of mechanoreceptors that were identified and studied.

Note that the number of vectors decreases
from the anterior teeth to the molar, indicating a decreasing number of receptors in
the periodontal ligaments distally along the
dental arch. Although the size of the teeth
(and their periodontal ligaments) generally
increase distally along the dental arch, the
number of periodontal receptors appears to
decrease. This finding attests to the importance of a well-developed mechanoreceptive
innervation for the anterior segment of the
dentition. The anterior teeth are involved in
the initial stages of taking food into the

mouth, and serve to guide the jaw into the
intercuspal position during the last phase of
the chewing cycle. Use of the anterior teeth assures that only bite-size pieces of food (e.g.,
segments of an apple) are taken into the
mouth and that they are then split, as needed,
into smaller pieces before being transferred to
posterior segments of the dentition. Sometimes the anterior teeth are even used as a
"third hand" in manipulative tasks, or as a
precision cutting tool. Proper execution of
these tasks relies heavily on sensory information as does the execution of comparably
exacting manipulative tasks performed by the
densely innervated finger tips of the hand.

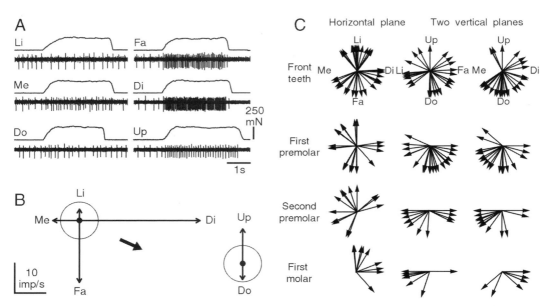

Figure 9. Directional sensitivity of human periodontal mechanoreceptors. A–B, Responses of a single periodontal receptor to forces applied in six directions to the lower central incisor (the receptor-bearing tooth). A, Examples of nerve recordings with the corresponding force records above each. B, Vectoral representation of the responses to sustained force application in the horizontal (left) and axial (right) directions. The length of each vector is pro-portional to the mean discharge rate evoked in each direction. The spontaneous discharge rate is represented by the circle with the radius indicating its intensity. Vectors longer and shorter than this radius illustrate increased and decreased firing, respectively. The thick arrow represents an estimate of the most efficient excitatory stimulus direc-tion in the horizontal plane, i.e., the calculated preferred direction. C, Preferred directions of individual receptors at different teeth projected to the horizontal plane and two vertical planes, respectively. (From Trulsson M, Johansson RS, Olsson KA: J Physiol 447:373–389, 1992 and Johnsen SE, Trulsson M: J Neurophysiol 89:1478–1487, 2002).

In the horizontal plane, the preferred directions of the mechanoreceptors supplying the anterior teeth and the premolars are quite evenly distributed around the circumference of the tooth (Fig. 9C). The receptors supplying the molars, however, have a clear preference for the distal-lingual direction. That is, other directions of the same magnitude of force do not evoke as great of responses as the distal-lingual direction. What anatomical and mechanical factors contribute to this directional preference have not

Although most clinicians today favor a canine-protected occlusion for the dentate patient, there is much controversy about the presence and significance of occlusal contacts on both the working (bolus side) and non-working sides of the dentition during mastication. Early studies suggested that during the final phase of the chewing cycle contact of the molars on the non-working side preceded occlusal contacts on the working side, including those on the canines. While guiding jaw closure, such contacts would result in the application of forces to the lower molar teeth on the non-working side in a mesial-facial direction, the direction opposite to that at which their periodontal mechanoreceptors are most sensitive. In contrast to early studies, more recent studies suggest that non-working side contacts often occur in a physiological occlusion during chewing, but only just prior to intercuspation. Thus, they do not serve a significant role in guiding the jaw into the intercuspal position.

been determined. In the vertical plane, there is a preference for downward-directed forces, but with fewer receptors responding preferentially in this direction with distance along the arch.

The shift from a high sensitivity to most directions at the anterior teeth to the distal-lingual direction at the molars meets the functional demands of the anterior versus posterior teeth. When the anterior teeth are manipulating food morsels and splitting them into pieces in the initial stages of food intake, forces are applied to them in all directions. The molars, on the other hand, grind food substances only during more forceful chewing. During the final phase of the chewing cycle, when the lower molars on the working side approach the intercuspal position from a posterior and lateral position, they are likely to experience distal and lingually directed forces upon contact with the opposing upper molar teeth. Given their directional preference for distal-lingual loading, the mechanoreceptors supplying the lower molar teeth are well suited to encode information about the forces that normally act on the posterior teeth during mastication.

The receptive field of human periodontal mechanoreceptors often extends beyond a single tooth. About half of the periodontal mechanoreceptors respond to loading of groups of adjacent teeth, typically two to four teeth. Each afferent always exhibits the highest response rates to stimulation of one particular tooth, presumably the tooth whose ligament bears the receptor ending (see above), with a gradual and rather sharp decline in responsiveness to loads applied to the adjacent teeth (Fig. 10). Moreover, the preferred directions of the different teeth strongly suggest that the multi-tooth receptive fields result from mechanical coupling between neighbouring teeth by interdental

Figure 10. Receptive field of a single periodontal mechanoreceptor showing steady state responses to maintained mechanical stimulation of five teeth, illustrated from a horizontal view (**A**) and a facial view (**B**). The vectors illustrate the receptor's response to a tooth load of 250 mN (corresponding to about 25 gm-wgt). The tested teeth: c1=contralateral central incisor, 1= central incisor, 2=lateral incisor, 3= canine, 4=first premolar. RBT, receptor-bearing tooth. (From Trulsson M: J Neurophysiol 69:474–481, 1993).

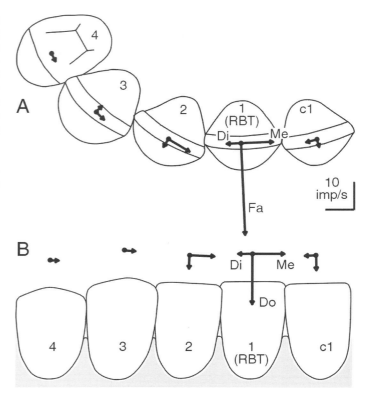

contacts and trans-septal collagen fibres, rather than by branching of axons to more than one tooth. Although one might predict that the multiple-tooth characteristic of the receptive fields makes it more difficult for the central nervous system to localize which tooth is stimulated, this does not seem to be the case. Overlapping peripheral receptive fields are characteristic of all sensory systems and have been shown to improve, rather than degrade, their spatial localization and resolution.

Coding of the intensity of loads applied to teeth

To determine how human periodontal mechanoreceptors encode information about the intensity of loads applied to the teeth,

forces of different magnitudes were applied to the receptor-bearing tooth in the most responsive of the six test directions (Fig. 11A). Each stimulus was applied for about 2 seconds. The relationships between the magnitude of the sustained force and the steady state discharge rate for a group of periodontal receptors supplying the anterior teeth is shown in Fig. 11B. Similar stimulus-response relationships were observed in less-responsive directions of stimulation, but with lower discharge rates. These stimulus-response relationships characterize the *static* sensitivities of the afferents to different forces applied to the teeth. The solid curves in Fig. 11B show that the response to a continuous force is a markedly downward-curved or hyperbolic relationship (see solid curves in Fig. 11B) for most of the human periodontal mechanoreceptors (about 80%). The slopes of the curves are steepest between 0 and 1 N, which indicates that these receptors are most sensitive to changes in sustained force levels below about 1 N in magnitude (1 N corresponds to 98 grams weight, which is about equal to half the weight of a disposable cup full of coffee). The corresponding value for the posterior teeth is slightly higher, about 3–4 N. In contrast to the steeply-inclined nature of the curves below these limits, the curves are almost horizontal for sustained force levels above the limits. This indicates that the individual afferents signal the presence of higher forces but provide the brain with no useful information as to their magnitudes. That is, the discharge of each afferent saturates and attains approximately its highest rate for all force levels above the limit.

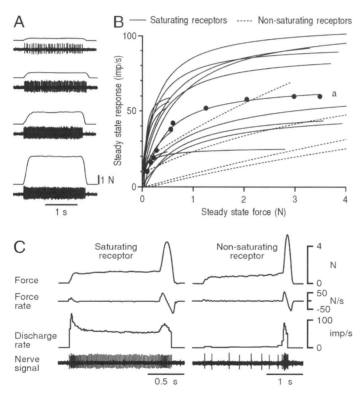

Figure 11. A–B, Responses of human periodontal mechanoreceptors to sustained forces of various amplitudes applied to the receptor-bearing tooth (an incisor or a canine) in the most responsive direction. **A,** Examples of force stimulation and nerve recordings of a single afferent during stimuli of four different amplitudes. **B,** Stimulus-response functions for 19 periodontal receptors. The curves fitted to the data are defined by the function F/(F+c), where F represents the force, and c the force at which half the estimated maximum discharge rate is attained. Solid and dashed curves refer to afferents showing saturating stimulus-response relationships (n=15) and non-saturating relationships (n=4), respectively. The curve labelled **a** refer to the same afferent as illustrated in **A**. **C,** Responses of a saturating and a non-saturating receptor to an abrupt increment in force superimposed on a sustained force (From Trulsson M, Johansson RS: J Neurophysiol 72:1734–1744, 1994).

In addition to their sensitivity to sustained forces, periodontal mechanoreceptors are sensitive to rapidly-changing forces, for example, during biting. Their sensitivity to rapidly-changing forces, or *dynamic* sensitivity, varies in parallel with their sensitivity to slow changes in sustained force. This is illustrated for a saturating receptor on the left of Fig. 11C. After about 1.5 seconds of exposure to a sustained force, the tooth was loaded further with a rapid increment in force. The rapid increase in force evoked an increase in the steady state discharge rate that was less than the addition evoked by the much smaller increment at the onset of the sustained force. That is, despite the fact that this force increment was larger and applied at a greater rate, the receptor discharged more strongly to the smaller increment in force and lower force rate at the initial contact with the tooth. This is because saturating receptors become progressively less sensitive to both the magnitude and rate of rapid changes in force as contact force grows in magnitude.

In contrast to the majority of human periodontal mechanoreceptors whose responses saturate at rather low forces, a minority (about 20%) do not saturate over the same range of forces. These non-saturating receptors exhibit stimulus-response relationships that are nearly linear (see dotted curves in Fig. 11B). The non-saturating receptors efficiently encode changes in sustained force levels at high, as well as low, force levels. As for the saturating afferents, the dynamic sensitivity of the non-saturating afferent parallels its static sensitivity. Thus, sensitivity to rapid changes in force is maintained at high force levels. This is illustrated for a non-saturating afferent to the right in Fig. 11C. The strong discharge evoked by the terminal, rapid increment in force was by far the largest component of the afferent's total response to the stimulation.

A bite block is desired to prop open the mouth of some patients during restorative procedures. However, such stimuli are highly effective in evoking undesirable salivation from the parotid gland. Salivation on the side of a bite block has been shown to increase in proportion to both the magnitude of the force exerted by the jaw and the frequency at which the patient clenches. In contrast, on the contralateral side of the mouth salivation is affected to a much lesser extent. These findings suggest that signals evoked in periodontal mechanoreceptors stimulate salivation in an adaptive manner. That is, the working side of the oral cavity receives a graded amount of saliva commensurate with the forces required to crush and soften hard food substances (see Chapter 1). The reflex is impaired by local anaesthesia of the sensory nerves to the mouth, and in particular, anaesthesia of the inferior alveolar nerve supplying the periodontal mechanoreceptors of the lower teeth on the working (bolus) side.

Loads during precise manipulative behaviours

Two criteria must be met to demonstrate that a population of receptors, such as the periodontal mechanoreceptors, contributes to the control of an oral motor behaviour. First, the receptors must provide reliable information about distinct phases of the behaviour. Second, there must be evidence that the information is actually used for regulation of the behaviour. The periodontal mechanoreceptors meet both criteria for precise manipulative behaviours involving the anterior teeth. Although technical limitations have prevented the recording of receptor activity while a subject bites or chews on food, their responses have been predicted. In short, the experimental data described above were used to develop a quantitative model of the force-encoding properties of the mechanoreceptors. Both the static and dynamic sensitivities of the afferents were incorporated in the model as they collectively determine the pattern of discharge evoked by loading the teeth.

To predict the mechanoreceptor discharge evoked by biting with the anterior teeth, the subject was instructed to manipulate and bite through a morsel of food resting on a bar equipped with force transducers (Fig. 12A). The transducers, like the periodontal mechanoreceptors, signalled time-varying information about the force from the teeth to a computer. The forces that were developed between the incisors when cracking a peanut (during a single phase "split task") and when first holding it briefly between the teeth (during a two phase "hold-and-split task") are shown in the top panels of Fig. 12B and C, respectively. Below each force recording is shown the predicted discharge rates from two periodontal mechanoreceptors – one saturating and one non-saturating in its response to sustained tooth loads.

The model predicts that the saturating receptor will respond distinctly to the small force produced by the initial contact with the peanut (shaded areas) and will provide an on-going response when the subject holds the peanut between the teeth (hold

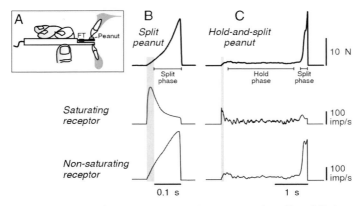

Figure 12. Simulated periodontal mechanoreceptor responses (viz., temporal profiles of discharge rate) to empirically recorded force traces (shown at the top) during a "split" task (**B**) and a "hold-and-split" task (**C**) with a peanut. The apparatus used to record the force profiles exerted on the food is shown in **A**. Subjects were instructed to position the bar so that the food morsel could be held and split by a pair of opposing central incisors. The food morsel rested on a horizontal plate of duraluminum equipped with force transducers (FT) for force measurement. Below the force traces in **B** and **C** are shown simulated receptor responses of a typical saturating and non-saturating receptor. Note that the two types of periodontal mechanoreceptors select out and signal different aspects of the forces generated during the behavioural tasks. (From Trulsson M, Johansson RS: Prog Neurobiol 49:267–284, 1996).

phase), thus signalling information about small changes in force and low levels of sustained force. However, during rapid exertion of the higher forces required to split the peanut (split phase), the receptor exhibits only a moderate and declining discharge rate. It is noteworthy that the highest discharge rates occur in response to the initial low force levels at tooth contact (shaded areas) and not to the higher amplitudes or force rates exerted during the split phase.

In contrast, the non-saturating receptor is predicted by the model to encode information about force throughout the split phase. Because dynamic sensitivity parallels static sensitivity, the small forces at the initial contact with the peanut (shaded areas) and during the hold phase result in much lower discharge rates than for the substantially higher forces generated during the split phase. Because of the receptor's dynamic sensitivity at high force levels, its discharge rates are predicted to provide a distorted reflection of the forces during the split phase. Fig. 12C shows that the rate of force recruitment was momentarily slowed during the split phase. This resulted in a "notch" in the discharge profile rather than two distinct levels of firing.

Together, these observations from the model simulations demonstrate that periodontal mechanoreceptors possess the capacity to signal information about the mechanical events that occur when humans manipulate and bite food with their anterior teeth. Receptors with different force-encoding characteristics capture and emphasize (and distort) different aspects of the mechanical events in their discharge. The simulations suggest that, just as different periodontal mechanoreceptors differ in morphology and in their stimulus-response relationships, they also exhibit diverse sensory functions during chewing.

Role in the control of jaw motor functions

Evidence supporting a role in motor control

It is well established that motor activity for chewing can be generated by neuronal networks in the brain stem in the absence of sensory information from the mouth and face (see Chapter 8). However, signals from mechanoreceptive afferents are required for an efficient and adaptive execution of the masticatory sequence, i.e., from the acceptance of food to the swallowing of it. Since the periodontal mechanoreceptors encode information about the temporal, spatial and intensive aspects of forces acting on the dentition, it is likely that their inputs contribute to the regulation of the muscle activity that generates masticatory forces and jaw movements. Indeed, four lines of investigation provide compelling evidence that periodontal mechanoreceptors are involved in the control of the jaw muscles. First, periodontal mechanoreceptors provide input to well characterized inhibitory and excitatory reflex pathways. These pathways and reflexes participate in the control of the jaw-closing muscles and are described in Chapter 8.

A second line of evidence that periodontal mechanoreceptors are involved in the control of the jaw muscles comes from behavioural experiments in patients with and without periodontal mechanoreceptors. Since most periodontal mechanoreceptors innervating the anterior teeth are highly sensitive to forces and changes in force levels of <1 N, it was hypothesized that their input is used for the regulation of precise manipulative actions involving application of low forces by the jaw. The "hold-and-split" task described above simulates the natural situation of positioning and holding food between the teeth prior to biting and provided a means to evaluate this hypothesis. Three separate observations suggested that subjects do use periodontal mechanoreceptive information to regulate the level of jaw force during the hold phase of the "hold-and-split" task (Fig. 13A). First, the distribution of hold forces coincided with the range over which periodontal afferents are most sensitive to changes in force. That is, subjects chose to exert jaw hold forces great enough to achieve a stable clasp (on average 0.6 N), but automatically avoided higher forces (>1 N) at which the sensitivity of most afferents (the saturating afferents) to force changes was compromised. Second, when the periodontal tissues were anesthetized, the hold forces employed were about four times greater (Fig. 13B and C). Finally, patients lacking periodontal receptors, i.e., who wore dental prostheses supported only by the oral mucosa (full removable dentures) or who had osseointegrated implants (Fig. 13D) used similarly high hold force levels. These higher hold forces provided a greater level of security in maintaining the clasp on the morsel and perhaps stimulated alternative, less sensitive mechanoreceptors in the tissues that were able to signal its engagement by the teeth. These findings demonstrate that periodontal mechanoreceptors are normally the receptors that dictate jaw-closing force levels when substances are manipulated and held lightly between the teeth.

A third line of evidence suggesting that periodontal mechanoreceptors are involved in the control of the jaw muscles comes from studies of jaw clenching forces. It has been demonstrated that both maximum jaw clenching force and the jaw forces employed during mastication depend on the number

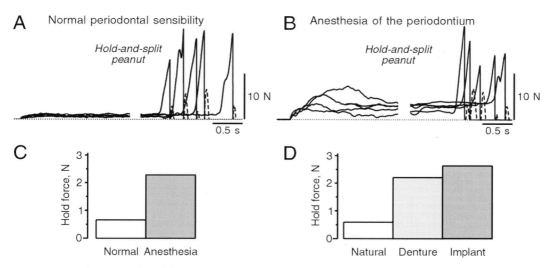

Figure 13. A and **B,** Examples of force profiles (five superimposed trials) obtained during the hold-and-split task with peanuts during normal periodontal sensibility and during anaesthesia of the periodontium, respectively. Note the considerably higher and more variable hold forces produced by the subjects during the periodontal anaesthesia. **C,** Bars show mean hold forces employed by subjects during normal conditions and during periodontal anaesthesia. **D,** Bars represent the mean hold force by subjects in three different groups: (1) Subjects with natural teeth, (2) subjects with full removable dentures supported only by the mucosa and (3) subjects with dental prostheses (in both jaws) supported only by osseointegrated implants. (From Trulsson M, Johansson RS: Exp Brain Res 107:486–496, 1996 and Trulsson M, Gunne HSJ: J Dent Res 77:574–582, 1998)

and stability of tooth contacts in the intercuspal position. This suggests that the central nervous system issues motor commands to the jaw-closing muscles in proportion to the total periodontal afferent discharge evoked by the teeth in occlusion. The aggregate discharge from the total population of periodontal mechanoreceptors presumably reflects the number of teeth in contact, particularly at the higher forces when the responses of most receptors are maximal. This simple regulatory process would protect individual teeth from being overloaded by excessively high occlusal forces.

The fourth line of evidence suggesting that periodontal mechanoreceptors are involved in the control of the jaw muscles comes from studies of the effects of tooth loading on masticatory muscle actions. These studies have shown that tooth contacts and forces exerted on the teeth during the power phase of the chewing cycle modulate the activity of the masticatory muscles. For example, contact of the working side maxillary canine by the opposing lower canine modifies the activity of the contralateral (non-working side) temporalis muscle. Final closure into the intercuspal position is thus under both mechanical, tooth-guided control from the canines and neuromuscular control mediated, in part, by periodontal receptor inputs.

Other studies have shown that pressure exerted on the posterior teeth by a bolus during closure alters masticatory muscle activity. The effect on the muscles varies with the posterior tooth that is loaded and the direction of the load. For example, loads directed buccally, but not palatally, on the maxillary first molar evoke increased activity in the contralateral temporalis muscle. Such loads occur during the wide lateral deviations of the jaw that occur when one is chewing hard food substances. The increased activity in the temporalis muscle probably results in more forceful grinding needed to crush the hard substances.

Predictive control of jaw function

During the course of normal mastication of food, jaw movements adapt to the gradually-changing mechanical properties of a bolus of food. Given their high sensitivity at low forces, most periodontal afferents are particularly well-suited to signal information about food while it is being positioned for biting and during the early contact phase of each chewing cycle. During this period when jaw closing forces are low, information about the spatial distribution of food particles and their intrinsic properties is collected, processed in the central nervous system and used to regulate subsequent jaw muscle activities. This has been shown in laboratory experiments on human subjects which found that anticipatory or predictive motor control mechanisms adjust jaw forces to the mechanical impedance of simulated food during chewing movements. That is, jaw forces during closure were determined, in part, predictively from previous sensory experience with the food substances. Sensory experiences which are no doubt partly of periodontal afferent origin were gained in the preceding chewing cycle and then helped determine the additional muscle activity required during the power phase of chewing to overcome the resistance of the food. This predictive control is considered to be *feedforward, open-loop* in nature, since it does not depend on continuous monitoring of the teeth's ability to crush the bolus of food. The predictive control lessens the demand on *feedback, closed-loop* motor control mechanisms that use signals from the muscle spindles in the jaw-closing muscles (see Chapter 8). In general, feedback, closed-loop motor control mechanisms are more accurate than feedforward, open-loop mechanisms but they require more time to function properly. During slow chewing, it has been estimated that predictive control explains

Adaptation to one's individualized dentition and occlusion is a sign of a normal, healthy neuromuscular control system. The findings reviewed in this section demonstrate that signals from the periodontal mechanoreceptors have a considerable effect in shaping jaw muscle forces and movements in a functionally adaptive manner. Although loss of adaptation occurs with loss of periodontal receptors, it is also a characteristic of patients who develop painful functional disorders of the masticatory system, e.g., the *myofascial form* of *temporomandibular disorders (TMD)*. Contemporary evidence suggests that sensory information may be normal in these patients, but not processed normally by their central nervous systems. For example, loads applied to the teeth do not necessarily result in the same modifications in the activity of the jaw-closing muscles of patients with TMD as they do in normal, healthy individuals. Although poorly understood, the abnormalities in central processing are thought to be a factor in motor changes, such as irregular jaw movements and pain in the masticatory muscles. Often, patients with signs and symptoms of TMD do not adapt easily to treatments that change the occlusion or alter chewing function.

only about 15% of the force adjustment to the toughness of a bolus of food. Feedback during jaw closure (i.e., reactive control) explains most, 85%, of the force accommodation when time is not a limiting factor. However, for fast chewing (about 120 cycles/minute) predictive control contributes over half, 60%, of the force accommodation.

The chewing behaviour of patients with prostheses supported by osseointegrated implants suggests that regulation of force during chewing depends on input from periodontal mechanoreceptors. In patients with natural teeth, the chewing forces and jaw movements decrease progressively as the bolus becomes softer and the food particles become smaller. However, implant patients who lack periodontal mechanoreceptors seem to chew with about the same pattern of muscle activity throughout the entire period of breaking down a given food bolus. Since signals from the muscle spindles should be normal in patients with implants, this lack of adaptation can be reasonably attributed to the absence of information from periodontal receptors.

Control of the direction of jaw forces

The predictive control described above uses sensory information from past chewing cycles to regulate the current cycle. Information acquired by periodontal afferents at the start of the current cycle may also serve to regulate the ensuing pattern of muscle activity. During closure, the activity in the masticatory muscles must be coordinated to generate a jaw movement in three dimensional space that takes into account the spatial distribution of food particles across the whole occlusal surface and their relation to the biting surfaces of the teeth. The periodontal mechanoreceptors can furnish spatial information about tooth-to-particle contacts when the bolus is first engaged during jaw closure. Hence, they are well-suited to specify the orientation and magnitude of the jaw-closing vector in space during chewing. That the receptors provide this information is attested by the experiments in which subjects held and split food morsels between anaesthetised teeth (see Fig. 13). These experiments clearly demonstrated the consequence of impairment in controlling the jaw action vector: The morsel often (in 14% of the trials) eluded the clasp of the teeth upon application of the hold or bite forces by the anaesthetised subjects. This rarely occurred in the absence of anaesthesia (in <2% of the trials). Hence, the necessary spatial contact information was not available for precise control of the directions and/or points of attack of the forces. Moreover, subjects reported the absence of distinct and reliable sensations of contact with the morsel and the position on the tooth at which contact was made.

Similarity of jaw and finger motor control
In previous sections of this chapter, it is shown that the orofacial and hand regions of the human body exhibit similarities in sensory innervations, tactile acuity, and tactile sensitivity. The two regions also carry out motor behaviours that are controlled in similar manners. For example, the control mechanisms described above for the precision manipulation of small objects with the teeth appear analogous to those used for precision manipulation of small objects by the thumb and fingers. For both, distinct responses are evoked in mechanoreceptive afferents at low contact forces. The responses of most afferents supplying the periodontal ligaments and finger tips saturate at higher forces of contact, signifying that firm contact has been made but providing no additional details about its nature. The responses of the mechanoreceptors evoked during low force

levels at both sites assure that fine manipulative forces are exerted in the correct directions at precisely the right times to maintain a secure and safe contact. These manipulative forces neither dislodge an object from the grasp of the teeth or fingers nor harm the object with excessive force. Working through feedforward motor control mechanisms, the responses of the mechanoreceptors trigger the release of central commands that initiate and drive subsequent phases of behaviour (e.g., the onset of the split phase and a stable contact between fingers and object during the precision grip). In addition, the responses of the mechanoreceptors provide information about the surface properties of the object (e.g., the intrinsic physical properties of food substances between the teeth and the friction between an object and the skin of the fingers). This information is used to determine predictively the magnitude of the forces that will be used in subsequent phases of manipulation to prevent the object from slipping. That the information contained in the responses of the mechanoreceptors is used for motor control is further attested by the behavioural impairment that occurs after anaesthesia of the periodontal ligaments and fingers. Manipulative forces are applied in the wrong directions and with inappropriate magnitudes, causing small items to escape the grip and making manipulation impossible (e.g., holding a morsel of food between the teeth and buttoning the shirt become extremely difficult). These observations, as well as others presented in this chapter, attest to a similarity of the mechanoreceptive innervations of the orofacial region and of the hand, of their exceptional perceptual sensibilities, and of the motor control systems serving these two important areas of the human body.

◼ Role in the tactile sensibility of the teeth

Psychophysical testing of human subjects has revealed that, in addition to their role in the motor control of the jaw, periodontal mechanoreceptors play an important role in the detection of objects between the teeth, as well as loads applied to the teeth. Detection thresholds have been measured both activity and passively from the teeth. For actively measurement, the subject's ability to detect thin metallic foils of different thicknesses placed between opposing teeth is measured, e.g., between stable occlusal contacts on the upper and lower incisors or premolar teeth. Ten or more foils graded in thickness from 10 to hundreds of μm are evaluated one at a time and on multiple trials. The minimum thickness of foil that the subject can detect on 50% (or 100% in some studies) of the trials is taken as the threshold thickness. For active measurement, the subject can base his/her response on all the available information regarding the presence of the foil. This includes information not only from the periodontal mechanoreceptors but from other sources as, e.g., subtle differences in the muscular effort required to occlude the teeth in the presence of the foil interference. With this approach, subjects with upper and lower natural teeth are able to detect foils only 20 μm in thickness, demonstrating an extraordinary level of dental tactile sensitivity. The minimum foil thickness detected by patients with conventional full dentures is 7 to 8 times thicker than this, and these patients are thus only 12–15% as sensitive as dentate individuals. Full denture patients with poor retention exhibit even less sensitivity, while the presence of retained, endodontically-treated teeth confers greater, nevertheless less than normal sensitivity to the overdenture patient. Of particular note

are edentulous patients with osseointegrated implant-supported prostheses. These patients are twice as sensitive as edentulous patients without implants. Foils only 3 to 5 times thicker than normal are detected, indicating that restoration of the edentulous ridge with implants restores near normal tactile sensitivity with the prosthetic teeth. For these patients the improved performance has been attributed to contributions from mechanoreceptors in the periosteum (osseoperception), the facial bones and sutures, and the ear through bone conduction.

Passive measurement of detection thresholds requires the controlled delivery of calibrated forces to individual teeth with the jaw at rest. The forces are delivered either steadily for estimation of *static* thresholds or periodically (vibrations) for estimation of *dynamic* thresholds. As for active measurement, the static thresholds for patients with dentures, without and with dental implants, are higher (by about 10 times, compared to 7 to 8 times for active measurement) than for dentate subjects. In the passive testing situation the subject must rely solely on information transmitted by the periodontal mechanoreceptors as there is no muscular effort by the subject to provide additional cues. This explains why the edentulous patients are more impaired upon passive measurement of sensitivity than upon active measurement.

In contrast to the ten-fold difference in the static thresholds across the different patient groups, dynamic (vibration) thresholds tend to be relatively similar. Implant patients without periodontal receptors have thresholds that are similar to dentate patients with periodontal receptors. The reason that both groups of patients exhibit the same sensitivity to tooth vibration becomes clear when the implants and teeth, respectively, are anaesthetised. Surprisingly, detection of vibration is impaired to a greater extent by anaesthesia of natural teeth than of dental implants, suggesting that the vibration is more effectively transmitted across the osseointegrated junction than across the periodontal ligament to receptors remote from the tooth. As such, the balance between the dynamic and static sensitivities of the mechanoreceptor systems available to the implant patients clearly differs from those of dentate patients with periodontal mechanoreceptors. A better understanding of these differences may lead to novel therapies for restoring more normal sensory function in patients with osseointegrated dental implants, improving further the quality of care we now offer patients who lose their teeth prematurely.

Summary

The orofacial region has a dense and diverse supply of mechanoreceptors. These provide the sensory input required for control and regulation of the expressive and manipulative behaviours that characterize orofacial function. They also underlie perceptions of tactile sensations from the mouth and face, and these surpass in detail sensations from other areas of the body. The mechanoreceptors in the orofacial soft tissues functionally resemble the four types described in the human hand: slowly adapting (SA) type I and type II receptors, fast adapting (FA) type I receptors and hair follicle receptors. Mechanoreceptors in the facial skin, lips and buccal mucosa respond not only to contact with environmental objects, but also to contact between the lips, to changes in air pressure generated for speech sounds, and to facial skin and mucosa deformations that accompany lip and jaw movements associated with chewing and swallowing. Hence, in addition to their role as exteroceptors, the afferents also provide proprioceptive information of importance to the control of orofacial motor functions. Human periodontal mechanoreceptors respond vigorously and adapt slowly to forces applied to the teeth. Populations of periodontal receptors encode information about which teeth are loaded and the direction of forces applied to individual teeth. Most periodontal receptors are most sensitive to changes in tooth load at very low force levels. Hence, they accurately encode the load on each tooth when subjects first contact, hold, and gently manipulate food with their teeth. In contrast, only a minority of the afferents encodes the rapid increase and stronger forces generated when biting or chewing on food. These periodontal receptors may contribute to the execution of high jaw forces required to carry the teeth through a bolus of food. Signals from both populations of periodontal receptors are responsible for the conscious detection of loads applied to the teeth (including, no doubt, the irritating sensation of food stuck between the teeth!), and are used in the fine motor control of jaw actions associated with the intraoral manipulation of foods. It is clear from studies of various patient groups that important sensory functions are lost or impaired when these receptors are removed during the extraction of teeth. This knowledge emphasises the importance of maintaining healthy periodontal function whenever possible, even if this means keeping at least the roots of badly-damaged teeth in place not only for use as future prosthetic supports, but also for use as sources of sensory information to support motor function.

Selected references

Linden RWA. Periodontal mechanoreceptors and their functions. In: Taylor A (ed). Neurophysiology of the Jaws and Teeth. New York: Macmillan 1990;52–88.

Rath EM, Essick GK. Perioral somesthetic sensibility: Do the skin of the lower face and the midface exhibit comparable sensitivity? J Oral Maxillofac Surg 1990; 48:1181–1190.

Trulsson M, Johansson RS. Encoding of tooth loads by human periodontal afferents and their role in jaw motor control. Prog Neurobiol 1996;49:267–284.

Trulsson M, Johansson RS. Orofacial mechanoreceptors in humans: encoding characteristics and responses during natural orofacial behaviors. Behav Brain Res 2002;135:27–33.

Masticatory muscles

Timothy S. Miles

Timothy S. Miles

Goals:
- To give a brief review of the general properties of skeletal muscles relevant to the masticatory system.
- To describe the particular adaptations of the muscles in the human masticatory system.
- To indicate clinical situations in which adaptations of the masticatory muscles may occur.
- To discuss the major pathological conditions that affect the masticatory muscles

Key words:
Skeletal muscle; masticatory; muscle fibre types; motor units; fatigue; histochemistry; force; isometric; isotonic; concentric; muscle plasticity; electromyography; muscle pathology.

■ Introduction

The masticatory muscles carry out a very wide range of functions. They are able to move the mandible very quickly and precisely to enable different speech sounds to be made in rapid succession, but they are also capable of exerting the enormous forces that are required to break down tough foods.

This chapter examines the properties of skeletal muscles that enable the masticatory system to carry out its diverse activities. The discussion is confined to a description of the human masticatory muscles (namely, the jaw-closing muscles masseter, temporalis, and medial pterygoid, and the jaw-opening muscles digastric and lateral pterygoid). However, it goes without saying that other muscles including those of the face and tongue and the infrahyoid muscles also play a vital role in mastication, swallowing and other functional behaviours of this system.

All of the masticatory muscles are skeletal muscles: that is to say, they contract only when a signal is sent to them along somatic motor nerves from the central nervous system. (In contrast, smooth muscles are either activated by the autonomic nervous system or by hormones, and/or they have intrinsic excitability that arises from the properties of their cell membranes.) Skeletal muscles are readily distinguished from smooth muscles when viewed under the microscope because of their distinctive, regular transverse striations, which are the result of highly regular organisation of the actin and myosin filaments that are responsible for the muscle's ability to shorten.

There are some notable differences between the masticatory muscles and other skeletal muscles of the limbs and trunk. Skeletal muscle is derived embryologically from mesoderm: however, the pattern of muscle formation is controlled by the connective tissue in which the myoblasts migrate during embryological development. For limb muscles, this connective tissue arises from somatic mesoderm, but for the muscles of the head, the connective tissue comes from neural crest cells in the first branchial arch: hence, they are innervated by the nerve of the first arch, the trigeminal. The type of myosin (a protein that is directly involved in muscle contraction) in the masticatory muscles is also unique: the so-called "superfast myosin" in the masticatory muscles has very high ATP-ase activity, which enables these muscles to contract very quickly and forcefully: this may be an adaptation that favours the aggressive biting behaviour of carnivorous mammals.

Organisation of skeletal muscles into motor units

All of the muscles of mastication are innervated by the trigeminal motor nerve, which has its origin in the trigeminal nucleus in the pontine area of the brainstem. The cell bodies of the motor neurones are located in the pons. Their axons form the motor root of the trigeminal nerve on each side, passing across the floor of the middle cranial fossa to leave the cranial cavity *via* the foramen ovale. The motor root then divides to give branches that proceed to each of the ipsilateral muscles of mastication to control their contractile activity. The motor nerve going to an individual muscle (e.g., temporalis) contains the axons from many motor neurones. When they reach the muscle, each of these motor axons branches many times to

form neuromuscular junctions with many muscle fibres. One motor neurone plus the skeletal muscle fibres that it innervates is called a *motor unit*. Figure 1 is a very schematic representation of a motor unit: in the masticatory system, each motor neurone innervates hundreds of muscle fibres (Table 1), not just the six shown! The organisation of muscle fibres into motor units is an essential feature of the way that a muscle's contractile activity is controlled by the nervous system.

Because each muscle fibre in a motor unit is innervated by the same motor neurone, and neuromuscular transmission is normally very secure, it follows that one action potential in one motor neurone will generate one action potential simultaneously in all of the muscle fibres to which it is connected. Consequently, all of the muscle fibres in a given motor unit contract at exactly the same time. This makes a motor unit the *basic functional contractile unit* of a skeletal muscle (note that this should not be confused with the smallest contractile element in an individual muscle fibre which is the sarcomere). In other words, the brain cannot control muscle fibres individually: rather, it

Table 1. Innervation ratios. The innervation ratio for a (whole) skeletal muscle is the ratio between the number of motor neurones that innervate it, and the number of skeletal muscles that it contains. This is of course indicates the average motor unit size; e.g., for temporalis, each motor nerve fibre innervates an average of 936 muscle fibres. However, the size of motor units is not uniform within temporalis (or most other muscles) and therefore different temporalis motor units contain different numbers of muscle fibres.

Muscle	Innervation ratio
Temporalis (jaw-closer)	1:936
Masseter (jaw-closer))	1:640
Gastrocnemius (ankle extensor)	1:1934
Anterior tibial (ankle flexor)	1:562
Lateral rectus (eye mover)	1:9

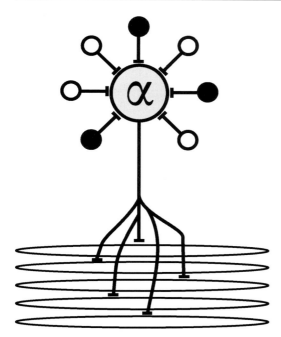

Figure 1. Schematic illustration of a single motor unit. A single alpha-motor neurone in the trigeminal motor nucleus gets inputs from many sources (motor cortex, sensory receptors in the skin and muscle, interneurons within the brain, etc.) and controls the activity of many skeletal muscle fibres. The number of muscle fibres controlled by one motor unit in different muscles can range from a single-digit number up to many hundreds. It is important to note that all alpha-motor neurones receive hundreds or even thousands of different inputs some of which are excitatory (represented as open circles) and others inhibitory (filled circles).

with a small number of muscle fibres. It follows that such muscles must be innervated by a relatively large number of motor neurones. This enables the brain to grade the force of contractions of these muscles very accurately by progressively increasing the number of motor nerves that are activated, thereby giving many small increments of force. This is essential to enable the tongue to make extremely precise movements during speech, for example. On the other hand, less-precisely controlled muscles such as those in the leg have more muscle fibres in each motor unit and relatively fewer motor neurones and, as a consequence, the brain cannot produce finely-graded force in these muscles.

Table 1 shows that, in comparison with other muscles, the size of motor units in the masticatory muscles is rather in the middle of the range. That is, these muscles have motor units that are, on average, neither very small (e.g., like lateral rectus that moves the eyeball) nor very large (like gastrocnemius, which extends the ankle). This middle-of-the-range size is consistent with masticatory muscle function which requires good control, but less precision than is required, for example, for the extremely rapid, flick-like movements of the eyes (saccades) that you will see when you watch someone who is reading.

controls groups of muscle fibres that are combined into motor units. The number of muscle fibres per motor unit therefore determines the size of the force increments that can be used to grade muscle force, i.e., motor units with fewer muscle fibres enable force to be graded more precisely.

The number of muscle fibres in a motor unit varies with the function of the parent muscle. Muscles that carry out highly precise contractions such as those in the tongue or those that move the eyes have motor units

Classification of muscle fibre types

Most whole muscles contain several different types of muscle fibres that have different functional properties. These are often classified crudely as "red" and "white" fibres, a classification that is evident to anyone who has ever looked through a butcher's shop window, or has seen a cooked turkey with its light and dark meat. (The colour difference is due to different amounts of myoglobin and different densities of capillaries and mitochondria in the different types of muscle fibres.) However, more precise classifications based on the functional characteristics and histological appearance of the muscle fibres are given later.

The production of force by muscle fibres is a complex process powered ultimately by ATP, in which the myofilaments (proteins) *actin* and *myosin* form cross-bridges which then pull the myofilaments along so that they slide over each other. The myosin acts as an enzyme to split the ATP to power the cross-bridge cycling, and the particular form of this myosin-ATPase in different muscle fibre types determines the maximal rate at which the muscle can generate force. This is one fundamental difference between different "fast" and "slow" muscles: another is a difference in their ability to release and reuptake Ca^{2+} quickly.

The biochemical processes that replenish the ATP used in this sliding process are different in different functional types of muscle fibre. Some muscle fibres (or more accurately, motor units) use aerobic mechanisms to replenish their ATP. These muscle fibres have many mitochondria for oxidative metabolism (Fig. 2). This process goes on continuously, and maintains a constant supply of energy in the muscle fibre. However, the rate of replenishment of ATP is slow, so such muscle fibres can contract only rather slowly and weakly. Nevertheless, because the replacement of ATP occurs continuously, they can continue to contract as long as they have a continuous supply of oxygen-bearing blood; that is, they are highly resistant to fatigue. Such fibre types are common in postural muscles such as those in the back and neck. These fibres called *Slow, fatigue-resistant*, or type S.

At the other extreme are muscle fibre types that contract extremely quickly (due to fast myosin-ATPase) and exert very large forces. It is not surprising, therefore, that they fatigue very quickly as their energy is rapidly consumed. These muscle fibres are thicker than type S fibres, and use anaerobic (glycolytic) mechanisms to restore their energy (ATP) stores. Glycolysis is a process that makes energy available extremely quickly to enable these fibres to produce large forces,

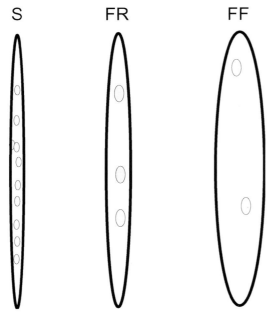

Figure 2. Schematic appearance of different muscle fibre types. Type *S* muscle fibres are relatively thin and have many mitochondria for aerobic oxidation of ATP. When stimulated, they twitch rather slowly, and are very slow to fatigue. *FF* fibres have relatively few mitochondria because they utilise primarily anaerobic metabolic pathways which enable them to generate large forces: as a consequence, however, they also fatigue quickly. Intermediate between these two are the *FR* fibres which use a mixture of aerobic and anaerobic metabolism that enables them to exert moderate forces for quite prolonged periods.

but only for very short periods of time. Even a brief, contraction of these powerful muscle fibres consumes all of their short-term energy supplies. The replacement of these energy sources then occurs relatively slowly, as does the return of contractile power of the muscle. Hence these fibre types are known as *Fast-Fatigable* fibres (usually abbreviated to type FF). Because they do not use aerobic metabolic pathways, they have rather few mitochondria compared with the type S fibres. However, they contain quite large stores of glycogen that can eventually be broken down anaerobically through glycolysis.

Finally, there are muscle fibres whose properties lie between those of types FF and S. These fibres have both aerobic and anaerobic enzymes, and are therefore able to exert reasonable amounts of force for long periods of time. That is, they are Fatigue Resistant and hence known universally as type FR muscle fibres.

The important point here is that the functional properties of muscle fibres are determined by the biochemical pathways that make energy available for them to contract.

The forces that are exerted by different types of motor units are usually described in terms of the force that they generate during a single "twitch" contraction. This twitch is produced artificially by giving a single electric shock to the motor neurone innervating the motor unit, thus causing all of its muscle fibres to twitch simultaneously. This is measured under isometric conditions, i.e, with the length of the muscle fixed so that it exerts its twitch force without shortening overall. (Note that, within a given motor unit, all of the muscle fibres are always of the same functional type, and therefore all contract at the same speed.) The force that a motor unit can exert varies greatly from the slowest to the fastest motor units. Figure 3 shows that the amplitude of a single twitch in a type S motor unit is small. At least in limb muscles, this is probably enough only to lift about a 2 g weight. A single twitch in a type FR motor unit is about 10 times greater than this, and a type FF motor unit twitch is about 50 times greater than a type S twitch. The data shown in Fig. 3 were obtained from muscles in the limbs where it is easier to obtain (because the motor nerves can more easily be dissected in experimental animals). However, there is compelling evidence from a small number of studies that type S motor units in the human masseter are much "faster" than those in the limbs, and exert substantially more force. This is probably a consequence of the different "superfast" myosin in the masticatory muscles.

The classification of motor units as "fast" or "slow" is based on the rate at which they develop force during a single isometric twitch, i.e., the mechanical response to a single action potential occurring simultaneously in all of the muscle fibres in the motor unit (Fig. 3). However, single twitches like

Glycolysis is a biochemical process consisting of a number of enzyme-controlled steps in which glucose is metabolised to pyruvate, which is then either transformed to lactate (under anaerobic conditions) or enters the Kreb's cycle. In both instances, ATP is regenerated from ADP. During anaerobic conditions, each glucose molecule consumed yields a net of only 6 ATP molecules. This is less efficient than aerobic metabolism in which a net of 30 ATP molecules is formed per glucose molecule consumed.

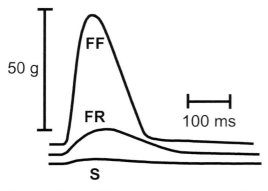

50 g

FF

FR

100 ms

S

Figure 3. Single twitches by motor units of the three major different muscle fibre types in a skeletal muscle. The muscle fibres in each of the three motor units were made to twitch isometrically by giving a single electrical shock to its motor nerve. In terms of their fibre types, type *S* motor units are Slow, *FR* are Fatigue Resistant, and *FF* are Fast, Fatiguable. Note that a single twitch in a FF motor unit yields about 50 times more force than a single twitch in a type S unit. The precise values of the force produced by single isometric twitches in the three or perhaps four different types of motor units in the human jaw muscles has not been established. However, it is likely that they are comparable with the twitch amplitudes (expressed in grams) of S, FR and FF motor units found in other muscles.

this occur only under laboratory conditions. Under normal circumstances, muscles contract when the nervous system sends continuous "trains" of action potentials down motor nerves to the active motor units. These result in a smooth contraction (sometimes called a fused contraction, or "tetanus" – which is nothing to do with the disease with the same name) of individual motor units and hence, of course, of the whole muscle. The action potentials in different motor units are relatively asynchronous during voluntary contractions, which further smoothes the force generated by the muscle as a whole. The higher the frequency of action potentials in the motor unit, the more force that it generates. Generally speaking, when a motor unit is in this state of continuous contraction, it generates about 2–

3 times as much force as it does in a single twitch. Thus, if we ignore biomechanical considerations such as direction of pull and leverage, a single type FF motor unit in masseter could probably support a weight of about 100 g – but only for a matter of a few seconds before it fatigues!

When whole skeletal muscles or smaller biopsy specimens are removed from the body and prepared for microscopic examination, they can easily be stained to show the enzymes that control the aerobic and anaerobic energy pathways. This enables slow (aerobic) muscle fibres to be distinguished by visual inspection from fast (anaerobic) fibres, so that the proportion of aerobic and anaerobic fibres in different muscles is easily determined.

Histochemical staining shows that, in addition to the slow and fast fibre types, there is a third type of muscle fibre whose properties fall between these two extremes. These fibres contain a mixture of aerobic and anaerobic enzymes, and consequently their functional properties also fall between those of the slow and fast motor units. These so-called "*Fatigue Resistant*" fibres (FR) are fast-contracting (due to their fast myosin ATPase), exert moderate amounts of force (because of their anaerobic capability), but can continue to do so for prolonged periods (because of their aerobic metabolic capacity).

Thus, muscle fibres can be characterised both functionally (in terms of strength, speed and fatigability) and histochemically (in terms of their metabolic pathways). Not surprisingly, there is a clear correlation between their functional and their histochemical properties, as shown in Table 2. However, because it is much easier to characterise the different types of fibres in a muscle histochemically by staining it than it is to determine their functional properties (especially in humans), most of what we know about the functional properties of human masticatory (and other) muscles is inferred from histochemical examination of the muscles.

One curious observation based on histochemical examination of human masticatory muscles is that they often contain finite numbers of muscle fibre types whose mixture of metabolic enzymes is intermediate between the major fibre types. These fibres have been called "IIC and ATP-ase – IM" fibres (18% of lateral pterygoid fibres are of this type). That is, they are a third variant of type II fibres (i.e., more aerobic than IIA and IIB) where "IM" is an abbreviation for intermediate to reflect their unique metabolic capabilities compared with the more common fibre types. These are common in developing limb and trunk muscles, during exercise training and in some pathologies, but rare in normal adult limb and trunk muscles. This raises the intriguing question whether the masticatory muscles are constantly in "training" compared with most other muscles. We have already recognised that any given muscle (such as temporalis) contains a mixture of different types of muscle fibres. Hence, the overall contractile capabilities of the whole muscle are the consequence of the numbers of each type of muscle fibre that it contains. Powerful muscles contain high proportions of fast-twitch fibres, while postural muscles that must continue to contract indefinitely without fatigue contain more slow fibres. Examples of the different proportions of different fibre types in specific masticatory muscles are given later in this chapter.

■ Force production

The fact that individual muscles contain these different fibre types raises the question of how the brain activates the right types of fibres at the appropriate time to produce the exact amount of force required, for example, to bite through a carrot. The control of the masticatory system is complex (Chapter 8); however, the way that the different types of muscle fibres (or, more accurately, motor units) in any given muscle are activated by the brain to produce force is very straightforward. When a muscle begins to contract,

Table 2. Relationship between histochemical properties of different types of skeletal muscle fibres and their functional capacities. Staining histological sections of whole muscles or biopsies shows the major metabolic enzymes that the different motor units use to generate force (i.e., histochemical type). These histochemical markers correlate closely with the different functional characteristics of the three major types of muscle fibres. (Of course, it makes more sense to think in terms of motor unit function than muscle fibre function, because the brain controls motor units, not individual muscle fibres).

Motor unit type based on function	Motor unit type based on histochemistry	General description	Twitch time	Aerobic capability	Anaerobic (glycolytic) capability	Susceptibility to fatigue
S (slow)	I	slow-twitch	slow	high	low	low
FR (fatigue resistant)	IIA	fast-twitch	intermediate	high	moderate	moderate
FF (fast, fatigable)	IIB	fast-twitch	fast	low	high	rapid

exerting a very weak force, the type S fibres are always activated first. As the brain calls for more and more force from the muscle, progressively more and more type S motor units are activated (or "recruited"). As the force continues to increase, the brain begins to recruit type FR motor units in addition to the S units and, when really large forces are called for, it recruits type FF last of all.

This system is beautifully adapted for optimal function. During weak contractions, the type S fibres continue to exert force indefinitely without fatiguing. Furthermore, during these weak contractions, the blood flow through the muscle is normal, so the delivery of oxygen and fuel can occur continuously. However, as the force level increases above about 20% of the maximum possible, the pressure inside the muscle increases. You can easily check this for yourself simply by palpating your masseter muscle while you clench your teeth together with increasing force. The rise in intramuscular pressure begins to interfere with the flow of blood through the muscle at about 20% of the maximal force that a muscle can produce. This reduction of perfusion interferes with the performance of the type S fibres which depend on a continuous supply of oxygen to maintain their aerobic metabolism. At about this stage, the brain begins to activate the type FR fibres in addition to the type S fibres. The anaerobic as well as the aerobic capability of the FR fibres allows the muscle to continue to exert force even when the perfusion of the muscle with blood is limited.

In a very powerful contraction, the brain activates the type FF fibres in addition to type S and type FR. In such contractions, the increase in intramuscular pressure prevents all blood from entering the muscle. Because they generate force by anaerobic metabolism, the FF fibres can continue to exert

force in the absence of blood flow, but contractions that obstruct blood flow totally can continue for only a short period before the force exerted by the muscle falls quickly. Hence, weightlifters can hold the heaviest barbells above their head only for a few seconds.

Thus the force that whole muscles generate at any particular time depends on:

- the number of motor units that are active
- the types of motor units that are active (remembering that the proportion of different types of motor units with different functional capacities differs from one muscle to another)
- the frequency of action potentials in the motor units that are active.

In multi-muscle systems such as the masticatory system, the total force exerted also depends on factors such as the relative activity of different whole muscles that are involved in the task. For example, during clenching, the masseter, temporalis and medial pterygoid muscles on both sides of the face are all contributing to the total force. When forceful clenches are applied to brittle food, the digastrics are also active (to stabilise the TMJ, see Chapter 8), which reduces the net force acting through the teeth.

Muscle fatigue

Muscle fatigue is a complex subject. Even the word "fatigue" means different things to different people, and has been defined in many different ways. However, a very general definition of fatigue in the context of human movements is that it is a reduction in a muscle's ability to maintain a desired contraction force.

It is now accepted that there are two major types of fatigue. Firstly, of course, the muscle fibres themselves can fatigue; this "contractile fatigue" is the inability of a muscle fibre to maintain the same force output with continued, repeated activity. The second type of fatigue relates not to changes that occur in the muscle, but to changes that occur in the central nervous system: this is so-called "central fatigue".

Let us first consider contractile fatigue. It has been widely believed for over 50 years that this type of fatigue is associated with the gradual accumulation of lactic acid in muscle fibres. This notion is reinforced constantly in the media in relation to sporting performance. However, this idea is based more on supposition than on fact, with the current consensus being that lactate, rather than causing fatigue, is a beneficial alternative substrate used to fuel muscle contraction.

If it is not lactic acid that causes muscle fatigue, what does? As yet there is no simple answer to this apparently simple question. What is certain is that contractile fatigue has a broad aetiology determined largely by the intensity and duration of muscle activity as well as the types of fibre that are involved. A simple way to class contractile fatigue is to divide it into two categories based on both its rate of onset and its rate of recovery. If the onset and recovery of fatigue occurs over minutes to hours, then the decreased force output is largely associated with metabolic changes in the cytoplasm and is termed "metabolic fatigue". If, however, the recovery from fatigue takes several hours to days, it is likely that functionally important proteins and structures have been damaged. This latter form of fatigue is often associated with low-frequency, long-duration activity, such as weight-lifting and long-distance running, and is aptly termed "low-frequency fatigue".

When a muscle is activated, an action potential propagates along the surface of the muscle cell and into the interior of the cell along the T-tubule system. This in turn leads to the release of Ca^{2+} from the sarcoplasmic reticulum, increasing the cytoplasmic $[Ca^{2+}]$. This free Ca^{2+} activates the contractile proteins myosin and actin, so that they slide along each other, causing the muscle to shorten and produce force. When the initial stimulus ceases, the Ca^{2+} is then quickly taken up again into the sarcoplasmic reticulum and the muscle fibre relaxes. While there is not full agreement on the precise mechanisms involved, it is clear that contractile fatigue involves a change in the Ca^{2+}-based coupling of the depolarisation of the muscle cell membrane to the activation of the contractile apparatus, a process known as excitation-contraction coupling. In short-term, metabolic fatigue, it is ATP and its metabolites that are thought to have the greatest affect on excitation-contraction coupling. During contraction, ATP is rapidly consumed to provide the energy required. Consequently,

In the human context, muscle fatigue is usually assessed experimentally as the ability to maintain the *maximal* force possible in a voluntary contraction. This is because it is difficult otherwise to ensure that:(a) the level of muscle activity remains constant throughout a sub-maximal, fatiguing contraction in each subject (i.e., if the muscle is fatiguing, the force will decline), and (b) similar numbers (and types) of motor units during the sub-maximal contraction are active in all of the different subjects who are being tested.

as the [ATP] falls, associated metabolites increase: these include inorganic phosphate, ADP, AMP and adenosine. All these factors decrease the sensitivity of the contractile proteins to Ca^{2+}, reduce the amount of Ca^{2+} that is released from the sarcoplasmic reticulum, and limit the rate of re-accumulation of Ca^{2+} back into this intracellular store and thus reduce the force-generating ability of a muscle fibre both directly and indirectly.

In contrast, longer-term, low-frequency fatigue is brought about by Ca^{2+} itself. This raises a rather interesting paradox. The amount of force a muscle fibre can produce is exquisitely dependent on the amount of Ca^{2+} released into the cytoplasm. Thus, Ca^{2+} is essential for contraction. However, if the $[Ca^{2+}]$ gets too high and remains in the cytoplasm too long, then both excitation-contraction coupling and the structural integrity of the fibre are compromised, a process termed Ca^{2+} uncoupling. It is thought that this mechanism provides a fail-safe switch important in preventing excessive and prolonged forces that could lead to more severe muscle damage.

In addition to these cellular processes which limit the force that muscle fibres can exert, central factors are particularly important in human fatigue. Many studies have shown that during a prolonged maximal contraction, the total muscle force exerted falls at a rate faster than it would as the result of contractile fatigue alone. This phenomenon, known as "central fatigue" is ascribed partly to motivational factors and partly to changes in the excitability of motor pathways in the brain.

Despite the extremely high forces that the jaw-closing muscles can exert and the presence of many fibres with primarily anaerobic metabolism, these muscles are apparently quite resistant to contractile fatigue. When you clench your jaw-closing muscles together as hard as possible, the force begins to decline quite quickly not because of contractile fatigue of the muscle fibres themselves, but because the pain arising from the hypoxic muscles prevents you from keeping them fully contracted. It is not surprising, therefore, that there is an inverse relationship between the force with which one bites and the length of time that one can sustain that force.

■ Types of muscle contraction

During the course of their normal function, muscles undergo several different types of contractions. For example, muscles often contract without actually shortening (the word *contract* here is misleading when the length is not changing, but this term is used universally despite this!). This is known as *isometric* (which literally means "same length") contraction. The masticatory muscles contract isometrically during a tooth-together clench (intercuspal position). The force exerted during such isometric contractions can be very high, and may account for the damage that is done to the teeth in people who brux, or forcefully grind their teeth together.

The jaw muscles also often shorten against a constant resistance, which is known as *isotonic* ("same force") contraction. For example, during speech, the jaw moves constantly, but the load during jaw-closing is virtually constant because the only force that must be overcome is gravity. Not surprisingly, muscles that are not loaded can shorten much more quickly than when they are loaded. The movements of the tongue during speech are an excellent example of extremely fast isotonic contractions that are made in the absence of external loads.

While it is convenient to think about isometric and isotonic contractions separately, most jaw movements are either a mixture of isometric and isotonic contractions, or switch quickly between the two. In these mixed contractions, there is a trade-off between force and speed.

Finally, muscles can exert force while their length is actually increasing. These movements are known as *eccentric* or *lengthening* contractions, a terminology that is even more peculiar. It is during this kind of activity that muscles exert their maximal force. If you grasp the front of your thighs when you bend your knees to squat down, you will feel the contraction in these antigravity (quadriceps) muscles while their length is increasing. The downward movement in a squat is much easier than the subsequent upward movement not only because the downward movement is going with gravity, but also because muscles exert more force for the same effort during the lengthening contraction.

Do the masticatory muscles ever undergo eccentric contractions? This is an interesting question in relation to pain syndromes in these muscles (see Chapter 4), as eccentric contractions are particularly effective at inducing muscle soreness that begins some time after the exercise. The conventional answer is that the jaw-closing muscles are only normally loaded when chewing and that there are no normal circumstances in which they contract while increasing in length. However, more careful examination reveals that some of the masticatory muscles do make eccentric contractions during some manoeuvres. For example, the lateral pterygoid muscle undergoes controlled lengthening when the condyle of the temporomandibular joint moves slowly back into its fossa. The powerful jaw-closing muscles masseter and temporalis on, say, the left side of the face are probably also lengthening when the teeth are ground from left to right, or from back to front. This may be important for the development of symptoms in the jaw-muscles and temporomandibular joint in people who brux, but there is no simple relationship between muscle activity and symptoms. However, it is important to note that many people brux without inducing symptoms of soft-tissue damage. In fact, people who brux the most during sleep have fewer symptoms than those who brux less!

Muscle force

The nature of the muscle contraction is very important in how much force a muscle exerts. However, another factor that affects the force that a contracting muscle can exert is its length. Muscles exert their maximal *active* force when there is a maximal overlap of their actin and myosin filaments so that the maximal number of cross-bridges can be formed between them. This maximal overlap occurs in muscles at their "resting length", shown schematically in Fig. 4. The resting length of a muscle is the length that it assumes when it is not contracting and not loaded. The masticatory muscles are probably at or near their resting lengths when the mandible is in its rest or postural position (although it has been claimed that different jaw-closing muscles have their resting lengths at different jaw positions).

However, it is not only the active force arising from muscle contraction that determines how much force a muscle exerts at different lengths. In the masticatory system, the biting force at different jaw openings also depends on the *passive* tension in the jaw-closing muscles which arises from elastic tissues primarily in the muscles themselves. In the combined jaw-closing muscles, the passive tension increases sharply with jaw

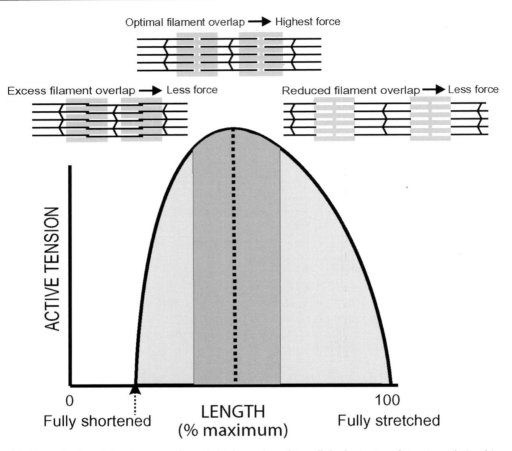

Figure 4. The active length-tension curve for a skeletal muscle and its cellular basis. Length-tension relationships are established by fixing the muscle length and recording the amplitude of the (isometric) twitch evoked by a single motor nerve stimulus, then increasing the muscle length slightly, and repeating the twitch measurement, and so on, from the minimal length at which the muscle normally functions to its maximal length. Muscle active tension results from an ATP-dependent interaction between the actin filaments and myosin filaments within myofibrils. In the presence of the appropriate stimulus, the myosin filaments shown here in grey draw themselves along the actin filaments (black) by forming and breaking cross-linkages. The amount of force that a muscle can exert depends on how far these two types of filaments can overlap each other, as this determines the number of cross-bridges that can interact. This is maximal at the resting length of the muscle (dotted line). However, when the muscle is stretched out, there is less interaction between the myofilaments and therefore less force. When the muscle is fully shortened, there is again less force because the actin filaments interfere with each other. Note that this graph does not show the passive component of the total force that a contracting muscle exerts.

opening to about 50 N. Hence, the total force exerted by the jaw-closing muscles is the result of active contraction (from the interaction of the actin and myosin filaments) plus the passive tension arising from elasticity.

The last factor that influences the amount of biting force is the biomechanics of the six jaw-closing muscles. Changes in the degree of jaw separation alters the geometrical relationship between the direction of pull of the muscles and the bones to which they are attached. This alters the mechanical advantage of the muscles, and therefore the net jaw-closing force.

Hence, the relationship between biting force and jaw opening does not flow simply from the length-tension relationship of a single muscle fibre. In practice, the only way that this relationship can be even estimated in humans is by recording the maximal biting force at different jaw openings (because this is the only force than can be standardised). The results of such studies are rather variable but the maximal biting force generally increases as the separation between the teeth increases, to an opening somewhere between 15 and 30 mm of occlusal separation, then decreases again.

The masticatory muscles

The masticatory muscles are *extremely* powerful. Most healthy people with sound dentitions are said to be able to bite with a force equivalent to lifting their own weight, and the record for the most powerful force recorded by any muscle group is held by the jaw-closers. One study reported a bilateral isometric bite force of 4,400 N: this significantly exceeds the current Olympic weight-lifting record of around 2,300 N for the "snatch"! The extraordinary force that the jaw-closing muscles exert is partly because of their fibre composition, and partly because of their biomechanics. Most other muscles act *via* long tendons and insert onto bones in a manner that gives them a poor mechanical advantage e.g., the muscles that flex and extend the elbow, knee, etc. However, the jaw-closing muscles act directly across the tem-poromandibular joint with a good mechanical advantage and without the need for a long tendon.

The masticatory muscles differ in composition from limb or trunk muscles: each has a distinctive histochemical profile. That is, each muscle is specialised in a manner that is adapted to its unique function. The lateral pterygoid consists mainly of type I (S) fibres, indicating a primarily postural stabilising role in which large forces are not often required. In contrast, the digastric muscle which one does not normally associate with forceful contractions, has many type II (FF and FR) fibres, which presumably confer the speed required for jaw movements during speech.

In addition to differences in fibre type composition between different muscles, there are also specialised regions within each of the masticatory muscles. For example, the superficial part of temporalis is rich in IIB (FF) to give acceleration and speed, and therefore precision, while the deep posterior part of this muscle is well endowed with type I (S) fibres, which suggests that it has a primarily postural role. The notion of functional partitioning in muscles is quite well accepted, and even the gross anatomy of muscles like temporalis suggests that different parts of the muscle (e.g., anterior compared with posterior) play different functional roles.

Examples of the different histochemical profile of several masticatory muscles are shown in Fig. 4.

"Plasticity" of muscles

There is now good evidence supporting the idea that the muscle fibres in motor units can be converted from one histochemical type to another by training. This response to

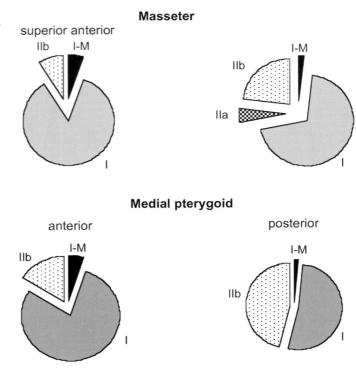

Figure 5. The composition of different muscle fibre types in different parts of the human masseter and medial pterygoid muscles. Note that these proportions are based on histochemical data, and the proportions are therefore expressed as Type I, IIA, IIB, and I-M. Type I-M is the intermediate type that in the limbs is found only in muscles during development, during exercise training, ageing and in some pathological conditions.

altered usage patterns is called muscle "plasticity", and is of clear importance in areas such as athletic performance, where athletes may wish to optimise their aerobic (endurance) performance for events such as long-distance running or swimming, or anaerobic (power) events such as weight-lifting or high-jumping.

It is now generally accepted that aerobic training can convert FF (type IIB) fibres to FR (type IIA). However, despite the wishful thinking (and belief) of many sports coaches and athletes, it is not possible to change between type I and type II fibres by training. Nevertheless, it is interesting that the metabolism of a muscle can be altered by changing the pattern of its motor activity. Therefore, it may well be that persons who brux or those who eat unrefined diets have different proportions of fibre types in their jaw-clos-

ing muscles. This has not been established because of the difficulties in measuring such changes, which can only be done accurately in a *post-mortem* histological examination. It is interesting, nevertheless, to consider the type of changes brought about by different patterns of use in other muscles, such as those in the limbs, where the proportions of various fibre types can be estimated from biopsy specimens examined histochemically.

Increased muscle use, or strength training based on *high-force isometric (resisted) contractions* results in an increase in the cross-sectional area of individual muscle fibres and also of course to the muscle as a whole. This leads to an increase in the maximal force that the muscle can exert, which is proportional to its total cross-sectional area. This certainly corresponds anecdotally with the hypertrophied masseter and often temporalis muscles that one sees in some patients who grind their teeth excessively.

There is no increase in the number of muscle fibres nor is there a change in the proportions of different fibre types with strength training. Minimal changes occur in intramuscular energy stores (with the exception of increased glycogen) and enzymes associated with either glycolytic or oxidative pathways. There is a *relative* decrease in capillary density in the muscle, indicating that the same number of capillaries now supply a bigger muscle, i.e., the overall blood supply probably does not change.

However, there is now good evidence that much of the increased force that comes with strength training is the result of changes in the pattern of motor unit activation by the brain. That is, the increased force is due to functional neurological reprogramming as well as structural change in the muscles themselves. There is even evidence that the strength of hand muscles can be increased by *imagining* forceful isometric contractions, without actually carrying them out!

Increased use or endurance training based on *lower-intensity, long-duration exercise* can convert FF (type IIB) to FR (type IIA) fibres, which confers increased resistance to fatigue. Again, there is no conversion of type II to type I. At higher intensities of exercise, enzymes associated with glycolytic pathways become elevated. Glycogen and fat stores in muscle increase, but these changes may also be the result of concurrent changes in eating and dietary patterns. Muscle fibre diameter is reduced, and capillary density increases.

At low intensities of activity, enzymes related to oxidative metabolism are enhanced. The changes can occur in all fibre types, but are restricted to the muscles being exercised. The effect on glycolytic enzymes is minimal.

The proportions of different types of fibres in the masticatory muscles appears to change with age, but in a manner that differs from one muscle to another, and that is different from what generally happens in limb muscles with age. In recent histochemical studies, for example, it has been found that, compared with young subjects, the masseter muscles of elderly human subjects have a reduced proportion of type I fibres and an increase of type IM and type II fibres. It is not clear to what extent these changes reflect general age-related atrophy or adaptive changes of the muscles. It is difficult to generalise about changes in the force exerted by the masticatory muscles with age, as this varies greatly with diet. Generally speaking, however, there is an overall diminution in the maximal force that most elderly people can exert with any of their muscles.

Biopsy specimens of skeletal muscle may be taken from either a living muscle or a muscle from a person who has died only a short time before. Biopsies from the muscles of living humans are usually obtained by use of a needle that removes a core of muscle, or from a small section of the muscle. While valuable information about the fibre composition of a given muscle can be gained from "live" biopsy specimens, there is a significant problem with sampling error. That is, the region of muscle from which the biopsy is obtained may not be representative of the muscle as a whole. In fact, most muscles, including those in the masticatory system, have different populations of the various types of motor units in different parts of the muscles. This is known as compartmentalisation.

Decreased use particularly with immobilisation has given very variable results in experiments with different muscles, species, duration of immobilisation, angle of fixation etc. Part of the apparent variability is no doubt due to the difficulty associated with controlling how much subjects contract muscles that have been immobilised by, e.g., a plaster cast. Some of the variability is also the result of the way in which the results are expressed. It is usually reported that immobilisation does not change the proportions of different fibre types, although different results have been obtained in studies of the masticatory muscles, as described below.

Immobilisation of many muscles has led to a reduction in the diameter of their type I fibres, and often their type II fibres as well. The capillary density per fibre is reduced, and muscle strength may be reduced, or unaffected. The glycogen content in muscle fibres is reduced, but there is no effect on glycolytic enzymes. The absolute oxidative enzyme capacity of an immobilised muscle decreases but, because of the atrophy that also occurs, this effect disappears when it is expressed as a proportion of muscle mass.

Immobilising the mandible by intermaxillary fixation in monkeys is reported to reduce both type I and type II fibre diameters by more than 50% in the masseter and temporalis muscles, although there was no change in the relative proportions of the two fibre types. In contrast, an increased proportion of type II fibres was found in the masseter muscles of patients 6–10 months after osteotomy to correct vertical maxillary excess overbite followed by 3 to 8 weeks of intermaxillary fixation.

Studies of altered usage patterns in the masticatory muscles have not given consistent results in monkeys or humans. It has been claimed that in monkeys made edentu-lous for periods of up to 4 years, the mean cross-sectional area of type I fibres was reduced in masseter and temporalis and there was overall a reduced oxidative capacity in jaw muscles. One study suggests that there is a reduced proportion of type II fibres in human subjects with ill-fitting dentures and that the cross-sectional areas of individual fibres is also reduced.

These studies do not really lead to any firm conclusions on the effects on the composition of masticatory muscles from manoeuvres that change the activity pattern of the masticatory muscles. The problem is likely to be inconsistencies in experimental methods and poorly controlled experimental data.

Despite the lack of specific evidence in relation to the jaw muscles, it seems fair to conclude from studies on other muscles that regular exercise of the masticatory muscles by chewing foods of firm texture is likely to be important to maintain their function particularly in the elderly.

■ Electromyography (EMG)

Electromyography is a specialised technique that is used to measure the activity of individual muscles. It is widely used in experimental analyses of the masticatory system, and it is also used in a small number of clinical environments to analyse patterns of masticatory activity in patients whose masticatory function is abnormal (see also Chapter 8).

The concept of electromyography is simple. The contractile activity of muscles is controlled by the central nervous system which sends action potentials along motor nerves to the neuromuscular junction of skeletal muscles. Here, acetyl choline is released into the cleft between the nerve ending and the motor end plate, and diffuses across to bind to specific receptors. This eventually leads to the generation of an action potential in the muscle fibre that passes along the surface membrane and triggers the sliding of the actin and myosin filaments along each other. It is these action potentials passing along the surface of the muscle fibres that are responsible for the electromyogram. In a contracting muscle, action potentials are occurring continuously in thousands of muscle fibres. These tiny electrical signals can be detected by attaching small electrodes to the skin above the muscle of interest, and amplifying them to produce an EMG record. However, the signal seen in the EMG looks rather complicated because it is the sum of many, many action potentials that are occurring in the population of active motor units at different times with respect to each other. Examples of EMG records are shown in Fig. 1 of Chapter 8. This shows the EMG recorded from the temporalis, masseter and

digastric muscles of a patient who was chewing on a piece of gum. The records show that the jaw-closing muscles are activated more or less at the same time as each other, and alternate with the activity of the jaw-opening muscles.

While it is comparatively easy to record the EMG of the superficial masticatory muscles, there are many pitfalls in its interpretation, and there are far too many reports in the dental literature that reflect the fact that their authors do not understand the limitations of the technique. It has frequently been claimed, for example, that the jaw-closing force can be estimated from the EMG of the jaw-closing muscles. Of course it is true that the force exerted by a muscle increases when the EMG increases (reflecting increased electrical activation its muscle fibres), if other conditions are kept constant. However, as we have seen earlier in this chapter, biting force is also determined by a number of other factors including muscle length. It is also influenced by the activity of other muscles that contribute to the force and those that oppose it. This relationship may also change with time. During muscle fatigue, changes may occur in the EMG and force capacity of the muscle fibres which weakens the relationship between them.

Muscle pathology

There is a range of pathological conditions that can affect skeletal muscles, most of which are mercifully uncommon. Some of these can be acquired but the most common are primary, genetically-determined myopathies and myotonias. While they can affect the masticatory muscles, this occurs sufficiently rarely that such cases are written up in medical journals.

It is relatively simple to record action potentials in single motor units in the human masticatory muscles. This is done by inserting very fine, insulated wires with only the tips exposed into the muscle. This method has revealed that motor units (and therefore motor nerves) discharge action potentials at much slower frequencies than sensory nerves. When the masticatory muscles are activated, their motor units discharge at frequencies in the range of about 5–25 Hz, compared with firing frequencies of hundreds of Hz in sensory nerves.

Despite its comparative rarity (prevalence about 3 in 10,000 people), *myasthenia gravis* is well-known to physiology students because it gives a striking illustration of one aspect of how the neuromuscular junction works. There are receptors at the motor end plate of all skeletal muscle fibre that bind the neuromuscular transmitter acetyl choline and cause the motor end plate, then the muscle to depolarise. Patients with myasthenia gravis develop antibodies which destroy these receptors so that when the motor nerve releases acetyl choline, there are fewer sites to which it can bind. As a result, the motor end plate and the muscle fibre membrane do not depolarise normally and hence will not contract. The result is muscle weakness and rapid onset of muscle fatigue. Myasthenia gravis commonly affects the function of facial muscles, including those of the masticatory system, producing difficulties in chewing and swallowing. It most often affects women younger than 40 and men older than 60. It is usually treated with drugs that slow the breakdown of the neurotransmitter (so-called cholinesterase inhibitors, such as neostigmine (prostigmine or pyridostigmine). This enables the neurotransmitter to remain for longer in the neuromuscular cleft, thereby increasing its opportunities to bind to the receptors.

The *muscular dystrophies* are rare, inherited muscle diseases in which skeletal muscle fibres are abnormal due to a genetic defect. The muscles, including those in the masticatory system, become progressively weaker and the muscle fibres may be replaced with fat and connective tissues. The more common dystrophies are caused by a deficiency or malfunction of the muscle protein dystrophin or of dystrophin-associated proteins.

The most common form of muscular dystrophy in children is *Duchenne's muscular dystrophy* which occurs in young boys. The muscles of pelvis and limbs are first affected, and the masticatory system can also be involved later. The abnormal patterns of force production arising from the weakness in the masticatory and facial muscles can lead to remodelling of the facial bones, and malocclusions are frequent in patients with long-standing dystrophies.

Myotonic dystrophy is the most common form of muscular dystrophy that affects adults. It is an autosomal dominant condition that affects approximately 5 persons per 100,000. This slowly progressive disorder is the result of abnormalities in the ion channels of muscle membranes that leads to muscle weakness along with muscle stiffness and the inability to relax the muscles rapidly after effort. It involves all skeletal muscles including those in the masticatory system.

The masseter muscle in particular is occasionally affected by a disorder known as *myositis ossificans traumatica,* which is an uncommon sequel to trauma (including surgery) or inflammation of the muscles. It is characterised by calcified lesions that appear in X-rays or other scans.

The functions of the masticatory muscles can also be adversely affected by disorders of the motor nerves either as the result of trauma, particularly during surgery, or because of more generalised neuropathies such as *Guillain-Barré syndrome.* This is an autoimmune condition that leads to inflammation of peripheral nerves (i.e., those outside of the brain and spinal cord). This condition is characterised by severe weakness and numbness usually in the legs and arms, but also in the face, where it affects the muscles used for mastication and swallowing and the external eye muscles. Its incidence is about 2 per 100,000 people, and increases with age. It is often triggered by a viral infection, or stresses such as pregnancy or surgery. While most people recover fully, up to 20% of patients who have had this disease have some residual sensory and or motor effects from it.

meat, and broke bones with their teeth. Individual muscles of mastication can be functionally subdivided into different compartments, and the motor units in these compartments are likely to have important roles in different tasks. While not unknown, it is comparatively rare for disorders of the muscles themselves to have an adverse affect on masticatory function.

Summary

The human masticatory muscles are superbly adapted to their primary function of breaking down food in preparation for its digestion. In particular, they contain a range of different fibre types that give an appropriate balance of force and endurance. The force that they are capable of exerting is probably inappropriately large for modern diets, but doubtless evolved when our distant ancestors ate raw

Selected references

Allen DG, Lannergren J, Westerblad H. Muscle cell function during prolonged activity: cellular mechanisms of fatigue. Exp Physiol 1995;80:497–527.

Close RI. Dynamic properties of mammalian skeletal muscles. Physiol Rev 1972;52:129–197.

Eriksson PO, Thornell LE. Histochemical and morphological muscle-fibre characteristics of the human masseter, the medial pterygoid and the temporal muscles. Arch Oral Biol 1983;28:781–795.

Miles TS, Nordstrom MA. Fatigue of jaw muscles and speech mechanisms. Adv Exp Med Biol 1995;384: 415–426.

Monemi M, Kadi F, Liu JX, Thornell LE, Eriksson, PO. Adverse changes in fibre type and myosin heavy chain compositions of human jaw. Acta Physiol Scand 1999;167:339–345.

Gandevia SC. Spinal and supraspinal factors in human muscle fatigue. Physiol Rev 2001;81:1725–1789.

Mastication

Timothy S. Miles

Goals:
- To describe the role of the masticatory pattern generator in controlling the rhythmical movements that occur during chewing.
- To understand the importance of sensory feedback in controlling chewing movements.
- To describe the contribution of muscle spindles and periodontal receptors to the control of chewing.
- To describe the control of the "rest" or "postural" position of the mandible.
- To understand the common disorders of the masticatory system.

Key words:
Mastication; chewing; central pattern generator; trigeminal reflex; stretch reflex; mandibular postural position; chewing cycle; bite forces; proprioception; neuromuscular diseases.

Introduction

The human masticatory motor system is a remarkable machine. While people may think of it mainly in relation to the chewing of food, it also carries out many different functions under a wide range of different conditions.

At one extreme the masticatory system is capable of exerting huge forces. Most people are able to exert more force with their muscles of mastication than with any other muscle system: in fact, many people can bite with a force equivalent to lifting their own weight! These high forces are usually required only for very brief periods to break down tough food and to perform such tasks as cracking nutshells. The existence of these high forces, and the fact that they are ap-plied through the teeth which are specifically adapted for breaking down tissue, gives the masticatory system a significant potential for self-injury. For this reason, it is obviously essential that the activity of the jaw-closing muscles is very tightly controlled.

However, the masticatory system is not only involved in high-force activities. It is also capable of great subtlety through the execution of extremely precise movements. Speech, for example, requires little power from the masticatory muscles, but extraordinary speed and accuracy to move the mandible rapidly from one precisely controlled position to the next. When forming speech sounds which follow one another very quickly indeed, the jaw moves with remarkable speed between these positions. This again requires the operation of very accurate, largely pre-programmed control mechanisms. You will find more on the roles of oral structures in speech in Chapter 10.

We are obviously not born with the ability to carry out these sophisticated motor tasks. Simple jaw and lip movements and swallowing are seen in the fetus and, by the time of birth, sucking is, not surprisingly, already well developed: this topic is dealt with in Chapter 9. The neonate is unable to chew (and normally has no teeth anyway!). However, within a few months after birth, coordinated chewing movements appear. Initially, these movements are largely reflex in nature, and occur in response to stimulation in or around the mouth. However, as the nervous system develops in the first months of postnatal life, these movements become increasingly less reflexive, and more under the infant's voluntary control. The eruption of the teeth is a significant landmark in the maturation of the infant's oral function, and accelerates the development of more structured mastication, eventually enabling solid foods to be chewed.

The nervous system continues to mature at a very rapid rate throughout the first year of life, enabling all motor functions to become increasingly skilled. This probably happens more quickly in the cranial nerve systems than elsewhere since, by the age of 12 months, some precocious infants begin to employ the most highly-developed oral function of all, speech, which involves the most elaborate interplay between trigeminal and facial sensory and motor mechanisms as well as the remarkable central programming that is required to drive the many muscles that are involved.

In this chapter, the neural mechanisms that control the movements of the mandible, particularly during mastication, are examined.

■ Control of mastication

It is first necessary to appreciate that there are several general classes of movements, which are controlled in different ways. *Voluntary* movements are of course those which are carried out as the result of a deliberate effort of will. These are primarily the result of the execution of a well-formed movement plan by the brain, although most voluntary movements are fine-tuned as they are carried out, through the action of reflexes. The final common output pathway from the brain for the execution of the plan for a voluntary movement is the motor cortex. Speech is perhaps the most refined example of voluntary movement, in which all of the components required to utter a series of complex sounds are read out by the motor cortex to a large number of muscles in a most complex sequence.

At the other extreme, some movements are purely *reflex*. That is, a given sensory input evokes a rather stereotyped motor response. Reflexes range from the very simple to the very complex. There are many examples of reflexes in and around the mouth. For example, tapping one's teeth briskly together activates a simple reflex that quickly stops the activity in the jaw-closing muscles – but only transiently. This is illustrated later in this chapter in Fig. 6. At the other extreme, swallowing is an extremely complex reflex response involving coordination of many muscles that is triggered by stimulation of the mucosa in the pharynx.

There is, however, another general class of movements. These are *cyclical movements*, like breathing or walking. Chewing is an excellent example of a cyclical movement involving the trigeminal system. The basic rhythm of cyclical movements is driven by a program that is hard-wired in the brain, and cyclical movements can continue without feedback. However, like voluntary movements, cyclical movements are normally fine-tuned by sensory signals acting through the action of reflexes. As we shall see, this is a good description of how rhythmical mastication is controlled by the nervous system.

The rhythmical nature of normal chewing movements is shown in Fig. 1. These records were obtained from a subject chewing gum on the right side of his mouth, with a cycle time of about one chew per second. The vertical, horizontal and sideways movements are shown at the bottom, and it is clear that these are all very similar from one chewing cycle to the next. The pattern of activity of some of the jaw-opening and jaw-closing muscles that produced these movements is shown as their electromyogram (EMG) records.

Note that all of the jaw-closing muscles on both sides are activated at about the same time during the closing movement. During opening, only the jaw-openers are active. The activity of the left masseter during the chewing stroke is less than the activity in the right masseter because most of the work is

The EMG is the result of the electrical activity that arises from the conduction of action potentials along muscle fibres, and is easily recorded from small electrodes glued to the skin above the muscles (Chapter 7). The amplitude of the EMG recorded in this way is very small, only about 0.001 V (compared with 1.5 V for a flashlight battery!). The record for the lateral pterygoid muscle was obtained by inserting a fine needle through the skin into the muscle.

being done by the muscles on the right-hand side.

There is very good evidence from experiments on reduced animal preparations that cyclical mastication like that shown in Fig. 1 is neither purely voluntary nor purely reflex. For example, delivering a long series (or train) of weak electrical shocks to any of several places in the brains of anaesthetised rabbits and guinea pigs can cause realistic chewing movements to occur. These chewing movements are the result of highly-coordinated activity of the masticatory, tongue and cheek muscles in a manner that closely resembles natural chewing. These movements are elicited at the same rate even when the frequency at which the electrical shocks are given is changed, which indicates that the stimulus is increasing the level of activity in some hard-wired circuits in the brain (i.e., a "pattern generator"), rather than directly driving the outputs to the masticatory muscles. Similar rhythmical "mouthing" movements are often observed when the lip or tongue is rubbed in anencephalic human infants, or adults whose brains have been so badly damaged by strokes that they are incapable of voluntary movements. This probably represents the output of the circuits that normally underlie the basic rhythm of chewing.

An ingenious experiment was used to prove beyond doubt that these rhythmical movements that are elicited in anaesthetised animals by electrical brain stimulation are the result of activity in a central pattern generator in the brain. In these experiments, rabbits were not only given a general anaesthetic but were also paralysed with a curare-like drug (based on the poison used by South American Indians on the tips of their arrows) that blocked neuromuscular transmission by blocking the nicotinic receptors on the skeletal muscle. That is, this drug did not interfere with the signals that travel out from the brain along motor nerves, but it did stop these signals from activating the chewing muscles. Hence, this drug prevented the jaw from moving in the normal rhythmical masticatory pattern when the animal's brain was stimulated. However, recordings of the activity of the motor nerves that innervate the masticatory muscles in this experimental situation revealed that the same protocol of continuous brain stimulation caused the nerves controlling the jaw-opening and the jaw-closing muscles to be activated in the same alternating pattern that occurs during normal chewing. Because the masticatory muscles could not contract, and the jaw did not move, it is clear that reflexes could not be contributing to the rhythmical activation under these conditions, which indicates that the underlying program for control of the masticatory muscles during chewing is centrally programmed.

While the following discussion will focus primarily on the muscles of mastication, it must be remembered that chewing also involves highly-coordinated movement of the tongue, lips and cheeks whose muscles are innervated by nerves other than the trigeminal.

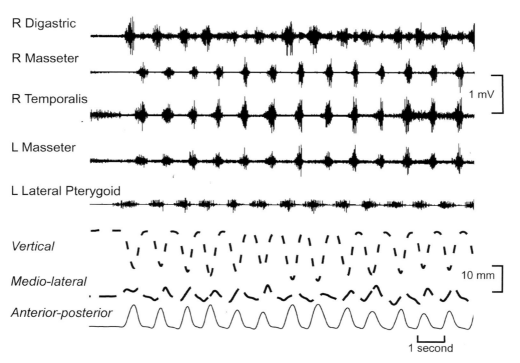

Figure 1. The pattern of jaw movements in a subject chewing gum on the right-hand side of his mouth. These very regular jaw movements were measured with a device glued to the teeth which gave a read-out in the three planes of movement. The electrical activity in some of the muscles of mastication (their electromyograph, or EMG) is also shown. The activity of, e.g. the right masseter during a chewing stroke appears as a burst of electrical activity in this muscle. (The vertical scale for the EMG signals is 1 mV for all muscles except lateral pterygoid: for this muscle the scale is 0.5 mV). These data were kindly provided by Dr Gregory Murray, The University of Sydney.

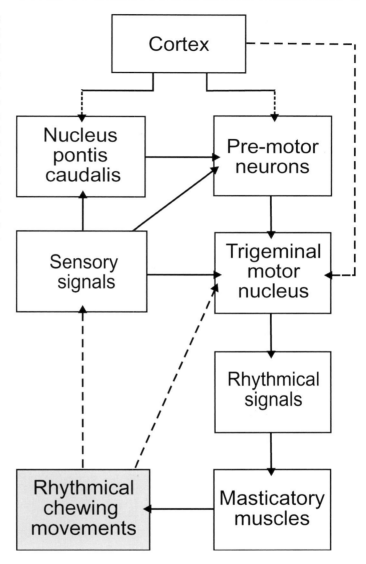

Figure 2. Schematic of the connections of various brain structures that control rhythmical jaw opening and closing movements. The central pattern generator (CPG) consists mostly of the brainstem nuclei and their interconnections. However, activity in the CPG can be triggered both from the cortex and from sensory signals from the masticatory system. However, the feedback signals from the masticatory muscles and other perioral structures shown as dashed lines are not necessary for activity of the CPG. The dashed line from the motor cortex to the trigeminal motor nucleus indicates the pathway that is responsible for voluntary control of jaw movements.

Fig. 2 summarises the important components of the central pattern generator. This shows that there are a number of structures in the central nervous system which interact in a rather complex manner to produce rhythmical activation of jaw-opening muscles alternating with the activation of jaw-closing muscles. The dashed lines are to remind us that the pattern generator can continue to send out its signals to motor nerves even when the rhythmical chewing movements are prevented pharmacologically: that is, the pattern generator does not depend on sensory feedback to continue.

However, this pattern generator is unable by itself to adjust the muscle force to deal with the changing conditions that occur when different foods are being chewed. For example, when one is chewing nuts, a high force must be generated in the first few chewing strokes to break the nuts into smaller pieces. After that, though, only relatively small forces are required to grind the nuts into a paste ready to be swallowed. How, then, is the activity of the masticatory muscles modified to produce the force required to break down food whose texture may be unpredictable, and is changing from one chewing stroke to another?

The answer is that the activity of the masticatory system is powerfully modulated by reflexes. These automatically fine-tune the centrally-generated masticatory movements to give the best possible control of position and force under all of the different circumstances in which the masticatory muscles must function. The reflexes that are responsible for this will be considered in turn.

■ Stretch reflexes from muscle spindles

The stretch reflexes in the trigeminal system function to adjust the force exerted by the jaw-closing muscles to compensate for changing resistance to closing that occurs during chewing. They also play a role in maintaining the posture of the jaw in its so-called "rest position" during vigorous head movements. Like other somatic reflexes in the body, they consist of a sensory receptor, an afferent or sensory pathway, an integrating centre in the central nervous system where the sensory neurones synapse onto motor neurones, and an output pathway consisting of the motor neurones and the skeletal muscles of mastication.

The receptors for stretch reflexes are muscle spindles. These complex sensory organs lie within the belly of most (but not quite

all) skeletal muscles, and in parallel with the normal muscle fibres. The jaw-closing but not the jaw-opening muscles are richly endowed with muscle spindles. These receptors are exquisitely sensitive to stretch which may occur either as the result of external forces acting on the jaw, such as gravity when one is running, or as the result of a more complicated scenario which is discussed later.

The sensory nerves that carry the signal from the muscle spindles to the brain are the largest myelinated nerve fibres found anywhere in the body, the so-called Ia afferent neurones. These nerve fibres are contained

Because both the nerve fibres that carry the action potentials from the muscle spindles to the brainstem and the fibres that bring action potentials from the brainstem back out to the muscles are large and myelinated, they conduct action potentials at very high velocities (about $50 \text{ m} \cdot \text{s}^{-1}$). Furthermore, because the distances over which the action potentials must travel in this reflex are quite short (about 90 mm in each direction), the stretch reflex occurs very quickly. In fact, if you tap on a person's chin, the signal from the muscle spindles gets up to the brainstem and back to activate the jaw-closing muscles in about or 7–8 ms (e.g., Fig. 4). The speed of this reflex response enables the muscles to react extremely quickly to changes in the resistance of the food being chewed. This chin-tap reflex is used by neurologists to test the normal function of the sensory and motor nerves in the trigeminal system.

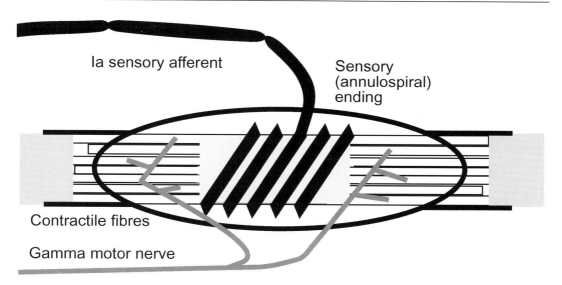

Figure 3. Innervation of the muscle spindle. The muscle spindle consists of a mechanoreceptor which is wound around the central part of the spindle, together with actin/myosin contractile elements (striated) at each end. When the spindle is stretched, or when the contractile elements are made to contract by means of their gamma motor nerves, the receptor is activated, and it sends out signals along its Ia sensory nerve to the central nervous system.

within the trigeminal sensory nerve. However, the trigeminal Ia afferents pass into the brainstem by an anatomically unique path. Although they are sensory fibres, they enter the brain in the same nerve trunk as the motor nerves that are leaving the brain, rather than with other sensory neurones as is the case in the spinal cord. Their cell bodies lie within the brain, in the mesencephalic trigeminal nucleus. (This arrangement also differs from that of the Ia afferents in spinal nerves, whose cell bodies are located outside of the spinal cord in dorsal root ganglia.)

They then pass to the trigeminal motor nucleus where they form a excitatory synapses directly onto the trigeminal motor nerves that innervate the jaw-closing muscles.

It should be noted that muscle spindles also have so-called "secondary" endings which are anatomically different from the "primary endings" shown in Fig. 3. Whereas primary endings are particularly sensitive to changes in muscle length and are therefore considered to be rapidly-adapting, the secondary endings give a continuous signal related to muscle length, i.e., they are slowly-adapting receptors. However, for simplicity, the functional roles of the primary and secondary endings will not be considered separately.

The operation of the stretch reflex in the jaw-closing muscles can easily be demonstrated by tapping on the chin with a tendon hammer. The brisk downward movement of the mandible stretches the jaw-closing muscles and their in-parallel muscle spindles. Stretching the spindles activates their sensory receptors, and sends a brief burst of action potentials along the Ia sensory nerves to their synapses which excite (depolarise) the motor neurones of the jaw-closing muscles. The burst of activity in the sensory nerves therefore elicits a brisk burst of activity in the motor nerves, which send action potentials back to the jaw-closing muscles, causing them to contract briefly, i.e., to twitch. This can be seen with the naked eye, but can be measured more accurately by electromyography, as shown in Fig. 4.

It has been argued that this stretch reflex operates continuously at a low level, to keep the mandible in its so-called "rest position" (or postural position) relative to the maxilla even when the head is stationary. This is an important issue because the rest position is a vital point of reference in prosthodontics, and this is a convenient time to consider how the jaw is normally kept in this position in a subject who is sitting or standing upright.

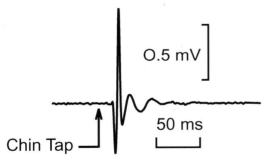

Figure 4. Reflex response to stretch of the masseter muscle. The record shown is an electromyogram (EMG), which was recorded by placing electrodes on the subject's masseter muscle to measure its electrical activity. A brisk downwards tap was delivered to the chin with a tendon hammer at the time shown by the arrow. This stretched the jaw-closing muscles and their muscle spindles, causing a burst of action potentials to be sent along the Ia sensory neurones to the brainstem where they activated the motor neurones that innervate the masseter (and other jaw-closers). This caused a brief, synchronous activation of the masseter muscle fibres which is seen as transient deflection in the EMG record about 8 ms following the tap.

Control of mandibular rest position

Every dentist knows that the occlusal surfaces of the teeth are separated by a distance of 3–8 mm when the jaw is in its rest position. The actual position can vary somewhat as the result of factors such as head posture, pain, and stress. Nevertheless, this distance (or small range of distances) is relatively constant throughout life, so it can be used, for example, to help decide where to place the teeth on artificial dentures. How then could this position be maintained by the stretch reflex in the jaw-closing muscles? The idea would be that the vertical position of the mandible is maintained by the continuous action of a stretch reflex that moves the jaw back up to its rest position every time that it moves down a little under the influence of gravity.

Despite the attractiveness of this notion, recent research has shown that stretch reflexes do not act in this way to maintain the posture of the mandible when the head is stationary. Rather, the mandible is held passively in place in this situation by elastic forces from the peri-oral soft tissues (which includes those in the muscles). It is actually more accurate to call these forces "visco-elastic", as the viscosity of the perioral soft tissues dampens down the springiness that would result from purely elastic recoil. These passive forces are sufficient to maintain the mandible in or near its rest position even when the head moves up and down during walking.

However, during more vigorous movements such as running or jumping on a hard surface, the brisker up-and-down movements of the head cause the mandible to move further and faster relative to the maxilla and, in this more challenging situation, the stretch reflex has recently been shown to play an important role in maintaining jaw posture. Consider a subject who is running. When he lands in each step, the mandible continues to move briskly downwards relative to the maxilla under its own momentum. This downward movement of the mandible relative to the maxilla stretches the muscle spindles in the jaw-closing muscles (rather as the chin tap did in Fig. 4) sufficiently to activate the stretch reflex pathway. The resulting burst of activity in the jaw-closing muscles stops the downward jaw movement and causes the mandible to move back up towards its rest position. Thus, with each step, the jaw-closing muscles are reflexly activated (then deactivated) in a manner that tends to reduce the vertical jaw movements that result from the inertia of the jaw. Hence, during running, the stretch reflex plays a key role in keeping the vertical position of the mandible reasonably constant with respect to the maxilla. By restraining excessive vertical movements in this way, this reflex stops the teeth from clashing together when one runs.

To summarise briefly: the vertical position of the mandible is maintained in its postural position by visco-elastic forces when the head is stationary or moving only slowly, but by stretch reflexes when the head is moving more vigorously up and down during running and jumping.

Mechanisms that modulate jaw-muscle activity during chewing

Let us now return to the control of the masticatory muscles during the chewing of food. The most important signals that help the chewing muscles to adapt to different types of food, and the changing texture of food as it is chewed come from muscle spindle receptors and from mechanoreceptors in the periodontal ligament. We will deal with these in turn.

Muscle spindle reflexes

To understand how the spindles operate in this situation requires insight into a more complex aspect of the organisation and operation of muscle spindles. So far we have considered only the sensory aspect of their function but, like skeletal muscle fibres, muscle spindles also have their own actin-myosin contractile system which is controlled by a special class of motor nerves called the "gamma motor" system.

The actual sensory receptor lies in the middle of the muscle spindle. This part of the spindle is elastic and can be easily stretched. The contractile parts of the spindle are at each end, and are innervated by the *gamma motor neurones* (Fig. 3). Thus, when the brain sends signals to the gamma motor neurones, the spindle contracts only at its ends. This stretches the middle of the spindle and the sensory receptor that is located there. Stretching the receptor activates it, causing signals to be sent along the sensory Ia neurones to excite the motor neurones in the brainstem.

How does this system work during chewing? During any normal muscle contraction, the brain sends signals along the motor neurones that innervate the normal muscle fibres (these are called "alpha" motor neurones) to make the muscle fibres contract: at the same time the brain also sends similar signals along the gamma motor neurones. These signals cause the ends of the spindle to contract, too, thereby preventing the muscle spindle from becoming slack when the muscle shortens. Fig. 5 shows what would happen in the hypothetical situation that the muscle were to shorten as the result of alpha activation of the normal muscle fibres, but with no gamma activation of the contractile apparatus of the muscle spindles.

Thus, the co-activation of alpha and gamma motor neurones normally maintains a steady level of tension on the sensory receptor of muscle spindles even when the muscle changes length during a normal contraction, which keeps the receptor ready to respond to small stretches.

To see how this mechanism controls biting force, consider what happens when you bite down onto brittle food such as a raw carrot. To begin the biting movement from the jaw-open position, the brain sends a stream of signals along the normal (alpha) motor neurones to your jaw-closing muscles. This causes the muscle fibres to shorten and move your teeth towards the surface of the carrot. This initial movement is an un-re-

sisted, *isotonic* (i.e. constant-force) movement. At the same time, the brain is also sending a continuous stream of signals along the gamma motor nerves innervating the muscle spindles in jaw-closing muscles: these cause both ends of the spindle to contract so that each spindle shortens at the same rate as the main muscle fibres, keeping the spindle receptor under steady tension. When the teeth touch the carrot, the resistance to closing suddenly increases sharply and the muscle fibres stop shortening because they are not contracting strongly enough to bite through the carrot. It is essential to note that, although they are prevented from shortening, the skeletal muscle fibres are still actively contracting; i.e., this has now become an *isometric* (constant-length) contraction. The brain continues to send signals to both the contractile part of the spindles and to the main muscle fibres. The main muscle cannot shorten, as it is

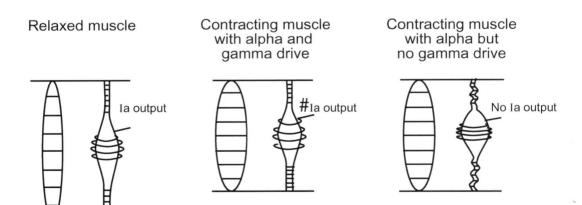

Relaxed muscle — Ia output

Contracting muscle with alpha and gamma drive — #Ia output

Contracting muscle with alpha but no gamma drive — No Ia output

Figure 5. Schematic illustration of the role of the gamma drive to muscle spindles in a skeletal muscles. In a relaxed muscle, there is steady, weak tension on the spiral receptor of the spindle so that it gives a continuous output of action potentials along its Ia sensory nerve. The centre panel shows that, when the muscle contracts normally, the brain sends signals along alpha motor nerves to the skeletal muscle fibres, and along gamma motor nerves to the contractile apparatus at both ends of the muscle spindle. This keeps some tension on the spiral sensory receptor in the muscle spindle so that it can respond to any stretches that may occur. However, if the muscle were to contract without gamma drive, the spindle would fall slack in the muscle, and would no longer send any outputs along its Ia sensory nerve. It would then be unable to respond to any stretches.

being resisted by the hard carrot. However, the contractile parts at both ends of the spindle can and do continue to shorten by stretching the elastic centre of the spindle. This activates the receptor in the centre of the spindle which of course causes more action potentials to be sent up the Ia fibres to the brainstem, where they activate the jaw-closer motor neurons more strongly. The increased activity of motor neurons then increases the activation of the muscle fibres, making them contract more strongly. The additional biting force generated as a result enables the teeth to bite through the carrot. All of this happens in a small fraction of a second and automatically, without any conscious intervention.

There is now evidence that this reflex response adapts quickly to changes in load in a given mouthful. When one first bites onto a tough food bolus, the reflex response in the jaw-closers is relatively small. However, in subsequent chewing strokes, the reflex response is greater. That is, encountering the high resistance informs the masticatory control system that the food is tough, and it then automatically resets the reflex responses accordingly. Hence, the masticatory control system rapidly "learns" about the texture of the food that is being chewed as the result of the signals coming from the sensory receptors in the chewing system, and modifies its activity accordingly.

Unloading responses of the jaw-closing muscles

It is equally or even more important for the jaw muscles to stop contracting when the resistance to closing suddenly decreases. A dramatic example of this is biting on a very hard, brittle object. Consider, now, trying to crack a tough nut shell with your teeth. The same spindle mechanisms are activated, but in the reverse direction. In this situation, while you are biting on the nut shell, the brain is sending ever-increasing signals to both the jaw-closing muscle fibres and to the contractile part of the muscle spindle to contract harder to bite down onto the shell. As the force builds up, the spindle receptors are stretched more and more because the intense gamma activity coming from the brain causes the actin-myosin apparatus at the ends of the spindle to contract while the whole spindle is prevented from shortening in length. The resulting Ia activity feeds more and more excitatory activity into the motor neurones supplying the jaw-closing muscles, making them contract still harder, as in the preceding example. When the force becomes large enough, the nutshell cracks without warning and the resistance to jaw closing suddenly falls to a low level or disappears altogether. At this point, the closing muscles are still active and contracting hard, and there is clearly the potential for the teeth to cause a lot of damage to intra-oral structures if they are slammed together. However, as you know from your own experience in this situation, this does not happen.

There are two reasons for this. First, when the nutshell cracks, the jaw begins to close as the muscles, now unresisted, begin to shorten at high speed. This shortening of the whole muscle removes the tension that was being applied to the middle of the spindle, and it falls slack within the muscle. As a consequence, the spindle receptor is suddenly no longer being stretched as it was before, and it therefore immediately ceases sending action potentials back to the brain along its Ia fibres. The sudden withdrawal of this powerful excitatory synaptic input to the jaw-closer motor neurones stops them from discharging action potentials, and the muscle is therefore deactivated very quickly. This "unloading reflex" mechanism helps to protect the peri-oral structures from damage when these potentially dangerous biting forces are being exerted by the masticatory system.

However, there is also a second important mechanism that acts to stop the teeth from crashing together when the jaws suddenly bite through a hard object. It has been shown that when the jaw-closing muscles make powerful isometric contractions, the jaw-opening muscles are activated at the same time. Then, when the hard object cracks and the jaw begins to close, the tension in the tonically-active jaw-opening muscles keeps the jaw from springing too far upwards. In this situation, the jaw-opening muscles act like a seat-belt in a motor vehicle, restraining unexpected rapid movements. The special advantage conferred by this mechanism is that it works instantly. The unloading reflex described above is extremely quick, but it still takes a fraction of a second to work and, when the teeth are only a couple of centimetres apart and the powerful jaw-closers are active, a speedy response is critical.

One important concept to emerge from this discussion is that a substantial amount of the excitatory input to motor neurones in the jaw-closing muscles (and to most other muscles) actually comes from peripheral sensory receptors rather than from the brain.

Finally, the afferent signals from muscle spindles also stimulate the secretion of saliva. You may have experienced or observed this when yawning, for example, when occasionally a spurt of saliva shoots out of the mouth!

In summary, then, the stretch reflex pathway acts to give automatic compensation for changes in the resistance to biting that are encountered during chewing. Stretch reflexes are equally effective in modulating the activity of the jaw-closing muscles when the load increases and when it decreases.

■ Periodontal reflexes

In addition to the stretch reflexes whose receptors lie in the masticatory muscles, there are reflexes whose receptors lie around the teeth. These are usually called the *periodontal receptors*. Chapter 6 gives a detailed description of how they are activated and how they contribute to conscious sensation. Here we will see that these receptors and their reflexes are also important in controlling the masticatory system during chewing.

The receptors themselves are located in the periodontal ligament and are oriented in directions that cause them to respond to any forces applied to the crown of the teeth. Other receptors are located in the bony socket. The receptors are directionally sensitive. Those around the anterior teeth are particularly sensitive to forces applied horizontally to these teeth. Almost all forces applied to a tooth during chewing have a vector that is horizontal. The teeth then act as levers which amplify the movement so that small tooth displacements cause (relatively) large changes in the shape of the receptors. Note, however, that the periodontal ligament around healthy teeth permits the tooth to move only a few microns in any direction, so the receptors respond to these extremely small movements.

These periodontal receptors play several functional roles. They give rise to subjective sensation about pressure on the teeth. This sensation is of course abolished by local alveolar anaesthesia. The periodontal ligament receptors signal only relatively small forces, and saturate when larger forces are applied.

Larger forces are probably signalled by the mechanoreceptors in the bony sockets. The signals from the periodontal receptors also contribute to the reflex control of mastication. Two different periodontal reflexes have been described. Firstly, brisk taps on a tooth elicit rapid and profound inhibition of activity in the jaw-closing muscles. This occurs, for example, when the teeth snap briskly together. The pathway for this reflex begins at the periodontal receptors (probably including those in the bone) and travels up sensory trigeminal nerves to enter the brainstem and continue to the trigeminal motor nucleus. Here, the signal is transformed by passing through one or two inhibitory interneurons, which then inhibit the motor neurones of the jaw-closing muscles. Inhibition of these motor neurones stops them from sending out action potentials to the jaw-closing muscles, which then cease to contract. Fig. 6 shows that this protective reflex response takes only about 0.01 seconds to act.

Periodontal receptors also contribute in a more complex manner to the control of the masticatory muscles. Pressing weakly on a tooth activates a different population of receptors in the periodontal ligament. When the signals from these receptors reach the trigeminal motor nucleus, the response is quite the opposite of that caused by the tap. Weak pressure reflexly excites the jaw-closing motor neurones and therefore increases the biting force.

The function of this excitatory reflex is not entirely clear. However, it seems likely that its role is to help the jaw-closing muscles to keep food between the teeth. When the teeth close onto a soft food bolus during chewing, the periodontal receptors are activated. The signals that they send to the trigeminal motor neurones reflexly activate the jaw-closing muscles to make them contract a little more strongly to hold the bolus between the teeth, ready to be crushed. The same reflex is likely also to be important in guiding the teeth into occlusion. At the end of the chewing stroke, the occlusal surfaces of the teeth come together to crush the food bolus, but then grind the bolus even further by sliding across each other towards the occlusal position. This sliding, grinding action is the result of the acti-

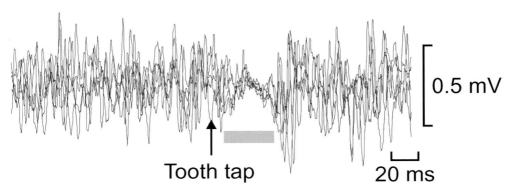

Figure 6. The "silent period" in the electromyograph of a human jaw-closing muscle. This record shows 5 superimposed EMG records from the masseter muscle. The subject was gently contracting onto a bite bar when a brisk horizontal tap was applied to an upper incisor tooth at the time shown by the arrow. After a brief delay, the muscle's activity decreased sharply and stayed "silent" for about 40 ms (shown by the grey line), before resuming its normal activity. This record was kindly provided by Drs Kemal Türker and Russell Brinkworth, The University of Adelaide.

vation of the appropriate masticatory muscles at the correct time when the teeth first touch during chewing. A reflex emanating from periodontal receptors is therefore well positioned to initiate and control this final grinding movement. It is also important that this grinding movement is made in the right direction, i.e., towards the occlusal position. Because the periodontal receptors are directionally sensitive, they may modulate the activity of the various jaw-closing muscles to ensure that the final grinding phase occurs in the correct direction.

The periodontal modulation of the masticatory muscles may be even more complex. For example, it may be necessary for these receptors to signal to the brain that the correct pattern of contact of opposing teeth has occurred before the grinding movement to the final occlusal position is reflexly initiated. That is, if the cusps of the upper teeth do not meet the occlusal surfaces of the lower teeth in the correct relationship, the grinding movement is not initiated. However, these higher-level functions have not yet been investigated carefully.

It must not be concluded from the foregoing that these (or any other) reflexes function in exactly the same way in all circumstances. In another form of rhythmical movement, walking, the activity of various reflexes that control the leg muscles are modulated continuously during the different phases of walking, and this is doubtless also true for the reflexes involved in rhythmical mastication.

The stretch reflex and the periodontal reflexes are undoubtedly the most important mechanisms for modulating or fine-tuning the activity of the masticatory muscles. However, several other receptors and reflexes can also affect jaw muscle activity. In some animal species, intense stimulation in the peri-oral region reflexly activates the jaw-opening muscles. Thus, if a cat or rat bites its lip or

tongue, the reflex activation of its jaw-opening muscles moves the teeth away from the damaged tissues, thereby minimising biting-induced injuries to soft tissues. This kind of protective withdrawal reflex response to painful stimuli is found in human limbs but not in the human masticatory system. Instead, painful stimuli in and around the mouth lead to reflex inhibition of the jaw-closing muscles but not activation of the jaw-openers. Strictly speaking, therefore, humans do not have "jaw-opening reflexes".

It is appropriate at this time to clarify one reflex response that is said to have diagnostic significance (see also Chapter 5). There are many papers in the dental literature describing aspects of the pattern of reflex response elicited in the human jaw-closing muscles by various intense stimuli such as snapping the teeth together, or by tapping on a tooth during clenching, or by electrical shocks applied to the lips. These stimuli cause the jaw-closing muscles to fall silent for a fraction of a second. This so-called "*silent period*" is usually measured in the electromyograph (EMG) of the jaw-closing muscles in response to such stimuli, as shown in Fig. 6. This is of course an inhibitory reflex response. It is unaltered by local alveolar anaesthesia and persists in edentulous subjects, so it does not depend on the periodontal receptors.

Much has been made of the potential for this reflex inhibitory response to be used as a clinical diagnostic tool. It has been claimed, for example, that the duration of the silent period is prolonged in certain temporomandibular disorders and other orofacial pain conditions, and that the duration of the silent period returns towards normal levels as the condition is successfully treated. In fact, the duration of the silent period depends on many interacting variables such as the nature, intensity and location of the stimulus, and on the level of muscle activity present at the time the stimulus was given. These variables are very difficult to control well enough to give reliable results even under the closely controlled conditions that are possible in research laboratories.

However, several trigeminal reflex responses are used for diagnostic purposes to detect abnormalities of both the peripheral nerve and brainstem functions in clinical neurophysiology. These include the jaw jerk referred to earlier, and other reflexes.

■ Tendon organ reflexes

In common with most skeletal muscles, the masticatory muscles contain other sensory receptors which are known as Golgi tendon organs. These are located in the junction between muscle fibres and tendons, and give a signal that is related to the force exerted by the muscle. Golgi tendon organs are known to be sensitive to small forces but their outputs saturate when the parent muscle contracts more strongly. There are various theories about how they contribute reflexly to muscle function but none is widely accepted, and there is no information at all about their functional role in the masticatory system. About all that we can say, by analogy with the spinal system, is that they monitor the force exerted by a number of different motor units during weak contractions.

■ Joint reflexes

The connective tissue in and around joint capsules contains many mechanoreceptors that are presumably activated when the capsule is distorted, i.e., when the joint is actively or passively moved. There is a substantial literature about the possible functional roles of these sensory receptors which are located

in and around the temporomandibular joint (TMJ) in health and disease. However, the conclusions reached in many of these reports do not stand up to close examination.

The difficulty in studying the receptors of the TMJ and their possible reflex functions arises primarily as the result of the anatomy of the nerves that innervate the joint. To measure the responses of joint receptors, it is necessary to record the activity of the sensory nerves that carry the signals from these receptors to the brain. Unfortunately, even in experimental animals, the nerves supplying the TMJ are very short and inaccessible: in humans, they are totally inaccessible for this purpose. Several investigators have attempted to study their function by blocking the sensory receptors by injecting local anaesthetic into the joint. The difficulty with this approach is that the local anaesthetic cannot be confined to the joint. Hence, some of the effects that have been ascribed to "joint anaesthesia" may be the result of blockade of other nearby structures, including the lateral pterygoid muscle.

Since we do not have specific information from TMJ receptors, it is necessary to extrapolate to the TMJ from what is known about joint receptors in other more accessible joints like the fingers (in humans) or knee (in experimental animals), from which unambiguous recordings from joint receptor activity can be made.

It was formerly thought from studies on the knee and other joints that the pattern of firing of joint receptors was able to give an accurate indication of the angle of the joint. However, the evidence overwhelmingly indicates that very few, if any, joint receptors accurately signal joint angle. In the case of the TMJ, a simple inspection of the anatomy of this joint and the remarkable complexity of the anatomy of both its capsule and the movements that it can make should have dismissed this argument before it was even made! While it is easy to see how the direction and amplitude of tooth movements can be coded accurately by mechanoreceptors in the periodontal ligament, just imagine how complex it would be for mechanoreceptors in the TMJ and its ligaments to signal precisely a combined rotation and hinge movement in which the jaw was moved to one side!

In fact, it is now accepted that most joint receptors are activated primarily at the extremes of movement. For the TMJ, this would be only the extremes of opening, protrusion or lateral excursion, as the joint capsule is not stretched when the teeth are in occlusion. The joint's anatomy suggests that receptors would also be activated in, say, the right joint capsule when an extreme movement to the left is made.

The role of joint receptors in the control of jaw movements is still unclear. However, since they signal extremes of joint displacement, it is at least possible that they could contribute to protective reflexes that prevent excessive joint displacement by activating muscles that oppose movements beyond a "safe" limit at which the capsule is tightly stretched. That is, receptors in the capsule of the TMJ may reflexly activate motor neurones of the muscles whose actions oppose excessive jaw-opening movements that threaten to dislocate the joint.

Painful stimuli in the TMJ area activate nociceptors which in turn cause strong co-activation of the jaw-opening and closing muscles. This has the effect of limiting the range over which the jaw and its joint will move, i.e., it is a sort of functional splint.

The chewing cycle

How then, do these various control mechanisms work together during chewing? While we know that chewing is cyclical, occurring at a rate determined by the central pattern generator, it is conventional to discuss the masticatory cycle in terms of a series of phases. In chewing, therefore, the pattern generator programs the following phases.

Preparatory phase
The chewing movement begins when the pattern generator causes the jaw-opening muscles to pull the mandible downwards from the rest or intercuspal position at about 7–$8 \ cm \cdot s^{-1}$. The pattern of jaw movements during a single chewing stroke is shown in Figure 7, beginning from the intercuspal position in A. The jaw may initially move away from its working side as it begins to open (shown in B), but then swings towards the working side (C), i.e., the side on which it will bite the food. This movement involves both a translation of the condyles primarily as the result of activity in the lateral pterygoid muscle pulling the non-working condyle forward and a hinge or rotary movement. When the jaw is open, the pattern generator ceases to activate the opening muscles, and activates the tongue and cheek muscles to position the food between the teeth. This cycle of the movement then continues without pause into the next phase, namely:

Food contact phase
As the pattern generator switches off the activation of the jaw-opening muscles, it almost immediately switches on the activity of the jaw-closing muscles to produce the initial closing movement (at about $10 \ cm \cdot s^{-1}$) that traps the food between the teeth (not shown in Fig. 7). It is in this phase of the cycle that the periodontal reflexes may assist in grasping the food in the correct position between the teeth, ready to be bitten through.

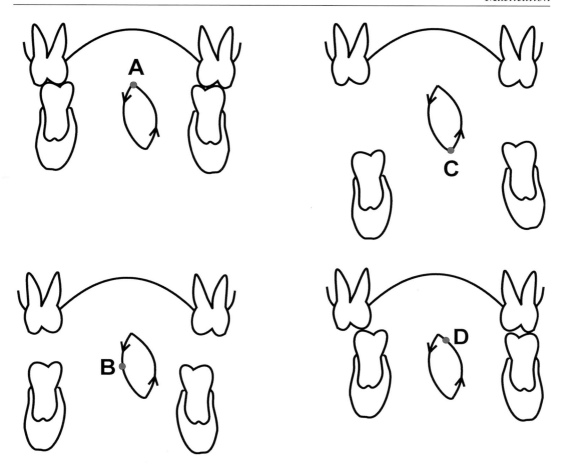

Figure 7. The movements made by the mandible during a single chewing cycle. The position of the upper and lower teeth are shown as coronal sections through molar teeth. The movement of a point located between the incisal surfaces of the lower incisor teeth is shown as the elliptical record, with arrows showing the direction of the movement. The position of the inter-incisal point at the four different phases of the chewing cycle is shown by the dots: in A it is in the intercuspal position; in B, during the initial phase of opening; in C at the point of maximal opening in this chewing cycle; and in D at the point of first occlusal contact of the posterior teeth during the closing stroke. From D, the teeth grind against each other to return to the intercuspal position. The food bolus that is being chewed is not shown in this figure.

Food crushing phase

In this phase, the output from the pattern generator to the closing muscles forces the teeth through the food bolus with the assistance of the load compensation reflex from the muscle spindle reflex system. For most western diets, the peak bite force during chewing is about 50–100 N, although tough food like nuts may involve much higher force levels transiently.

Tooth contact phase

Activation of the jaw-closing muscles continues as the opposing teeth come into contact (D), and while they slide from the working side into the intercuspal position.

Such tooth contacts occur in 30–90% of chews. During this phase, the outputs from the periodontal ligament receptors reflexly control the jaw-closing muscles (and probably lateral pterygoid, too) to ensure that the teeth slide in the correct direction towards the intercuspal position (A), thereby grinding the food into a paste. At the end of this slide, the pattern generator switches off the jaw-closers, and reactivates the jaw-opening muscles to move into the next chewing cycle.

Most people with natural teeth favour the same side for chewing throughout their lives, although some denture wearers change to a bilateral chewing pattern. No doubt this helps to prevent the dentures from twisting in the mouth when forces from the food tend to displace them. Bizarre chewing patterns can sometimes be observed in patients with abnormal occlusion. Painful teeth, joints and muscles temporarily alter the chewing pattern usually in a manner that minimises stimulation of the painful area. Even with healthy natural teeth, some people make the first few chewing strokes bilaterally, after which the bolus is shifted to one side for unilateral chewing.

■ Voluntary control of the masticatory muscles

The main focus of the discussion in this chapter has been on the control of the masticatory muscles by the pattern generator and by the various reflexes that fine-tune the output of the pattern generator to meet the changing forces that must be overcome during chewing. However, like most other skeletal muscles, the masticatory muscles are also subject to highly precise voluntary control. When one wills a particular mandibular movement, the movement plan is output through the motor cortex, and passes directly to the trigeminal motor neurones. This direct corticobulbar pathway is indicated by the descending dashed line in Fig. 2. The appropriate combination of trigeminal motor neurones is activated, and these send the signals to the muscles to execute the movement. This is essentially the process that controls other skeletal muscles as well, but with one important difference. While it is common to move, say, just one finger on one hand, the masticatory muscles on both sides are activated during almost every voluntary jaw movement. This is the result of the way that they are controlled by the motor cortex, which can be demonstrated with the help of some new technology.

It is now relatively easy to stimulate the human motor cortex painlessly in the experimental laboratory. This is achieved by discharging a very large current through a coil held next to the scalp. This indirectly induces activity in the motor cortical neurones, which send signals down to the motor neurones that activate the muscles controlled by that part of the cortex, causing the muscles to twitch. When, for example, the coil is held over the part of the scalp overlying the motor cortex that controls the hand muscles, it induces a twitch in the muscles in the hand on the opposite side of the body. However, when one discharges the coil over the part of the motor cortex that controls the jaw muscles, a twitch is evoked in the masticatory muscles on both sides of the face. Notwithstanding this, when given appropriate feedback of the muscle's activity, most people can voluntarily activate only one masseter muscle. That is, they can suppress the bilateral cortical control circuit.

Bite forces during normal mastication

One study has reported that chewing peanuts can involve bite forces of up to 350 N, which is roughly equivalent to the force required to lift a large child! However, such forces which involve activation of all of the muscle fibre types in the jaw-closers occur only for fractions of a second during normal chewing, so fatigue of the masticatory muscle does not occur during normal function. It also is important to note that the masticatory muscles are like most other muscles in that they only very rarely contract maximally. When chewing normal western diets, the jaw-closing muscles exert only about 30–40% of their maximal force of which they are capable.

It is stated in Chapter 8 that isometric training increases the maximal forces that can be exerted by skeletal muscles. One study found that the maximal bite force of subjects who chewed sticky wax for 1 hour per day for 7 weeks increased by about 20%. This clearly explains the greater-than-normal maximal bite forces found in people who repeatedly grind or clench (brux) their teeth at night. It is entirely possible, or even likely, that the jaw-closing muscles do fatigue during prolonged, high-force, primarily-isometric contractions that may occur during bruxing, although most jaw-muscle activity during sleep is relatively low-level and often phasic.

The maximal bite force of subjects who have lost all of their natural teeth is decreased by about 50%, even when they wear well-fitting full dentures. The loss of force depends roughly on how many posterior teeth have been lost: hence partial-denture wearers usually lose less maximal biting force. This decrease in maximal biting force may be insufficient to break down foods such as meat and fresh vegetables. Chewing efficiency is also substantially diminished, with denture-wearers usually requiring 3–6 times the number of chewing strokes to break down a given food load. If the dentures do not fit well, the diet may be limited to foods such as fats and carbohydrates which are easily chewed: this clearly has adverse consequences for their nutrition and general health.

The subject of bite forces is dealt with in more detail in Chapter 7.

Role of individual muscles in chewing

There are many detailed reports of the patterns of activity in masticatory muscles and the direction of the forces that they exert during chewing. This level of descriptive detail lies outside of the scope of this chapter, which will comment on only a couple of aspects of the kinematics of chewing. The role of the major jaw-closing muscles masseter and temporalis during chewing is for the most part fairly obvious. The direction in which the muscle fibres run in these muscles indicates the direction in which they apply force to the mandible. The pattern of arrangement of the muscle fibres is quite complex in the temporalis muscle with the fibres converging in a fan-like manner on the anterior ramus of the mandible, so that the most posterior fibres pull posteriorly, and the most anterior fibres pull upwards and anteriorly.

The lateral pterygoid muscle plays an important role in several phases of the chewing cycle. It not only pulls the mandible forward during jaw opening, but also controls the rate at which the condyle returns to its fossa during jaw closing. The jaw-opening muscles are not normally required to exert much force during chewing because there is rarely much resistance to opening. Hence the role of the fast muscle fibres in lateral pterygoid is probably to help change the position of the mandible quickly during speech.

Finally, it should not be forgotten that, in jaw opening, contraction of the digastric muscles is not in itself sufficient to pull the mandible downwards. It is also necessary that the hyoid bone is held in a stable vertical position so that the digastric has a stable platform against which it can pull, and this is achieved by contraction of the infrahyoid muscles. Hence, mastication can proceed normally only when they, as well as the digastric muscles, are appropriately activated.

Role of tongue in mastication

Everyone knows that despite its proximity to the teeth and its role in positioning food between the teeth, the tongue is usually not bitten while food is being chewed. However, it does not require a conscious effort to keep the tongue out of harm's way. It is clear that the position of the tongue during chewing must be highly coordinated with the activity of the masticatory muscles through linked control of the motor nerves to the intrinsic and extrinsic tongue muscles from the masticatory pattern generator. It should however be noted that patients will very often bite their tongue when it (or half of it) has been made anaesthetic by the lingual nerve block that usually accompanies a mandibular block injection. This emphasises the role of sensory receptors in fine-tuning masticatory control.

In addition to its other important roles in speech, breathing and swallowing, the tongue plays a vital role in the positioning of food between occlusal surfaces of the teeth for chewing, and for forming the chewed food into a bolus and pushing it into the oropharynx where swallowing is initiated.

Masticatory efficiency

People with intact and healthy dentitions take for granted the efficient and automatic mastication, or breaking down, of their food. However, measurement of masticatory function by a variety of different approaches indicates that masticatory efficiency can vary widely particularly in people who have incomplete dentitions. When masticatory ability has been assessed simply by asking subjects how well they can chew, it is usually reported that chewing ability is perceived to be substantially impaired when the number of well-positioned teeth falls below 20. In other studies, masticatory efficiency has been measured more objectively by determining people's ability to break down a test meal into smaller pieces. These studies have confirmed that chewing efficiency is reduced in most people who have lost posterior teeth and in those who wear removable dentures.

It has also been claimed that age, maximal biting force and saliva secretion rates may also influence masticatory function. However providing that the dentition is intact, age has been found not to be an important variable. Maximal bite force appears to be a factor in masticatory efficiency in people with an intact dentition but is apparently less important in edentulous subjects. This is surprising, because the inability of people with full dentures to generate relatively high biting forces is a factor that limits what they can eat. As described in Chapter 1, saliva may soften the food as it is being chewed and is important for forming the food into a bolus ready to be swallowed.

Proprioception

It is appropriate to consider proprioception of the mandible at this point. Proprioception is the sense of position in space or, for the limbs, their positions relative to other body structures. For the mandibular system, it is an awareness of the position of the mandible relative to the maxilla. This sense is particularly important in some clinical situations. It is this proprioceptive sense that tells a patient that her mandible is in its normal rest position, for example, or perhaps that it is open a little wider than the rest position. The best example of the importance of proprioception in dentistry is the everyday observation that patients can accurately detect even very small "high spots" on the occlusal surfaces of a restoration. In careful studies, it has been shown that people can detect objects between their teeth that are less than 20 μm thick when they close carefully onto them (see also Chapter 6). This obviously poses an extraordinary challenge to dentists who are restoring an occlusal surface, to get the height of the restoration correct.

Despite its importance clinically, the proprioceptive sense of the masticatory muscles is not fully understood. Hence, to understand the mechanism underlying the sense of the position of the mandible relative to the maxilla, we need again to extrapolate from studies on the limbs, where the mechanisms of proprioception have been studied carefully. It turns out that the proprioceptive acuity of the limbs is very high even at very complex joints like the shoulder which has many degrees of freedom in which it can move. Changes in the position of the shoulder joint of even a degree or so in any direction are easily detected. What mechanisms are responsible for this extraordinary level of proprioceptive acuity? In this brief discussion, we will consider proprioception only in the context of the sensory receptors that signal it, as the central processing of these signals by the nervous system that results in the conscious awareness of the joint's position is immensely complex.

Most recent studies have concluded that proprioception in the limbs arises largely from muscle spindles, although inputs from cutaneous receptors can be quite important, particularly in the fingers and in the face

The removal of natural teeth removes a valuable source of proprioceptive information from the central nervous system. What happens, then, when the natural tooth is replaced by an artificial implant which is firmly fixed into the bone and obviously has no periodontal ligament? It has now been shown that sensory signals can be activated by pressure applied to implants: indeed, the term *osseoperception* has been coined to describe the perception of mechanical stimulation applied to a bone-anchored prosthesis. The replacement of full dentures with implant-supported prostheses results in improved tactile ability (as well as improved motor function). However, these capabilities are still less than those in people with their normal dentition. (Note that the expression "osseoperception" is a little misleading as there is no evidence that sensory receptors in bone itself are responsible for the sensation.)

(Chapter 6). Joint receptors appear to play a very minor role. Even when the normal hip joint and its capsule including the joint receptors is completely removed and replaced with an artificial joint, there is little or no detectable decrease in the proprioceptive acuity at the hip joint.

In the masticatory system, therefore, proprioception is also likely to arise primarily from the muscle spindles in the jaw-closing muscles (remember that the jaw-openers have no spindles), as well as from other mechanoreceptors in and around the mouth. Muscle spindle receptors are exquisitely sensitive to stretch, and have the ability to signal the length of the jaw-closing muscles and, by inference, the vertical position of the mandible relative to the maxilla.

It is likely that other sensory receptors also contribute something to the sense of jaw position. For example, mechanoreceptors in the skin of the face are activated when the perioral skin is stretched during jaw movements. It has been claimed that receptors in the TMJ are important in conscious awareness of the position of the jaw, but for reasons given earlier in this chapter, this is almost certainly not the case except when the jaw is stretched wide open.

In the light of the knowledge that muscle spindles and cutaneous receptors are largely responsible for proprioception in the limbs, let us return to the question of how patients are able to detect a restoration that is only a few microns too high. As mentioned above, most normal subjects can detect the presence of metal foils that are only 20 μm thick when they close gently down onto them. Even when both the upper and lower teeth (and therefore their periodontal mechanoreceptors) have been locally anaesthetised, patients are still able to detect foils that are only about 80 μm thick. Hence, while the detection of a high spot on a restoration is assisted by the mech-

anoreceptors in the periodontal ligaments of the teeth that are in contact, other proprioceptors must also play an important role.

In fact, it is not been shown definitively which receptors are responsible for detecting high spots when the opposing teeth are locally anaesthetised. It is possible that the some of the signals that give rise to the recognition of the high spot come from other teeth particularly on the other side of the mouth which are not anaesthetised: these are presumably signalling that the force being applied to them is different from what occurs when the teeth come fully into occlusion. However, it is equally likely that the muscle spindles are signalling to the brain that the jaw-closing muscles on one side of the head are a tiny bit longer than they are when the teeth are fully occluding. This idea is supported by the observation that even patients with full dentures can still detect quite thin foils, perhaps 7–8 times thicker than those identified by patients with natural teeth. A definitive answer to this intriguing question awaits an answer from some well-designed experiments.

■ Disorders of mastication

The most common disorder of the masticatory system is, of course, the chewing inefficiency that is the result of the loss of teeth. Chewing efficiency falls particularly sharply when posterior teeth are lost. To compensate for the decreased chewing efficiency, people with depleted dentitions chew for longer periods and swallow larger food particles. The good news is that a substantial improvement in chewing efficiency in the partially edentulous patient can be obtained by appropriate prosthodontic treatment.

The loss of all of the teeth leads to an even more dramatic reduction in chewing ability.

Even well-fitting full dentures restore only a fraction of the functional efficiency of a natural dentition. It was mentioned earlier that the ability of patients with full dentures to break down test meals is greatly diminished: commonly, they needed to chew each mouthful 3–6 times more often than people with natural teeth to reduce the food particles to the comparable sizes. Their ability to chew is reduced even further when they consume tougher food.

Part of the reduction of function in the denture-wearer is the result of a decrease in the maximal amount of force that they have available to chew. A number of studies have reported that the maximal unilateral bite force of denture wearers is between 75 and 140 N, compared with the forces produced by the dentate subjects in those studies that ranged from 350 to 550 N. This level of reduction in maximal bite force is sufficient to limit the range of foods that edentulous people can eat, as foodstuffs like meat and even hard bread may require bite forces of more than 150 N. Thus, the inability of full-denture wearers to generate sufficient chewing forces clearly has the potential to lead to dietary deficiencies.

The reason for the diminished maximal bite force has not been established. It is likely that it results partly from the lack of mechanical stability of the artificial teeth on their supporting platform, and partly from the atrophy of their jaw-closing muscles that results from diminished use.

Although it is difficult to quantify, it is certain that the loss of important sensory signals from the periodontal receptors in edentulous people also contributes to the loss of chewing ability by reducing the fine control of the masticatory muscles.

Chewing ability is substantially improved when a mandibular denture is supported by oral implants. Such patients can bite up to twice as hard than patients with a conventional full denture, although even this force is still only about 70% of what can be generated by subjects with natural dentitions.

Temporomandibular disorders

Orofacial pain syndromes are dealt with in Chapter 4, but the topic of temporomandibular disorders (TMDs), which is a family of clinical problems that involve the masticatory musculature, the TMJ and associated structures, or both, will be touched on briefly here for completeness. Despite variations in the clinical presentation of these musculoskeletal disorders these disorders have three cardinal signs, namely, pain, joint sounds such as clicking and crepitation, and functional interferences such as restriction and deviations during jaw movements. The aetiology of the TMDs is largely unknown and the management will therefore be mainly symptomatic. Pain from the musculoskeletal tissues will influence the mastication probably both at a conscious level, i.e., the patient is careful not to chew too hard or open the jaws too wide, but also at reflex level involving the coordination of nociceptive signals from the painful site in the central pattern generator and other pre-motor neurons in the brainstem. As a consequence, pain is associated with limited jaw-opening, less forceful contractions and generally longer chewing cycles. This change in coordination of mastication has been termed an adaptation to pain.

Once it was believed that excessive grinding or clenching teeth, which commonly is referred to as bruxism, was the cause of TMD problems: today, however, sleep bruxism is viewed as a disorder which involves excessive activation of the central pattern generator. Many studies have shown that bruxism alone not can explain the TMD problems but that it may be a risk factor. Factors like stress, medication, alcohol and personality traits may predispose to bruxism, but it is generally accepted that occlusion or high contacts in the occlusion do not initiate bruxism. The anatomical and pathophysiological origin of the muscle and joint pain in people who brux has not been clearly established, and may have many causes. Even factors such as the personality of the patient may contribute to susceptibility to this disorder. Interestingly, it has been shown that the people who brux the most have the fewest pain symptoms, although of course, their teeth wear badly. In this case an occlusal splint is an effective approach to protect the teeth from further wear.

Rather surprisingly, the different therapeutic interventions that are used, ranging from wearing mouthguards to antidepressive medication have similar success rates in most forms of TMD. This points to a significant psychogenic component in this disorder that responds to "being treated" in a general way rather than to the specific efficacy of a particular treatment.

Neuromuscular diseases

In marked contrast to swallowing (see Chapter 10), chewing is relatively immune to most neurological disorders. Even strokes usually do not have a profound impact on the masticatory system: this is doubtless the result of the strong, bilateral, cortico-bulbar control of the masticatory muscles.

The masticatory system is often adversely affected in *myasthenia gravis*, an auto-immune disorder of the neuromuscular junction that affects all skeletal muscles (see Chapter 7). The disease is characterised by an abnormal feeling of weakness and loss of muscular strength, which can adversely affect chewing. A recent study of patients with this disorder reported that maximal bite forces were reduced to about 50% compared with those of matched control subjects: however, the level of decrease in biting force will continue to deteriorate as the condition advances.

Persons suffering from *bulbar myasthenia gravis*, which affects only the cranial nerves, may also have difficulty swallowing.

Damage to the neural mechanisms that control the tongue can certainly impair chewing by reducing the ability to position food accurately between the occlusal surfaces of the teeth. The motor nerve to the tongue is the hypoglossal (XII). It can be injured during neck or intracranial surgery (so-called lower motor neuron lesion) but it is more common for higher centres that control the hypoglossal motor nucleus to be damaged (upper motor neuron lesion). As one would predict, loss of unilateral control of the intrinsic and extrinsic muscles of the tongue results in significant deficits in tongue control which then impair the positioning of the food bolus between the teeth during chewing.

The lingual nerve (trigeminal) is more susceptible to damage where it courses through the mouth near to the mandibular foramen. Most commonly, damage occurs during the extraction of third molar teeth, which results in unilateral loss of sensation from the surface of the tongue. Most dental patients will have experienced this sensation on a temporary basis when the lingual nerve is blocked together with the mandibular nerve with local anaesthesia. Strictly speaking, the effect of unilateral lingual anaesthesia on masticatory efficiency is relatively slight, although the anaesthetic tongue, lacking protective reflexes, is very prone to be bitten.

Summary

Chewing is the first step in the digestion of food. It is a complex process that involves the precise control of a number of muscles including those in the tongue, and is integrated with swallowing. Mastication is a semi-automatic, cyclical process in which a basic rhythmical signal originating in a pattern generator in the brainstem alternately activate the jaw-opening and the jaw-closing muscles. This basic opening and closing movement is fine-tuned by a number of complementary reflexes which automatically adjust the activity of the motor neurones controlling the muscles to compensate for unexpected changes in the texture of the food, and to ensure that the teeth come correctly into occlusion in each closing movement.

Selected references

Bakke M. Mandibular elevator muscles: physiology, action, and effect of dental occlusion. Scand J Dent Res 1993;101:314–431.

Lund JP, Kolta A, Westberg K-G, Scott G. Brainstem mechanisms underlying feeding behaviours. Curr Opin Neurobiol 1998;8:718–724.

Takada K, Yashiro K, Sorihashi Y, Morimoto T, Sakuda M. Tongue, jaw, and lip muscle activity and jaw movement during experimental chewing efforts in man. J Dent Res 1996;75:1598–1606.

Türker KS Reflex control of human jaw muscles. Crit Rev Oral Biol Med 2002;13:85–104

Woda A, Piochon P, Palla S. Regulation of mandibular postures: mechanisms and clinical implications. Crit Rev Oral Biol Med 2001;12:166–178.

Swallowing

Timothy S. Miles

Goals:
- To understand the physiology of swallowing and vomiting in adults.
- To point out how infantile swallowing differs from adult swallowing and to discuss the possible significance of this in dentistry.
- To describe some of the major common disorders of swallowing and vomiting.

Key words:
Swallow; gag; vomit; nausea; retch; infantile swallow; tongue thrust; swallowing centre; dysphagia; aspiration.

■ Introduction

All dentists must deal with patients who swallow or, worse, gag or even vomit during treatment. This is inconvenient for the dentist and uncomfortable for the patient. What triggers these behaviours, and what can the dentist to control them? This chapter looks in detail at swallowing and the closely related activity of vomiting from the dentist's perspective.

The primary function of swallowing is of course to move food and liquid from the mouth to the stomach. However, while this is the context in which we usually think about swallowing, it is much easier to understand the sequence of events that occur during swallowing if one considers this activity in terms of its role in protecting the airway from the potentially catastrophic ingress of food and fluid. In the course of transporting food through the pharynx, the highly-coordinated swallowing response seals the back of the nose and the entrance to the trachea to prevent the entry of foreign bodies into these vulnerable areas. Fig. 1 shows that these mechanical barriers to the entry of food and liquid into the airways (particularly the lungs) are vitally important because the respiratory tract and gastro-intestinal tract cross over each other in the pharynx, and there is clearly a substantial risk that food might pass into the airway and, worse, into the delicate tissue of the lungs.

The complexity of the swallowing response is illustrated by the fact that it involves 25 pairs of skeletal muscles in the pharynx, larynx and oesophagus, as well as the smooth muscle in the oesophagus. It is absolutely essential for the timing and sequence of activation of all of these muscles to be correct for the act of swallowing to

Figure 1. Schematic diagram of the human head and neck, showing the airways and the gastro-intestinal tract crossing in the pharynx. The powerful, feedforward swallowing reflex prevents food passing into the larynx by pulling the epiglottis downwards to cover it (respiration also ceases and the glottis closes) and elevates the soft palate to prevent the food from entering the rear of the nose.

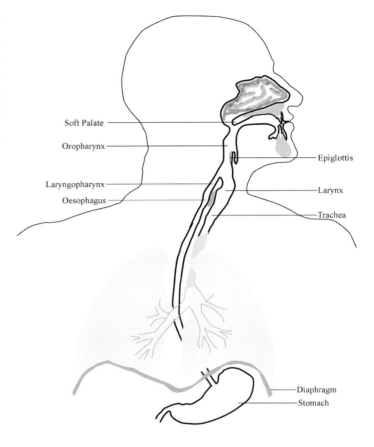

Soft Palate

Oropharynx

Laryngopharynx

Oesophagus

Epiglottis

Larynx

Trachea

Diaphragm

Stomach

proceed normally. This is achieved by a control centre in the brainstem which not only controls the responses that comprise swallowing but integrates them with both mastication and with respiration. The neural circuits that control swallowing are complex, and involve interactions between a number of nuclei that lie just deep to the floor of the fourth ventricle of brainstem. A schematic illustration of some of the important nuclei and their connections is shown in Fig. 2. This shows that swallowing can be initiated by sensory signals arising in the area of pharyngeal mucosa of pharynx that is innervated by the superior laryngeal nerve. These signals pass to the nucleus of the solitary tract, where the complex interactions between the brainstem nuclei then occur, resulting in the activation of nerves that control various muscles in the larynx and pharynx, and the initiation of swallowing. Swallowing can of course be initiated voluntarily, as by the descending inputs to the swallowing circuits shown schematically in Fig. 2.

Despite its complexity, swallowing can be considered to be a reflex response, because the appropriate stimulus will cause it to occur in a highly stereotyped manner. In engineering terms, this would be called a "feedforward" response because, once initiated, the complex pattern of responses is carried out without the need for modification from sensory signals. Indeed, once the pharyngeal phase of swallowing begins, it cannot be voluntarily stopped. Obviously, it is very different from mastication in this regard.

The normal swallowing frequency in healthy individuals is about 600 times during a 24 hour period; however, this varies widely. The frequency decreases to about six times per hour during sleep when the production of saliva is minimal. With a normal dentition and salivary flow rate (see chapter 1), swallowing will happen after about 20–30 chews. After a swallow a small volume of saliva of about 0.8 ml will remain in the mouth. Most of these swallows are to dispose of mucus and saliva, and the number of swallows that transport a chewed food "bolus" (which means, literally, a "ball") is

relatively low. In experiments in which water has been infused into the mouth, it is found that a volume of 1–3 ml of water elicits a swallow. However, when eating, the number of chewing strokes before the food is swallowed depends on the size of the food particle and the concentration of particles in the bolus.

Because the events that comprise swallowing are so complex, it is usual to consider this integrated response as a series of overlapping phases. Note that the pattern of adult swallowing described below differs in some important ways from the infant swallowing pattern which is described later in this chapter.

Oral preparatory phase

In this stage the food is chewed and mixed with saliva to form a moist, cohesive bolus ready to be swallowed. The time taken for chewing depends on many factors including the efficiency of chewing and the eating habits of the chewer. Some people deliberately linger over this oral phase in order to savour the food that they are eating.

True swallowing begins when the tongue pushes the chewed bolus, which is by this stage coated with lubricating mucus from the salivary glands, into the pharynx. This is the only part of this complex response that can be interrupted voluntarily. A similar sequence of events occurs when a liquid is swallowed. Cine-radiographic studies have shown that each swallow that occurs during normal feeding is imbedded in the chewing cycle; that is, swallows are integrated with normal rhythmic chewing movements so that the latter are interrupted only transiently when swallowing is initiated, and then resume quickly after the pharyngeal stage of swallowing is completed.

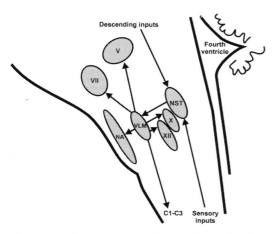

Figure 2. Brainstem structures involved in swallowing. Many brainstem nuclei are involved in the control of swallowing including the trigeminal (V), facial (VII), vagal (X) and hypoglossal (XII) nuclei, the nucleus ambiguus (NA), and other groups of neurones in the nucleus of the solitary tract (NST) and ventrolateral medulla (VLM). These are interconnected in a complex pattern. Swallowing is initiated by sensory inputs from mechanoreceptors in the pharynx or voluntarily, by descending pathways from higher centres in the brain.

To stabilise the mandible so that the swallow can begin, the teeth are brought together by the jaw-closing muscles, and the lips usually seal. The intrinsic tongue muscles then push the tip of the tongue against the palatal surface of the upper (or sometimes the lower) incisor teeth and form a groove in the tongue along which the muscles push the food bolus. This process is aided by the cheek muscles such as the buccinators, which help to propel the bolus towards the pharynx.

Pharyngeal phase

When the food bolus comes into contact with the mucosa of the pharynx and larynx (including areas such as the soft palate, uvula, dorsal surface of the tongue, faucial pillars, dorsal pharyngeal wall, particularly around the epiglottis (an area innervated by the inferior laryngeal nerve), it activates mucosal mechanoreceptors that send sensory signals along the glossopharyngeal and vagus nerves to the nucleus of the solitary tract, from where they are sent to the nucleus ambiguus in the brainstem. These and other interconnected nuclei in the medulla near the floor of the fourth ventricle comprise the so-called "swallowing centre" that controls the sequence of the events manifest as a swallow (Fig. 2). After appropriate processing of the sensory signals, these motor nuclei send out signals along the glossopharyngeal and vagus nerves to activate the many muscles that are involved in swallowing. The sequence of activation of these muscles is complex and must be very precisely timed in order to prevent the food or liquid from entering the airway, and to move the bolus into the oesophagus. For simplicity, we will consider these events to be happening sequentially, although in reality there is considerable overlap in the timing of the activation of the various muscles and their related biomechanical events.

The next event in this complex sequence of events is the inhibition of respiration. The soft palate is elevated to seal the back of the nasal cavity. This is the result of contraction of the levator palatini (innervated by the vagus nerve) and tensor palatini (innervated by the trigeminal nerve). The glottis (vocal cords) closes and seals the entrance to the trachea. The entrance to the larynx is pulled upwards into the pharynx to a level at which food is less likely to enter it. This is achieved through the combined action primarily of the trigeminally-innervated mylohyoid muscle, and to a lesser extent by the thyrohyoid and geniohyoid muscles (both innervated by the first cervical nerve) which pull the larynx anteriorly.

Champion beer drinkers (known as "scullers" or "chug-a-luggers" in diferent parts of the world) can "scull" or "chug" a full glass (or in some cases a jug) of beer extremely quickly. These people, most of whom seem to be University students, have learned to swallow without the usual elevation of the hyoid bone and larynx. Their pharynx expands as a reservoir and the cricopharyngeus relaxes to allow liquids to enter directly into the oesophagus. Sword swallowers have also learnt to overcome the normal pattern of swallogwng, and can swallow a sword by voluntarily relaxing their cricopharyngeus muscle and keeping the oro-pharyngeal passage open. In this situation, descending inputs have over-ridden the powerful reflex responses of the brain stem.

The vocal cords are adducted by the intrinsic laryngeal muscles (lateral cricoarytenoid, interarytenoid, transverse arytenoid and cricothyroid), all of which are controlled by the vagus. The epiglottis tilts backward over the larynx (aryepiglottic muscles innervated by vagus nerve), which has the effect of deflecting food or fluid so that it flows around the sides of the entrance to the larynx.

The so-called pharyngo-oesophageal sphincter then opens, and the food bolus or liquid passes into the entrance to the oesophagus.

Once the food or liquid passes, this sequence of events is reversed. The glottis reopens, the openings to the back of the nose and the trachea are restored by relaxation of the appropriate skeletal muscles, and breathing resumes. The next and final phase of swallowing then ensues.

(A fringe benefit of the pharyngeal phase of swallowing is that the activation of the pharyngeal muscles pulls open the entrances to the Eustachian tubes, thereby unblocking them and enabling the pressure in the middle ear to equalise with the pressure in the pharynx. Swallowing can therefore be used to relieve the pressure difference across the eardrum during the change in atmospheric pressure that occurs when an aeroplane is taking off and landing, or during scuba diving).

Oesophageal phase

Once in the oesophagus, the food bolus is propelled towards the stomach by *peristalsis* (partly controlled by the vagus nerve). This consists of a wave of contraction of the circular smooth muscle of the oesophagus which is preceded by a wave of relaxation. This wave of relaxation-in-front-of and pressure-from-behind the food bolus propels it along the oesophagus to the stomach.

When the bolus nears the entrance to the stomach, the gastro-oesophageal sphincter opens and food enters the stomach.

It is instructive to note the pressures involved in the oesophageal phase. Because the oesophagus passes through the thoracic cavity, the pressure within its lumen varies with the breathing cycle, and is frequently less than atmospheric (-5 to -10 mmHg). However, the pressure in the lumen of the stomach is $+5$ to $+10$ mmHg: hence, a functional sphincter is required to prevent the contents of the stomach (which are very acidic and rich in digestive enzymes) from being pushed back into the oesophagus. Intra-abdominal pressure increases in the fifth to the eight month of pregnancy: this accounts for the tendency of pregnant women to experience "heartburn", which is the irritation of the oesophagus by the acidic contents of the stomach.

Gravity does contribute to the movement of liquids during swallowing: normally, water reaches the stomach before the wave of oesophageal contraction, but it is possible to swallow liquids (and solids) while hanging upside down.

Clinical implications

It is believed that the teeth are positioned by the balance of forces exerted by the tongue, lips and cheeks. Clinically, a large, hyperactive tongue can push the teeth outwards, whereas a small or absent tongue can cause the mandible dentition to collapse inwards. However, forward pressure from the tongue during normal swallowing is unlikely to play a major role in this because the tongue/lip force ration only 2:1 during swallowing, and pressure on the teeth during swallowing would occur for only about 30 min/day. Note that swallowing can be abnormal (*dysphagia*) in some neurological disorders which affect motor function, including strokes and motor neurone disease. Special precautions must be taken during dental procedures in such instances to avoid aspiration into the lungs of fluids and solids from the mouth. This occurs because of the patient's impaired ability to prevent premature spillage of the oral contents into the pharynx, and abnormalities of the airway protection mechanism. Aspiration commonly also occurs after the swallow, if the swallow has been weak and unswallowed material remains in the hypopharynx close to the entrance to the larynx. There is now evidence that aggressive oral hygiene regimens may be a very effective means of lowering the incidence of pneumonia and respiratory infection in patients who are known to aspirate.

Cerebral palsy is another disorder in which swallowing is often abnormal. The incidence of dysphagia in children with severe cerebral palsy is reported to be as high as 70%, which doubtless contributes to the high incidence of lung infections in patients with this disorder.

Generally speaking, the basic sequential motor pattern of swallowing seems to remain nearly normal as long as the nervous structures located between the first cervical segment of the spinal cord (C1) and the trigeminal motor nuclei are intact.

■ Infantile swallow

Swallowing develops early during fetal development. The normal human fetus can swallow by the twelfth week of gestation, which is before most cortical and subcortical structures have developed in the central nervous system. By the time of birth, of course, it essential that the swallowing response is robust, so that the infant can begin to suckle immediately. However, the swallowing response is purely reflex in nature in the newborn; that is, it is not initiated "voluntarily" as it is in the more mature infant.

The pattern of activity in the newborn swallow is very different from that of an adult, and this has important implications in some clinical situations. Infantile swallowing is clearly adapted to suckling where the diet is fluid only, and the swallowing must occur with the jaws apart because the nipple of the breast (or bottle) is held between the alveolar pads. This differs from adult swallowing in which the teeth are clamped together: this stabilises the mandible and keeps the entrance to the pharynx in a stable posture. Neonates do not have teeth, and they must seal their lips onto the breast in order to extract milk, so a different strategy has evolved for this. Infantile swallowing is characterised by swallowing with the jaws (alveolar pads) apart, with the mandible stabilised by the muscles of facial expression (innervated by the facial nerve) and the tongue (innervated by the hypoglossal nerve). The infant suckles by sealing the lips around the nipple of the breast or feeding bottle and drawing the nipple well back into the mouth. The tongue protrudes through the lips and literally "milks" the milk from the breast with powerful thrusting movements. At the same time, the mother's milk ejection reflex causes the milk to spurt from the nipple so that the milk is deposited directly into the pharynx.

As in adults, the infant's swallowing reflex leads to precisely-timed repositioning of structures in the pharynx and larynx, but the outcomes of these movements are quite different. The anatomy of the infant pharynx allows the laryngeal complex to be elevated so that the epiglottis sits behind the soft palate. In swallowing, therefore, the entrance to the infant larynx is elevated so that the epiglottis sits behind the soft palate which is then positioned in the vallecular space just in front of the epiglottis. In effect, this arrangements forms a functionally continuous tube from the nose through the larynx to the bronchi and enables uninterrupted breathing even during swallowing. Milk then passes around the sides of the larynx into the oesophagus, and respiration is not inhibited during swallowing.

As the infant matures, its swallowing pattern is progressively modified in response to a number of important changes. Firstly, the anatomy of the pharynx changes. It becomes progressively more elongated so that the epiglottis can no longer be locked-in behind the soft palate during a swallow. Secondly, the consistency of the food changes from liquid to semisolid and solid; and finally the teeth erupt. As a result of these changes, the tongue no longer protrudes between the teeth during swallowing, but rather is positioned with its tip near the incisive foramen. The position of the mandible is now stabilised by the jaw-closing muscles holding the teeth in occlusion rather than by the tongue and cheek muscles. This transition occurs gradually until, around 18 months of age, the adult swallowing pattern is well established. Note, however, that one study found that 11% of adolescents continued to protrude their tongues during swallowing in order to make a good lip seal.

Tongue thrust

There is a continuing debate about the extent to which a continuing, infantile-style, tongue-thrust swallow may damage the occlusion and possibly even influence mandibular growth. The arguments in favour of the damage model point out that people may swallow 600 times per day or more and that, if the tongue continues to be thrust forward with each swallow during the phase of rapid growth, it will prevent the anterior teeth from growing into their normal occlusal relationship, producing an anterior open bite with protruding teeth.

Opponents of this model argue that even though the tongue may press on the anterior teeth with forces of up to 20 N during a swallow, the total duration of tongue thrusts is not sufficient to cause an open bite. Each swallow lasts for about one second, so 2000 swallows will result in tongue thrust pressure against the teeth for only about 30 minutes per day. However, teeth will normally move only when a force is applied to them for 8 to 14 hours per day. Furthermore, of all the children who do have tongue-thrusts, only about one in ten develop this form of malocclusion.

At the other end of the age spectrum, older denture-wearers and those who have worn full dentures for a long time often swallow without tooth contact and without the tongue applying much force to the denture.

Dysphagia

Dysphagia is the subjective sense of difficulty in swallowing which is caused by impaired progression of food or liquid from pharynx to stomach. Most patients with this condition complain that food "gets stuck" on the way down, a sensation that may be painful. Dysphagia can be the result of lesions of the pharynx, oesophagus and adjacent organs resulting, for example, from cancer or surgery. It is also a common symptom in a number of functional disorders of the neuromuscular system, including stroke, cerebral palsy, multiple sclerosis, Parkinson's disease and scleroderma.

Dysphagia is a complex topic in its own right. For example, dysphagia may be *pre-oesphageal*, resulting from abnormal function proximal to the oesophagus. This is usually caused by neurological or muscular disorders that affect skeletal muscles, such as motor neurone disease. Patients with pre-oesophageal dysphagia often suffer regurgitation into the nose, or aspiration into the trachea followed by coughing.

Patients with *oesophageal dysphagia* have difficulty moving food through the oesophagus. This may be the result of obstructive disorders (e.g., cancer or strictures of the oesophagus) or motor disorders. Patients with this condition may have difficulty swallowing solids, but be able to swallow liquids without difficulty.

Dysphagia is sometimes confused with "globus" sensation, which is the feeling of having a lump in the throat that is unrelated to swallowing and occurs without impaired transport of food or liquid. Globus sensation is emotional in origin, and often associated with feelings of anxiety or grief. The current view is that a thorough investigation will find a motility disorder in the majority of individuals with this complaint. Most commonly, there is a problem in the oesophagus which appears to cause referred sensation of discomfort to the pharynx.

The treatment of dysphagia usually involves specially-trained allied health professionals: in different parts of the world, these may include speech-language pathologists, occupational and physical therapists and registered dieticians.

Vomiting, gagging and retching

Vomiting is a response which is very closely analogous to swallowing although, of course, the liquids and solids travel in the opposite direction! Vomiting is induced by gastric distension or irritation, mechanical stimulation of the pharynx, or some drugs (including narcotics and chemotherapeutic agents). Like swallowing, vomiting is a highly-coordinated response involving many muscles, which is coordinated by its own specialised area in the brainstem.

Vomiting is usually preceded by pallor, sweating and salivation, reflecting the activation of the sympathetic nervous system.

Vomiting is usually said to have three stages (although would seem reasonable to consider the prodromal autonomic phase to be an additional, first stage). Conventionally, though, the first stage is *nausea,* characterised by a sudden feeling of "sinking" in the epigastrium, which is due to a loss of the normal tone of the smooth muscle in the wall of the stomach. This may (or may not) progress to the second stage of *retching* or *gagging.* Retching or gagging consists of unpleasant spasmodic and abortive respiratory movements with the glottis closed. The words retching and gagging seem to be used rather interchangeably, although most clinicians would probably agree that retching is a slightly more violent version of gagging. Whether or not this is so, the responses are sufficiently similar to be treated as the same thing from the functional perspective. Retching/gagging is a reflex which can be triggered by mechanical stimulation of the faucial pillars, the base of the tongue, the soft palate and the posterior pharyngeal wall. A common stimulus for patients reclining in a dental chair is the accumulation of fluid in the pharynx which cannot be swallowed. The taking of dental impressions can also lead to gagging if the impression material overflows from the back of the impression tray and comes into contact with the pharyngeal trigger areas.

Stimulation of salivary secretion occurs during retching. Saliva confers some protection against the corrosive effects of the acids and digestive enzymes that are found in the stomach contents, if these are subsequently ejected into the mouth.

The pharyngeal stimulation sends signals to the vomiting area in the brainstem, which triggers simultaneous contractions of the pharyngeal constrictor muscles, as well as the inspiratory muscles of the chest and the diaphragm and activation of the anterior abdominal muscles. Together, these squeeze the stomach between the diaphragm and the anterior abdominal muscles. The smooth muscle of the stomach also contracts.

The gag reflex is easily conditioned. A subject who has gagged when having a dental impression made may on subsequent occasions begin to gag at the sight of the impression tray or even just the smell of the impression material. However, subjects may also learn to inhibit their gag reflex with appropriate training.

Gagging may or may not continue to the ejection phase of vomiting which is called *emesis*. This occurs when the gagging movements are accompanied by the sudden relaxation of the cardiac sphincter of the stomach. The increased intra-gastric pressure resulting from the contraction of the abdominal muscles and descent of the diaphragm then ejects the contents of the stomach up through the oesophagus into the pharynx and mouth.

Thus, vomiting is an orderly sequence of events beginning with inspiration, in which the sequence of events seen in swallowing is reversed.

Finally, there are drugs that can be used to control vomiting which are known as *antiemetics*. These range from comparatively mild agents that are used such as antihistamines that are available without prescription for the alleviation of the symptoms of motion sickness, to more powerful agents that are used during and after treatment carried out under sedation or general anaesthesia, or to reduce one of the most unpleasant side effects of chemotherapy treatment for cancer.

> The gagging and vomiting that occur in response to mechanical stimulation of the pharynx or as the result of conditioning can often be suppressed by distracting the patient's attention. Perhaps the most widely used technique is to make the patient focus on breathing slowly and continuously, as gagging and vomiting require that respiration cease. Hypnosis is also said to be an effective method for suppressing gagging and vomiting when they cannot be controlled by simpler means. Other methods including acupuncture/acupressure have their exponents, but the success of these is mostly anecdotal. In cases where gagging is intractable, usually as the result of a psychological condition, it may be necessary to consider sedation in order to conduct even routine dental treatment: propofol (2,6,-diisopropylphenol) is an agent that has been used for this purpose, although its use in children has been the subject of considerable controversy. It is also possible in some instances to manage gagging by spraying a topical local anaesthetic onto the trigger areas of the pharyngeal mucosa or by having the patient gargle with an appropriate local anaesthetic solution.

Disorders

Bulimia (often called *bulimia nervosa*) is a disorder characterized by repeated bouts of overeating and an excessive preoccupation with the control of body weight, which leads to the adoption of extreme measures to prevent the weight gain that this binge eating is likely to cause. It is often a sequel to the related eating disorder *anorexia nervosa*. One of many strategies used by patients with bulimia to prevent weight gain is to induce vomiting after binge eating. Most patients do this at least twice a week. These eating disorders occur overwhelmingly in women, with only about 10% of patients being male. The American Psychiatric Association estimates that 0.5–3.7% of American women experience anorexia and 1.1–4.2 percent experience bulimia in their lifetime.

Repeated vomiting has many consequences including disturbances of electrolyte balance and cardiac arrhythmias. However, there can also be oral complications arising from the repeated presence of vomitus in the mouth. These include acid dissolution of enamel particularly on the lingual surfaces, and break-down of metal restoration and orthodontic appliances. There is often also a decreased in salivary flow resulting in dry mouth, soreness of the mouth, throat, tongue and gums, and swollen lymph glands. The presence of these clinical signs may lead the dentist to suspect the presence of this emotional disorder. Dentists should certainly assist in the management of this disorder by minimising the oral consequences of repeated vomiting. There are other disorders in which vomiting occurs sufficiently frequently to led to intra-oral damage. For example, many people occasionally experience gastric reflux, in which the contents of the stomach are regurgitated. However, this can occur sufficiently often to lead to oesophagitis, in which case the diagnosis of *gastro-oesophageal reflux disease* (GERD) is made. If the stomach contents reach the mouth, they will have predictable oral consequences.

The sequence of events in swallowing and vomiting and the neural mechanisms that control them are now fairly well understood. A clear understanding of these will give dentists a rational basis not only for the management of issues related to these responses in normal patients, but also of patients with neurological and other disorders that affect them.

Selected references

Ertekin C, Aydogdua I. Neurophysiology of swallowing. Clin Neurophysiol 2003;114:2226–2244.

Grélot L, Miller AM. Vomiting – its ins and outs. News Physiol Sci 1994;):142–147.

Jean A. Brain Stem Control of Swallowing: Neuronal Network and Cellular Mechanisms. Physiol Rev 2001;81:929–969.

Speech

Tim Bressmann

Goals:
- To describe the physiology of speech.
- To describe the oral mechanisms in speech.
- To describe speech disorders pertaining to dentistry.

Key words:
Speech sounds; language; phonation; articulation; resonance; phonetics; prosthodontics; orthodontics; malocclusion; cleft palate.

Introduction

Almost any intervention that a dentist undertakes in the oral cavity of a patient can have varying degrees of temporary or permanent effects on oral kinaesthetic perception and oral motor control, and therefore speech production. For instance, every orthodontic or prosthodontic device that is brought into the oral cavity is a mechanical obstacle to normal movement of oral structures and speech. Most people adapt surprisingly well to structural modifications to their oral cavity. However, sometimes an intervention may leave the patient with a marked speech articulation impediment. In this case, it is important that the dentist can appreciate what has happened and remedy the problem as efficiently as possible. On other occasions, patients may seek help from their

dentist in order to improve their speech if the speech problem is related to dentition or occlusion. A basic understanding of how speech sounds are produced in the human vocal tract is therefore paramount for every dentist.

Although speech is only a secondary function of the human upper aero-digestive tract (as it is known amongst speech professionals), there are a number of special features in the human vocal tract that make it particularly apt for speech. One of these features is the relatively low position of the larynx in the neck, compared to other hominids. This enables the human vocal tract to achieve the optimal resonance across a range of differentiated vowel sounds. Although the low position of the larynx in our necks is advantageous for speech (or song), it is a natural disadvantage when it comes to swallowing: humans often gag or choke on food, which is something that rarely occurs in other mammals (Chapter 9).

Another feature that indicates that we are predisposed for speech and language is our well-developed control of the velopharyngeal mechanism that allows us to produce differentiated oral speech sounds (most consonant and vowel sounds) without having air escape out of our noses. Finally and most importantly, our brain is pre-wired to develop language, if there is linguistic input in the environment.

Speech vs. language

Human language is a complex topic, but it can be broken down into several basic components. The most important distinction is that between *language, speech* and *hearing. Language* comprises the central functions that are associated with language comprehension and use, i.e., the processing of linguistic information in the brain. *Speech* and *hearing* denote the peripheral

It is difficult to appreciate how many different languages and dialectal variations there are in the world and there is some debate between researchers about how they should be counted. There are probably close to 1,000 languages that are spoken by groups of 10,000 speakers or more but researchers who also include smaller languages and dialects in their counts arrive at over 5,000 different languages. Language is truly a human universal characteristic.

processes that are needed to produce spoken language and to receive spoken utterances. This chapter will focus mostly on speech since this is of direct relevance to the dentist. However, since speech production is inseparably interwoven with language, there will be occasional references to linguistic abilities. We will neglect hearing in this chapter because it pertains less directly to dentistry.

The neurophysiology of speech and language

The localization of language functions in the brain is a fascinating research topic for neurologists and neurolinguists. However, there are still many more questions open than answered. Because the brain is such a complex structure, research about the localization of cognitive functions focuses mainly on acquired brain injuries such as strokes or traumatic brain injuries. These injuries can result in highly localized neurological lesions and the resulting functional impairments may speak to the responsibilities of the affected structures. Generations of stroke and accident victims have contributed to a basic understanding of the role of different areas of the brain in language. According to the general consensus, acquired disorders of language processing and production (aphasias) are mostly the result of lesions in the cerebral cortex of the left hemisphere. While the right hemisphere probably contributes to speech melody (prosody), most linguistic processing takes place in the left hemisphere in the majority of people. Isolated lesions in the inferior aspect of the left frontal lobe (Broca's area) often result in slow, laboured language production with only rudimentary grammatical structures. However, such patients usually have relatively good language comprehension. Isolated lesions around the posterior end of the left sylvian fissure (Wernicke's area) can result in speech that is more fluent but sometimes devoid of meaning. Patients with lesions in this area usually have comparatively poorer language comprehension.

When the linguistic form for a word or a phrase has been found, speech production begins in the motor areas of the brain. The main structures responsible for motor coordination of the articulators are found bilaterally in the pre-central gyri. From there, nerve impulses are fed to structures in the midbrain through the pyramidal system where the articulatory gestures are fine-tuned. The main cranial nerves that are responsible for voice production and articulation of speech sounds are the trigeminal (V, control of jaw movement and cranial facial sensation), the facial (VII, lip movement), the vagus (X, pharyngeal and laryngeal muscles, pharyngeal and laryngeal sensation) and the hypoglossal (XII, tongue movement). Speech production is a highly coordinated fine-motor task that involves a multitude of muscles. In order to facilitate understanding and help with diagnoses, motor speech is usually broken down into several functional subsystems.

Functional subsystems of motor speech

Speech is a motor activity and consequently can be mapped onto anatomical structures of the articulatory tract. Operationally, speech production is broken down into five separate, but interacting functional subsystems:

1. *Respiration*: Airflow from the lungs is necessary to drive the larynx and generate voice and speech. The main muscle of inspiration is the diaphragm which increases the volume of the thorax and compresses the abdominal cavity as it contracts. This creates a negative (i.e., sub-atmospheric) pressure in the chest, causing air to flow in and fill the lungs. During a normal passive expiration, the diaphragm relaxes and its recoil reduces the volume of the thorax, leading to expiration. In more forceful inspiration and expiration, a number of other costal and abdominal muscles may be recruited. It follows from this that respiratory disorders can result in inefficient or insufficient breath support for speech.

2. *Phonation (sound production)*: When the vocal folds in the larynx are in position for phonation, the air-stream from the lungs makes the soft cover of the vocal folds vibrate. This generates a sound that is raw and unmodulated. In order to become speech, this raw signal must be filtered in the pharynx and oral cavity. Voice disorders are marked by a change in voice quality (hoarseness, roughness, breathiness of the voice) or voice quantity (pitch, loudness) that is unacceptable to either the speaker or those listening.

3. *Resonance*: As the sound passes from the larynx into the pharynx, the raw signal that has been produced by the vocal folds is amplified and filtered. The pharynx provides a resonating cavity that helps shape the sound for speech or song. The velopharyngeal sphincter mechanism also regulates the nasality of a speech sound. To form nasal sounds such as /n/ or /m/, the velopharyngeal sphincter is opened by lowering the velum or soft palate so that the sound goes through the nose. However, most speech sounds are produced as oral sounds. For these sounds, the velum

must be elevated to close the velopharyngeal sphincter so that no air goes through the nose. Disorders of resonance disrupt the normal nasal-oral balance in speech. Speakers can present with excessive nasal airflow (hypernasality) or a blocked, stuffy nose (hyponasality). These disorders can be congenital and are frequently seen in cleft lip and palate and other congenital craniofacial syndromes. Acquired resonance disorders can be caused by neurological impairment of the central and peripheral nervous structures involved with velopharyngeal control. Structural defects of the velopharynx can also result from head and neck cancer and its treatment.

4. *Articulation*: In order to produce the large variety of different speech sounds that we use to convey linguistic information in the languages used around the world, the sound stream that has been emitted from the vocal folds and filtered in the pharynx is further modified through multiple quick movements or "gestures" by the articulators in the oral cavity. Most consonant sounds are oral speech sounds, i.e., produced in the oral cavity. However, many languages of the world also use laryngeal and pharyngeal consonants. For instance, some British dialects of the English language substitute a little laryngeal clicking noise for word-medial and final "t"-sounds, so that "butter" is pronounced "bu'er".

Disorders of articulation must be distinguished from linguistic deficits such as phonological disorders. In patients with phonological disorders, the linguistic speech output planning is disrupted, which is obviously not something that the dentist could influence. However, articulation disorders that are related to structural defects of the vocal tract such as malocclusions, cleft palate, or partial tongue resections pertain very much to the dentist's work. Some articulation disorders that are related to structural anomalies can be improved by orthodontic or prosthodontic appliances as will be detailed below.

5. *Suprasegmental characteristics*: This comprises features of speech such as pitch, inflection and rhythm of speech and is also referred to as prosody or "speech melody". Beyond the linguistic content of a phrase, the emphasis that a speaker puts on words gives important information about his or her emotional and physical state. Obviously, suprasegmental characteristics are the compound result of events in the other four areas of motor speech and cannot be mapped onto any particular organs.

Most suprasegmental speech disorders are related to speech fluency. In *stuttering*, the speaker experiences sudden blocks that prevent him or her from speaking a syllable or a word. In *cluttering*, the speaker blends sounds and syllables together with quick and undershooting articulatory movements, often rendering speech unintelligible.

▪ Speech articulation and the oral cavity: Active and passive articulators

When speech sounds are formed in the oral cavity, the air and sound stream from the larynx is modified by a number of articulating organs. We can distinguish structures that move actively (active articulators) and structures that provide a passive counterpart to the movement of an active articulator (passive articulators). The active articulators that move during speech are the lips, the mandible, the tongue and the soft palate. Passive articulators are the front teeth, the alveolar ridge, and the hard palate (see Fig. 1). The soft palate serves as both an active and a passive articulator: On one hand, it has an active function because it regulates the nasal-oral balance during speech. On the other hand, it can serve as a passive counterpart for the tongue when we say a sound like "k".

Description of speech sounds: The International Phonetic Alphabet

Most languages use alphabetic systems to write down speech. These alphabets are based on the speech sounds of the particular language and allow a writer to record an almost endless amount of words with very few

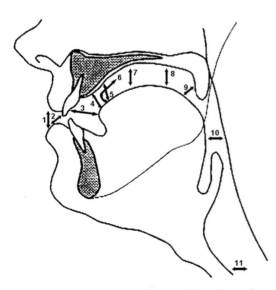

● **Figure 1** .Schematic representation of the places of articulation: (1) bilabial, (2) labio-dental, (3) dental, (4) alveolar, (5) post-alveolar, (6) retroflex, (7) palatal, (8) velar, (9) uvular, (10) pharyngeal, (11) laryngeal.

symbols. In comparison, writing systems like Chinese that are based on a symbolic notation are much more difficult to learn and to use because they require a unique symbol for every single word of the language. Most Western languages use alphabets that are very similar because they are all derived from the same Latin alphabetic system. However, while people speaking English or French may use largely the same letters, they will pronounce them differently. The phonological system of French is highly regular: Letters in a certain order will always be pronounced in the same way. For example, "-eaux" looks complicated but it will always be pronounced as "o". English, on the other hand, has an system of spelling that is irregular and complex. Take, for instance, the words "ghost", "rough" and "dough": In "ghost", the "gh" is pronounced as "g", in "rough" as "f" and in "dough" the "gh" is not audible. Consequently, transcriptions of different languages cannot really be trusted when we want to compare speech sounds. Therefore, phoneticians have developed a unified system for the transcription of speech called the International Phonetic Alphabet (IPA). The IPA uses normal typographic symbols that are found in common alphabetic systems and associates each symbol with a speech sound. This means that one writing system can be used to transcribe all the languages of the world.

Fig. 2 shows the symbol inventory for pulmonary consonants. In the remainder of this chapter, we will use a mix of orthographic and phonetic transcriptions ("orthographic" refers to conventional spelling, which is not necessarily related to pronunciation). IPA symbols that directly represent sounds of English are written between dashes without additional explanations, e.g., /p/. IPA symbols that are less intuitive are explained with an additional orthographic transcription in inverted commas, e.g., /ʃ/ ("sh").

Place of articulation

	bilabial	labio-dental	dental	alveolar	post-alveolar	retro-flex	palatal	velar	uvular	pharyn-geal	glottal
plosive	p b			t d		ʈ ɖ	c ɟ	k g	q ɢ		ʔ
nasal	m	ɱ		n		ɳ	ɲ	ŋ	ɴ		
trill	ʙ			r					ʀ		
tap/ flap				ɾ		ɽ					
fricative	ɸ β	f v	θ ð	s z	ʃ ʒ	ʂ ʐ	ç ʝ	x ɣ	χ ʁ	ħ ʕ	h ɦ
lateral fricative				ɬ ɮ							
approxi-mant		ʋ		ɹ		ɻ	j	ɰ			
lateral approxi-mant				l		ɭ	ʎ	ʟ			

Manner of articulation

Figure 2. The International Phonetic Alphabet: Pulmonary consonant chart.

Consonants

In all spoken languages, most of the linguistic information is conveyed through consonant sounds. These are also the sounds that are usually most affected by dental or occlusal anomalies, or by interventions of dentistry. Consonant sounds can be produced in a number of different ways. In this chapter, we will discuss only the main classes of English consonant sounds. Every consonant sound can be classified by three parameters: The place of articulation (i.e., the passive articulator), the manner of articulation, and whether it is "voiced" or not. For instance, the sound /f/ is produced by bringing the lower lip close to the upper incisors. If you then "switch on" your vocal folds in addition, you get the sound /v/. So, /v/ is a voiced sound while /f/ is an unvoiced sound. These subtle phonetic contrasts are important linguistically because they allow us to differentiate different words.

Classes of consonant sounds
- *Plosives*: In plosive sounds, the air stream is interrupted and then suddenly released in a little burst or explosion, hence the name. Plosive sounds of English are the bilabial /p/, the alveolar /t/, and the velar /k/ and their voiced counterparts /b/, /d/ and /g/.
- *Fricatives*: In fricative sounds, the air stream is forced through a constriction in the vocal tract, which results in turbulent, noisy airflow. Fricative sounds of English are the labiodentals /f/ and /v/, the interdental unvoiced and voiced "th" sounds /θ/ and /ð/, the alveolar fricatives /s/ and /z/ and the palatal "sh" and "zh" sounds (/ʃ/ and /ʒ/).
- *Nasals*: In nasal sounds, air exits the vocal tract through the nasal cavity, not the mouth. The extra resonances from the nasal cavities are modulated by the positions of the articulators in the oral cavity. /m/ is formed as a bilabial nasal, /n/ is an alveolar nasal and /ŋ/ (the "ng" sound in "long") is a velar nasal. The nasal sounds in English are voiced.
- *Retroflexes*: In retroflex sounds, the tip of the tongue is bent backwards. The "r" sound /ɻ/ is the main retroflex sound in English.

- *Laterals*: In lateral sounds, the body of the tongue is raised in the oral cavity and air streams past to the right and the left of the tongue. The constriction of the airflow is not tight enough to create noisy turbulences but the airflow around the tongue is accelerated (laminar). The /l/ sound is a lateral sound of English.
- *Affricates*: Affricates can be thought of as combinations of plosive and fricative sounds. Affricate sounds of English are /ts/, /tʃ/ (as in "cheese") and /dʒ/ (as in "jungle").
- *Approximants*: Approximants are consonant sounds that are similar in sound quality to vowels. Approximant sounds of English are /w/ and /j/.

Vowels

Vowels are continuous, harmonic sounds that are produced with different degrees of tongue elevation, jaw opening and lip rounding. Every syllable in speech is constructed around a vowel. Vowels amplify certain resonance frequencies of the raw glottal sound. If you say "aaaa-eeee-uuuu", you notice how the sound that comes from your larynx stays pretty much the same but the resonance of the vowels that you produce in your mouth changes. Indeed, /a/ (as in "car"), /i/ (as in "beet"), and /u/ (as in "boot") are the most "extreme" positions of vowel articulation that you can assume. In /a/, the tongue is flat against the floor of the mouth and the jaw and lips are opened maximally. In /i/, the tongue is elevated towards the hard palate. The jaw is elevated relatively high and the lips are slightly spread. In /u/, the tongue is raised towards the velum. The jaw is elevated again but this time, the lips are rounded. All other vowel sounds that we

can produce such as /e/, /o/ etc. are somewhere in between these extreme positions.

Motor coordination in speech

It is easy to see from the description of the different speech sounds that there are many degrees of freedom for the active articulators during speech production. Perceptually, it makes a big difference whether the tongue approximates the alveolar ridge or goes to the post-alveolar region, which is just a few millimetres posterior. Although this is only a small difference in articulatory place, the resulting sounds will be markedly different (/s/ vs. /ʃ/, the "sh" sound). The exact articulatory gestures require precise fine motor control and coordination of the motor speech subsystems respiration, phonation, resonance and articulation as well as the suprasegmental characteristics. On top of the precision that is required, speech gestures also have to be fast. An adult can produce speech rates of up to 250 words per minute, which corresponds to 3–5 syllables per second. As an example, say the words "spring sprouts". This takes you well under a second. However, if you look at the phonetic transcription of the same words (/spɹɪŋ spɹaʊts/), you will realize that you have just produced ten different speech sounds (the diphthong /aʊ/ and the affricate /ts/ count as single sounds). One reason why you were able to produce so many sounds so quickly is that you blended them together. You did not say "sss-p-rrrr-i-ng" by pronouncing every speech sound one at a time. This process of hitting different articulatory places in one swift movement is called co-articulation. To give you an example how far co-articulatory processes can go, say the word "handbag" out loud.

Chances are you are saying something like "hambag" (/hɛmbɛg/). The /n/ and the /d/ sound in "hand" are alveolar sounds but the /b/ is a bilabial. Because your lips had to make a closing gesture for the /b/ anyway, you saved your tongue tip a little work by assimilating the alveolar /nd/ into the bilabial nasal /m/. In fluent speech, we do not always enunciate every single speech sound but sometimes take these little short cuts. Obviously, the acquisition of a motor skill as complex as speech cannot take place over night: it takes children years to develop the speed and accuracy necessary for speech.

Milestones of speech and language development

All children are different and they may show accelerations or lags in their individual development of language abilities and speech motor skills. This means that children of the same ages can show considerable variation in their speech and language development. Even siblings of the same family may show considerable variation. For instance, it is a common phenomenon that the second child in a family often appear to lag behind the first child in terms of language and speech development. Girls are generally faster and more adept in their acquisition of speech and language skills than boys. Children who grow up in bilingual environments may show minor delays until they work out how to learn two languages simultaneously. Although some variation across different children is normal, there are some milestones that are usually met at particular ages. These milestones are summarized in Table 1. If you notice that a child lags considerably behind the expected development, further assessment by a speech-language pathologist or otolaryngologist is warranted.

◼ Normal development of articulation

In newborn babies, the oral space is very small. The tongue fills the mouth almost completely and newborn babies are predominately nose-breathers. Because the tongue of the newborn is too large for the oral cavity, the initial vocalizations of the baby are glottal and pharyngeal and marked by hyper-nasality. At six months of age, the oral cavity has grown considerably and the tongue no longer fills the whole mouth, the larynx starts to sink down in the pharynx and the function of the velopharyngeal sphincter matures. As the velopharyngeal closure mechanism improves, the child can start to produce oral speech sounds. At this point, the development of the consonant sounds begins with coordinated movement of the lips and mandible. The infant starts babbling in simple, repetitive consonant-vowel sequences (/mamama …/, /bababa …/). From there, articulation development progresses towards more posterior articulatory places first on the alveolus, then the palate and finally the velum.

Consonant sounds differ in their articulatory complexity. Children learn easier sounds such as /m/ or /b/ first. Sounds that require more refined motor control such as /r/ or /s/ are usually developed later. For children learning English, researchers have identified a hierarchy of developing sounds, which holds for most children. As a convenient way of explaining this hierarchy, researchers sometimes refer to the "*early 8*", the "*middle 8*" and the "*late 8*". The *early 8* are the sounds /m/, /b/, /j/, /n/, /w/, /d/, /p/ and /h/. These are the consonant sounds that are typically used in advanced babbling and in the first words. As children grow, they start mastering the more complex *middle 8* sounds /t/, /ŋ/, /k/, /g/, /f/, /v/, /tʃ/ and /dʒ/.

Table 1. Developmental milestones for language and speech.

At the end of the first year, the child should be able to ...	• lick a spoon with tongue and lips • keep the mouth predominately shut when at rest and swallow saliva • cough, shriek, coo, imitate simple sounds • babble simple syllables • modulate his or her voice to indicate mood
At the end of the second year, the child should be able to ...	• chew solid food • imitate sounds (animal or environmental noises) • speak words with simple consonant sounds • address caregivers by name • use two-word utterances • use some adjectives/adverbs • indicate basic needs using language
At the end of the third year, the child should be able to ...	• use verbs and personal pronouns (I, you, he, she etc) • refer to him- or herself by first name • ask questions • talk to him- or herself and to animals and toys • use sentences with multiple words (with occasional grammatical errors) • name pictures (e.g., in a picture book) • be understood my family members most of the time
At the end of the fourth year, the child should be able to ...	• be understood by strangers most of the time • relate events in a coherent way • produce simple, grammatical sentences • produce past tense and plurals correctly • recognize and describe complex events in picture books
At the end of the fifth year, the child should be able to ...	• produce most speech sounds and sound combinations of the target language with only occasional minor distortions • speak grammatically with only occasional minor errors • name colours correctly

Finally, the *late 8* sounds have the highest degree of articulatory complexity. These are the sounds /ʃ/, /θ/, /ð/, /s/, /z/, /l/, /r/ and /ʒ/. Even normally developing children can sometimes exhibit mild distortions on these sounds until school age.

Children (but also adult speakers) who experience difficulties producing speech sounds will commonly use one of three strategies to compensate for their inability to pronounce the sound. The simplest strategy is the *omission* of sounds. For example, the omission of final consonants or consonant clusters can be observed on many first words (/kɛ/ for "cat", /mɪ/ for "milk"). A child may also use a *substitution* in the place of a target sound that is too difficult (/dɛd/ instead of "bed"). Finally, a child could make a brave but unsuccessful attempt at producing the target sound. In this case, a *distortion* is observed. Omissions, substitutions and distortions are developmentally normal phenomena that children usually outgrow as their speech matures. However, dentists should be aware of persisting articulation errors that may indicate a speech or language disorder and consider referral to a speech-language pathologist. Special attention has to be paid to patients with congenital malformations since these patients are at a higher risk of developing speech and language disorders.

Speech disorders related to cleft lip and palate

There are many more congenital craniofacial syndromes than can be discussed in this short chapter. However, cleft lip and palate deserves some special attention because it is the most frequent craniofacial syndrome and it is also characterized by very salient and unique disorders of articulation and resonance. In cleft lip and palate, the patient is born with a cleft of the lip, alveolus, hard palate, soft palate or any combination of these. A cleft results from a disturbance of the craniofacial development sometime between the 4th and 12th week of the pregnancy. This cleft has to be repaired surgically. There are different treatment concepts but according to most treatment plans, all primary repairs are completed by the first year in order to ensure that the child has the proper oral mechanisms by the time he or she starts to speak.

However, many patients with clefts that involve the soft palate have persisting difficulties with their velopharyngeal closure mechanisms. We saw in the section on the subsystems of motor speech that the velopharyngeal sphincter is important for speech because most speech sounds are produced as oral sounds. When the velopharyngeal sphincter does not close properly during speech, air and sound escape through the nose. Many patients with cleft lip and palate exhibit hypernasal speech. We saw in the section on the normal development of articulation that velopharyngeal closure is an important prerequisite for the development of oral speech sounds. Because air pressure is

escaping through the dysfunctional velopharyngeal sphincter in patients with cleft palate, they compensate by relocating their articulation contacts below the level of the velopharynx. This is a phenomenon that is qualitatively different from the regular omission, substitution and distortion errors that are found in other speech disorders because the patients with cleft lip and palate employ speech sounds that are not found in the phonological system of their language. The result is the typical cleft palate *compensatory articulation*, which is characterized by glottal and pharyngeal speech sounds. This articulation disorder requires intervention by a speech-language pathologist.

Speech disorders related to dentition or occlusion

For speech articulation, the most crucial teeth are the front teeth. These serve as important passive articulators for the alveolar fricatives (/s/ and /z/) and the interdental fricatives (/θ/ and /ð/). Missing or misaligned teeth will often cause sound distortions ("lisps"). The often-pronounced misalignments of teeth that occur in skeletal malocclusions can interfere with the same sounds. Severe skeletal malocclusion may also interfere with bilabial closure for sounds such as /p/ and /b/. Patients with marked class III malocclusion sometimes develop alternative labiodental closure patterns because they cannot close their lips quickly enough for speech. Malocclusions may also affect labiodental approximations for /f/ and /v/. Because the lower lip is not always able to reach the upper incisors, some patients with class III malocclusions present with an inverse articulation pattern, in which the upper lip approximates the lower incisors. The severity of the malocclusion and the extent of the alveolar and dental compensation for the malocclusion will determine the extent of the speech problem. As a rule of thumb, patients with class II malocclusions are usually more successful at compensating than patients with class III malocclusions. Patients with class IIa malocclusions usually do better than patients with class IIb malocclusions. Inverted bites and crossbites usually do not interfere with speech unless they are so severe that they restrict the movement of the tongue.

Cosmetic modifications of the oral cavity

Lip and tongue piercings are relatively new fashion trends but they are probably here to stay. The main concerns for the dentist are tooth fractures and gingival recession that are often associated with intraoral piercings. However, depending on their size and location, large or multiple lip piercings may interfere with bilabial closure or labiodental approximation. Large tongue piercings can lead to distortions of alveolar and dental sounds, especially /s/, /z/, /l/, and the "th" sounds /θ/ and /ð/. If a speech problem is observed, it can usually be fixed by removing the piercing or substituting it with a smaller piece of jewellery.

Iatrogenic speech disorders relating to dentistry The Greek word "*iatros*" means "physician"; iatrogenic disorders are disorders that are a direct negative consequence of medical treatment. Iatrogenic speech disorders can be expected to occur as a result of many dental interventions but, interestingly, we have almost no information about the frequency of their occurrence and their persistence. Since these speech disorders are currently

not counted and monitored, it is also impossible to decide how many of them could be prevented.

Nerve damage following dental or orthognathic surgery will usually affect only the patient's oral sensation but not interfere with speech motor control. Speech disorders may result from loss or extraction particularly of the front teeth. These "lisps" are normal after the loss of primary teeth in children and resolve when the permanent teeth erupt. In adults, it is important that a regular frontal occlusion be restored as soon as possible.

Orthodontic appliances especially for the maxilla can be quite large and may interfere with speech. When moulding a dental retainer, the orthodontist should take care to make the palatal plate as thin as possible in order to interfere with the passive articulators as little as possible. Palatal expanders of the hyrax or the quadhelix type cover a substantial part of the palate. These appliances will usually significantly interfere with the patient's speech. This can be particularly critical in patients with articulation disorders because these patients will not be able to make gains in speech therapy while the palatal expander is in place. If a patient is already undergoing speech therapy for an articulation disorder, it is important that the orthodontist discusses the palatal appliance with the speech-language pathologist and other members of the patient's team in order to ensure that all professionals involved coordinate their timelines for treatment and that the expected benefits are carefully weighed against potential disadvantages.

Prosthetic appliances that cover the palate or the alveolar ridge can sometimes interfere with the articulation of the alveolar fricatives /s/ and /z/ as well as with the palatal fricative /ʃ/ ("sh"). It is important that the prosthodontist makes the palatal part of the prosthesis as thin as possible. If the patient finds that he or she cannot adapt to the prosthesis and that the alveolar and palatal fricatives remain distorted, a small midsagittal groove of 1–2 mm width can be cut into the palatal prosthesis. This "s-canal" has been reported to improve speech in some patients.

Throughout the life span, the motor speech systems retain some degree of plasticity and the tongue can adapt to many structural alterations of the passive articulators. However, there are physiological limits as to what can be reasonably expected of a patient. As an analogy, imagine that you had only ever worn running shoes. If you were then for some reason required to wear shoes with high heels, you could probably tolerate one or two centimetres without much difficulty, and walk and run like you did before. However, if really high and thin stiletto heels were added to your shoes, it would take you considerable time to relearn your gait for walking and you could probably never run in these shoes. Patients undergoing orthodontic or prosthodontic treatment face a very similar challenge. Intelligible and acceptable speech is invaluable for your patient and constitutes an important outcome measure for your treatment.

Prosthodontic interventions for the improvement of speech and tongue function

The insertion of a prosthesis into the velopharynx is one form of therapy for hypernasality in cleft palate patients as well as in other individuals with velopharyngeal dysfunction resulting from neurological injury or tumour surgery. In these prostheses, a palatal extension is attached to a dental retainer. There are two types of prostheses:

Speech bulb prostheses are shaped in such a way that they completely fill a residual velopharyngeal opening during speech. *Palatal lift prostheses* help to elevate a palate that is long enough but does not move enough to achieve complete palatal closure during speech. Both types of prostheses can be very successful at eliminating hypernasal speech.

Orthodontic and prosthodontic appliances can also be helpful to improve the function of the tongue in swallowing and speech. One such application is the control of the tongue position in patients with Trisomy 21 (Down syndrome). Trisomy 21 patients tend to have relatively flaccid tongues in combination with an open mouth posture that makes the tongue appear too large. In order to achieve better muscle tone and a correct rest position of the tongue against the alveolar ridge, orthodontists sometimes use retainer plates with little geometrical shapes or movable pearls moulded onto the alveolar ridge. These little modifications are usually quite successful at redirecting the movement of the tongue at rest and during swallowing in Trisomy 21 patients.

Oral cancer patients with partial tongue resections (glossectomies) may have a markedly reduced lingual movement range, which can affect speech and swallowing. Dentists can assist by "lowering" the palate or modifying the shape of the palate with a prosthodontic appliance (sometimes referred to as an "inverted tongue") so that the patient's tongue can make contact with the palate again.

Prosthodontic appliances for the improvement of speech and tongue function are usually the result of the combined effort of a dentist and a speech-language pathologist. Successful outcome must be determined not only in terms of the success of the device fabrication but also with regards to speech intelligibility, speech acceptability and quantitative acoustic measures.

How to interact with a person with a language or speech disorder

As a dentist, you will sometimes interact with patients who have speech or language disorders. It is essential that you treat these patients with respect and allow them to preserve their dignity despite the communication impairment.

Referral to specialists

As a dentist, you have the responsibility of recognizing speech and language disorders that may require further diagnosis and treatment by a qualified professional. Obviously, it is not your responsibility to undertake specific diagnostic speech and language assessments or provide therapy but it is important that you make an appropriate referral decision in order to ensure that a patient will receive timely and adequate treatment. Professions that are involved with the diagnosis and assessment of speech and language disorders are the following:

- Speech-Language Pathologists/ Speech-Language Therapists (also called Logopedists a number of European countries): These professionals assess and treat speech, language, and swallowing disorders.
- Audiologists: Audiologists are experts in the assessment and management of hearing disorders.
- Otolaryngologists: This is the main medical profession that deals with people with speech, language, and hearing disorders. The otolaryngologist will be responsible for the medical diagnosis of a patient, which usually cannot be made independently by the speech-language pathologist.

Things to remember when you are communicating with a person with a language disorder (or any person who does not understand or speak your language well):

- Adjust your language level and speak in short and simple but grammatically correct sentences. Never use "baby talk" or "foreigner's talk" ("You go radiologist – he make picture of teeth") as this will not facilitate the communication with your patient in any way. It will, however, reflect poorly on your own communication skills.
- Use frequent questions to check that the patient is understanding.
- Do not pretend to understand if you do not. Indicate to the patient how you can understand him or her better (e.g., slow down etc).
- In developmental or acquired language disorders (just like in second language learners), receptive language is usually stronger than productive language. Remember that the patient will understand more than he or she can say.
- Avoid complex linguistic constructions and long sentences as well as irony or sarcasm.
- Unless the patient also has a significant hearing impairment or asks you to speak up, you do not need to shout!

In many European countries, you may also find professionals called Phoniatricians (literally "voice doctors"). These are otolaryngologists who are specialized in speech, language and hearing disorders.

- Neurologists: These specialists should be involved in any case of speech, language or hearing disorders related to the nervous system. This includes neurodevelopmental disorders as well as acquired brain injuries or neurodegenerative processes.

Conclusions

When a dentist and a speech-language pathologist look into a patient's mouth, they see very different things. The dentist sees a complex stomatognathic system that needs to be maintained and kept it in good order. The speech-language pathologist sees a resonating cavity that allows the formation of a multitude of differentiated speech sounds through fine-motor adjustments of the articulators. Whenever necessary, both professional disciplines must seek each other's advice and input and maintain open lines of communication in order to achieve optimum treatment outcomes for every patient. No matter which area of dentistry you will specialize in, it is important for you to realize that the structures for which you are responsible play a vital role not only for chewing and swallowing but also for speech communication. It is one of your responsibilities to minimize detrimental effects of your therapeutic interventions on speech articulation.

Selected references

Crystal D. The Cambridge Encyclopedia of Language, 2nd edition. Cambridge: Cambridge University Press, 1997.

Shames GH, Anderson NB. Human Communication Disorders, 6th edition. Boston: Allyn & Bacon, 2002.

Van Riper C, Erickson RL. Speech Correction: An Introduction to Speech Pathology and Audiology, 9th edition. Boston: Allyn & Bacon, 1996.

Protective mechanisms

Timothy S. Miles

Goals:
- To emphasise that dental practitioners treat not only the entrance to the gastrointestinal tract but also the entrance to the respiratory tract.
- To describe the series of protective mechanisms that protects the respiratory tract against the entry of foreign matter particularly from the mouth.
- To point out the relevance of these protective mechanisms in dentistry.

Key words:
Inspired gases; sneeze; cough; laryngospasm; mucociliary escalator; clinical considerations.

Introduction

All patients would of course be well aware that their dentist specialises in maintaining the health of the entrance to the gastrointestinal system. However, it probably does not occur to them that their dentist is also maintaining one of the major portals to their respiratory tract. The mouth is just as important for breathing as it is for mastication, and this has important implications for dentists, their staff and their patients.

It also goes without saying that it is critical that dentists have a clear understanding of respiratory mechanisms. They need to understand the implications of manoeuvres that they perform in the mouth for the health of the respiratory tract, and they must also understand the implications of some disorders of the respiratory system to the practice of dentistry. In particular, they need a clear understanding of the mechanisms that prevent foreign objects that they introduce into the mouth from entering the respiratory tract. Virtually any object placed into the mouth by the dentist may be aspirated. There are reports in the literature of, amongst other things, rubber dam clamps, dental instruments, restorative materials, implants, broken bits of teeth and impression materials entering the airways. The risk of foreign body aspiration is increased by the conventional practice of lying the patient virtually supine for treatment. Indeed, it has been reported that dental procedures are the second most common cause of aspirated foreign bodies. Disorders such as Parkinson's disease and drugs that alter consciousness including those used in intra-venous sedation, and old age also increase the likelihood of aspiration.

The short-term consequence of foreign object aspiration is decreased ventilation of the lung: this may be compounded by laryn-gospasm (see later) if the object lodges in the larynx. Longer-term consequences include, predictably, infection of the area of the lung supplied by the obstructed bronchi-ole, and atelectasis.

The main issue dealt with in this chapter is the series of complementary mechanisms that prevent foreign particles from entering the airways, particularly from the mouth.

These are many and complex, reflecting the importance to health of maintaining a clear airway.

■ Composition of inspired air

However, before beginning, we should consider just what it is that the airways normally need to be protected against. First, there is the normal inspired air. Even so-called "clean" air contains many types of particulate matter, including dust, pollen and airborne carbon particles (which are visible as smoke). The presence of these particles can

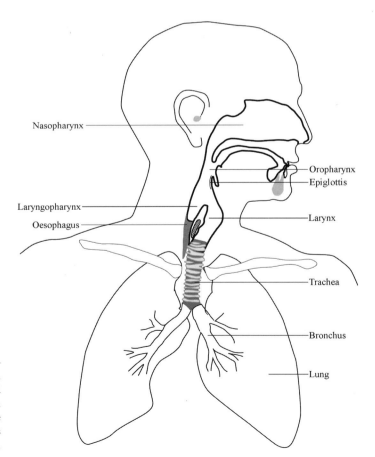

● **Figure 1.** The airway and the gastrointestinal tract cross over in the pharynx, so that the possibility exists that food or liquids which are swallowed can pass into the airway. An elaborate series of reflex responses prevents this from happening almost all of the time.

easily be confirmed by looking in a shaft of sunlight coming through a window, in which you can see the larger of these particles floating in the air. These particles do not only exist in the shaft of sunlight, of course, but are everywhere in the air!

There are also many smaller particles in the air that cannot be seen with the naked eye, including bacteria, viruses and spores.

Inspired air, particularly in cities, also contains gaseous pollutants, the largest by weight being carbon monoxide (CO) which comes chiefly from internal combustion engines, as well as oxides of sulphur and nitrogen (mainly from burning coal) and various hydrocarbons. Many of these gases are highly irritating to the mucous membranes of the respiratory tract and eyes.

The air that is inspired by dentists and their staff and patients has some special hazards. For example, unusually high concentrations of heavily-infected aerosols are generated when drills (particularly water-cooled, air-turbine drives) and sprays are used in the mouth. (Aerosols are tiny droplets of liquid that remain suspended in the air for several seconds because they are so small).

For the same engine conditions and load, diesel engines emit about 100 times more sooty particles than gasoline engines. Chronic inhalation of diesel exhaust has been linked to increased hospital admissions for respiratory diseases, chronic obstructive lung disease, pneumonia, heart disease and up to 60,000 premature deaths annually in the USA. There is also some evidence to suggest that lung cancer is linked to this pollutant.

Moreover, operative dentistry or intra-oral surgery can dislodge large particles of tooth or restorative materials that may be inhaled by the patient. These and many other dental procedures often stimulate an increased flow of saliva that tends to run into the pharynx in patients who are in a reclined or even supine position. The taking of dental impressions can provide an even greater threat of airways invasion when semi-solid impression material drips from the tray into the pharynx near to the entrance to the larynx.

So it is clear that the world in general is a dangerous place for the lungs, and that this is even more so in the dental clinic. However, despite the fact that the air inspired with every breath is laden with particulate pollutants, the alveoli of healthy lungs remain free of foreign particles and infective micro-organisms almost all of the time. The maintenance of this sterility is clearly vital since the air in the alveoli is only a micron or so from the blood in the pulmonary capillaries. It follows that protective mechanisms must operate to keep the lungs clean. In fact, most lung diseases are the result of break-down or by-passing of these defensive mechanisms, leading to the passage of inhaled foreign particles to the airways or alveoli. Viable particles may give rise to respiratory infections, and non-viable particles or gases can lead to other diseases such as bronchial carcinoma, asbestosis, etc. Allergic disorders such as asthma may result from the inhalation of either viable particles such as pollen, or non-viable particles such as smoke.

Notwithstanding the rich cocktail of pollutants that we all inhale with every breath, some people choose to supplement them still further with cigarette smoke in which pollutants such as CO, nicotine and aromatic hydrocarbons (tars) as well as unburnt carbon particles are present in very high concentrations in aerosol form. Even people who have spend much time in the vicinity of a smoker may be exposed to relatively high concentrations of these pollutants: they become so-called "passive smokers", whose risk of smoking-related diseases is higher than normal.

The relationship of smoking to various diseases is now universally accepted, but it is worth quickly recounting some of the statistics for lung cancer (which vary from one society to another). Smoking is believed to be responsible for about 30% of cancer deaths: Lung cancer is the most common cause of cancer death in western males and the third leading cause in women: About 80% of lung cancers in men and 70% in women can be directly linked to smoking. Overall, smokers are 10 times more likely to die from lung cancer than non-smokers and the risk of dying from lung cancer is 15 to 25 times higher for heavy smokers than it is for non-smokers. Cigarette smoking is also a major cause of cancers of the oral cavity (tongue, lips, gums), oesophagus and larynx. Oral cancers account for 5–10 percent of all cancers diagnosed, and 2–3 percent of all cancer deaths are from oral cancer. Long-term passive exposure to smoking increases the risk of cancer by 20–30%, and the risk of ischaemic heart disease, serious respiratory illness, asthma, and the sudden infant death syndrome in babies is also increased.

◼ Site of deposition of inhaled particles

When a mixture of particles is inhaled, the size and shape of the individual particles determine where they are deposited in the respiratory tract, and hence where various disease processes arising from their presence begin. However, many particles that are inhaled in one breath are simply exhaled in the next.

The very largest objects that are aspirated, for example during eating or during dental procedures, will lodge in areas of the airways whose diameter is too small to enable them to pass further. Objects such as artificial dentures or crowns may lodge in the larynx, or may travel further to lodge in one of the larger airways.

However, most objects that enter the airways are much smaller than this. These include airborne particles, the largest of which lodge in the nose, where the anatomy of the turbinate bones and nasal hairs causes highly turbulent airflow during inspiration and expiration. This turbulence throws the bigger particles onto the mucosa where they are trapped by its mucus coat. This mechanism is not available to people who breathe through their mouths, and consequently more inhaled particles pass into their tracheas and beyond.

Medium-sized particles (1–2 μm) which pass through the nose or mouth usually settle out gradually in the small-diameter bronchioles under their own weight and are again trapped by the mucus lining the airways. Note that there is time for them to settle out because the gases move through these airways quite slowly: this is because the total cross-sectional area of the airways after the first few branchings of the respiratory tree is very large relative to the area of the trachea.

The rate of airflow continues to decrease as the inhaled air moves closer to the alveoli. Here, the very smallest particles suspended in the air (including the smaller bacteria and viruses) are moved along primarily by diffusion, which may carry them as far as the alveoli.

Despite the large particulate load that is inhaled, the alveoli are usually both sterile and free of foreign particles. This indicates the effectiveness of the mechanisms which prevent infectious and other particulate material from reaching the alveoli. In addition to the physical barriers such as the nasal hairs and the small diameter of the bronchioles, there are a number of complementary physiological, biochemical and immunological defence mechanisms that protect the alveoli from the entry of potentially dangerous particles. There is no mechanism that protects against the entry of gaseous pollutants, however.

Sneezing

The first line of physiological defence, particularly for large particles, consists of a series of powerful neural reflexes, the first of which is *sneezing*. Sneezing is a coordinated reflex that expels foreign objects that have lodged in the nose. Sneezing is triggered by irritation of receptors in the nasal mucosa. The stimulus can be either particulate matter that activates mechanoreceptors, or chemicals such as ammonia or histamine (i.e., if the mucosa is inflamed) that irritate chemoreceptors. The large volumes of nasal mucus produced in upper respiratory tract infections can also trigger sneezing.

The stiff hairs in the nose not only physically trap particles, but also act as levers that amplify the effect of particles that alight onto them. Bending of these hairs powerfully activates mechanoreceptors in the nasal mucosa. These receptors send signals through the anterior ethmoidal branch of the trigeminal nerve to the medulla to trigger the series of reflex events that we know as a sneeze. This begins with a deep inspiration, at the end of which the glottis closes (i.e., the vocal cords adduct), and the uvula and the soft palate are depressed: this helps to direct air primarily through the nasal passages, although a considerable amount still passes out through the mouth. The expiratory muscles then contract forcefully against the closed glottis which leads to a marked increase in the pressure in both the abdomen and the thorax. Then the glottis suddenly opens, and this high pressure forces air through the nose and mouth at remarkably high speeds which often forcefully dislodges the particles from the nose and may propel them a considerable distance from the nose. It has been claimed that some particles leaving the nose during a sneeze travel at speeds of more than 150 km/hour, thus accounting for the extraordinarily loud noise made by a sneeze!

Swallowing

Surprising at is may seem on first sight, swallowing is undoubtedly the most important reflex that prevents foreign objects from entering the airways. Its importance is underlined by the fact that it is one of the first reflexes to develop in the fetus, and it is one of the last to disappear during general anaesthesia. Swallowing is discussed in detail in Chapter 9. However, it is timely to remind ourselves in this respiratory context that, while swallowing is usually thought of in terms of moving liquids and semi-solids from the mouth to the stomach, the coordinated swallowing response reflexly seals the back of the nose and the entrance to the trachea to prevent the entry of foreign bodies and fluids into these vulnerable areas. These mechanical barriers to the entry of food and liquid into the airways (particularly the lungs) are vitally important.

■ Coughing

The next major reflex that protects the airways is coughing. This is an important defence mechanism of the body that clears the larynx and upper airway of excessive secretions and foreign matter. It can be either voluntary or reflex. Reflex coughing is triggered by the presence of either foreign particles or liquid (including large amounts of mucus) on that part of the mucosa of the larynx or pharyngeal mucosa that is innervated by the inferior laryngeal nerve. Chemoreceptors that are activated by noxious gases and fumes that are located in the mucosa of the larynx and bronchi can also trigger coughing.

Again, the sensory signal is transmitted to the medulla where the motor events mechanism of coughing are triggered. The efferent pathways are primarily cranial nerve X and the cervical spinal motor nerves, including the phrenic nerve (C3,4,5).

The cough reflex consists of a series of coordinated events that is qualitatively similar to, but less violent than a sneeze. Like sneezing, coughing occurs by the establishment of a high intra-thoracic pressure which is then suddenly released. Coughing begins with an inspiration of about 2–2.5 L of air (in an adult). The glottis closes, and the abdominal muscles contract quickly and forcefully, increasing the intra-abdominal pressure and forcing the abdominal contents upwards against the diaphragm, thereby increasing the intrathoracic pressure. The internal intercostal muscles also contract forcefully. These two events cause the pressure in the lungs to in-

crease to about 100 mm Hg. The glottis is then opened, and the high intra-thoracic pressure forcibly expels the air from the lungs, sweeping the contents of the airways upwards through the larynx towards the mouth. This tends to sweep along with it the foreign object in the upper airway that triggered the cough, so that it reaches the pharynx or the mouth, where it is swallowed.

Coughing can also be triggered by irritation of the mucosa which often happens in the "dry" phase of upper respiratory tract infections. Coughing may occasionally also be the result of a centrally-initiated signal in the absence of peripheral stimulation.

The cough reflex is markedly depressed by several drugs, a factor which should be kept in mind during dental treatment. Narcotics including codeine and morphine strongly suppress coughing, and are often used clinically for this purpose as well as for pain control. Coughing is also suppressed by alcohol at a blood concentration of 0.08%, which accounts in part for the increased susceptibility of alcoholics to pneumonia. In dentistry, it is not uncommon for patients to present for treatment after taking codeine and/or alcohol to help alleviate a painful in-

It may seem surprising that up to 20% of people who drown are found to have no water in their lungs. This phenomenon is often called "dry drowning" and occurs because the initial entry of water into their larynx causes reflex laryngospasm which persists for many minutes so that they asphyxiate through being unable to breathe rather than as the result of having their lungs fill with water.

tra-oral condition. The depression or even absence of a cough reflex that these drugs induce increases in the susceptibility of these patients to the invasion of the respiratory tract by foreign particles, including those that are the result of dental treatment. One of the worst possible outcomes in this situation is the aspiration of vomit in people who are intoxicated by alcohol or who have taken narcotics either for pain relief or recreation.

The cough reflex (and/or the gag reflex discussed under swallowing) may be absent in patients suffering from severe cerebral palsy. This doubtless contributes to the high incidence of chronic lung infections in this disorder, and special precautions must be taken to avoid aspiration of the contents of the mouth during dental procedures with patients who have this condition.

Therefore, while sneezing effectively clears the nose, coughing clears the larynx and upper airways, but in a less violent manner.

If a patient inadvertently inhales a foreign particle into the airway (almost always from the mouth) and is unable to expel it by coughing, they will begin to choke, that is, to make spasmodic, forceful and unsuccessful respiratory exertions. This response is almost invariably associated with a feeling of profound panic, and is potentially life-threatening. The accepted approach to expel the object in this situation is called the *Heimlich manoeuvre* which forcefully increases the intra-abdominal and hence the intra-thoracic pressure. This is achieved by standing behind the choking person and wrapping your arms around his or her waist. Bend the person slightly forward. Make a fist with one hand and place it slightly above the person's navel. Grasp your fist with the other hand and press hard into the abdomen with a quick, upward thrust. Repeat this procedure until the object is expelled from the airway. If this fails, the final (and extreme) course of action possible is an emergency tracheotomy, in which an incision is made in the cricothyroid membrane, and a tube inserted.

Laryngospasm

This is another reflex that appears to have evolved to protect the respiratory tract, but in fact it often acts in a highly counterproductive manner that is dangerous to the patient. Intense, mechanical or irritant chemical stimuli may trigger reflex *laryngospasm* in which the glottis closes tightly, and remains closed for a long period after the stimulus is removed. If, for example, a fragment of tooth is inhaled and lodges in the larynx itself, it may trigger laryngospasm which will cause the glottis to close, leading to extreme difficulty in breathing. Laryngospasm is usually recognised by the characteristic choking sound, known as *stridor,* that it induces, particularly during inhalation. This is the result of trying to force air past the tightly-closed glottis. Laryngospasm may also result from abrasion of the vocal cords during the insertion or removal of an intubation tube, particularly if undue force is used. Laryngospasm is a life-threatening event, and must always be treated as an emergency. An ambulance must be called, and, if it is the result of aspiration of a foreign body, one should attempt to remove it by means of the Heimlich manoeuvre. Oxygen should be administered to minimise hypoxia.

Local airways reflexes

The last group of neural reflexes that help to protect the airways against particulate invasion are the so-called local airways reflexes that are activated by mechanical or chemical irritants, or antigens. These activate receptors in the bronchioles and cause a vagus-mediated reflex bronchoconstriction in the area stimulated. This tends to shunt air away from airways in which small foreign objects have lodged, or where there is inflammation. However, this can be counterproductive when the airways become sensitised to antigens, as in asthma, and the diameter of airways remains inappropriately reduced. This of course increases the work of breathing, particularly during exhalation when the airways are partially compressed by the higher intrathoracic pressure.

Mucociliary escalator

In addition to the various neural reflexes, there are other mechanisms that remove small particles and liquids from the airways. The airways are lined with mucous membrane, the most superficial layer of which consists of ciliated epithelial cells. Each epithelial cell in the mucosa has about 200 cilia which are 5–6 μm in length and gain the energy that they need to beat from ATP.

Mucus is a tough, disposable, sticky mucopolysaccharide that can bind large quantities of water, and forms stringy, sticky fibres. Its elastic recoil tends to make it form a continuous film over the surface of the airways. The sticky, viscous surface layer traps particulate matter including micro-organisms. Fig. 1 shows that the mucus lining the respiratory tract is arranged in two layers about 15–30 μm thick.

This is secreted by seromucous glands that lie deep in the in the bronchial walls and by goblet cells in the bronchial epithelium.

The seromucous cells are multicellular glands whose walls of contain both mucus-secreting and serous-producing cells. They are responsible for producing the layer of mucus that surrounds the cilia, deeper more fluid keeping them moist. The low viscosity of this more serous fluid allows the cilia to beat slowly within it. The more superficial layer of mucus is secreted by the goblet cells, which are single cells with an exocrine function. This layer is much stickier and more viscous, and traps any particulate matter that settles on it. Hypertrophy of these mucus-secreting glands is one of the cardinal

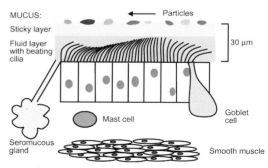

Figure 2. The "mucociliary escalator" in the airways consists of a layer of ciliated columnar epithelial cells that lines the whole of the respiratory tract, together with its overlying mucus layer and the exocrine glands that secrete mucus into the lumen of the airways. Goblet cells are single cup-shaped cells that secrete mucus. The mucus has a superficial layer that is sticky and viscous, and a deeper, less-viscous layer in which the cilia can readily move. The cilia constantly wave back and forth in a manner that moves the layers of mucus and any foreign particles that it traps, towards the pharynx where it swallowed.

signs of chronic bronchitis, when large amounts of mucus are secreted.

The cilia in both the nasal mucosa and the airways beat continuously towards the pharynx, moving the mucus lining of the airways together with any particulate matter trapped in it at about 5 mm/min. This continuous process clears the nasal mucosa from front to back every 10–15 minutes but, because the distance from the terminal bronchioles to the pharynx is much greater, the time taken to clear the bronchial mucosa may be as long as 24 hours.

The sheet of mucus and trapped particles is moved by the constantly beating cilia to the pharynx where it is swallowed. Any infective matter that has been moved from the lungs or the nose is then sterilised by the acid and proteolytic enzymes in the stomach. This arrangement is often called the muco-ciliary system or, more evocatively, the muco-ciliary escalator.

In healthy humans, 7–21 ml of mucus is secreted by the mucous glands in the airways every day. The amount secreted is controlled partly by the autonomic nervous system, primarily through the vagus nerve in the bronchioles, the facial nerve in the nose and glossopharyngeal nerve in the pharynx).

The function of the muco-ciliary escalator is adversely affected by inhaled pollutants or disease. Inflammation of the mucosa may kill the cilia. Most heavy smokers have chronic bronchitis in which the number of cilia is sharply reduced. At the same time, the rate of mucus formation is increased by the irritation arising from the smoke, which can lead to overloading of the escalator. Mucus that is not expelled into the pharynx may flow back down into the airways and alveoli, with the consequent risk of pneumonia.

■ Cellular defences

The next line of defence of the respiratory tract is at the cellular level. While these cellular mechanisms operate throughout the respiratory tract, they are particularly important in the alveoli, which have no mucous membrane and no cilia. Like most other tissues, the lungs have macrophages and leucocytes which leave the blood and enter the airways and alveoli through their walls. They are able to engulf most particulate matter and carry it to the mucociliary escalator for removal from the lungs, usually via the lymphatic system. The function of these cells is depressed by cigarette smoke, hypoxia, radiation, steroids, and alcohol.

Finally, of course, there is the immune system with its cell- and antibody-mediated defences, but these mechanisms lie within the province of immunology.

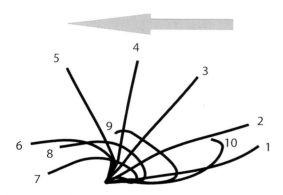

Figure 3. The action of a single cilium in a bronchiole is shown here in more detail. The ciliary process "waves" from right to left in this picture, propelling the mucus layer towards the pharynx, then rolls back to begin a new working stroke.

■ The diving reflex

We will end this review of the mechanisms that protect the respiratory tract with a brief description of perhaps the oddest of the many trigeminal reflexes. Although it is not particularly relevant to dentistry except in one small group of patients and, strictly speaking, does not act primarily to protect the respiratory system, the *diving reflex* in humans is worthy of mention if only for its curiosity value as an relic of evolution. As its name suggests, this response actually consists of a complex series of reflexes that prepares the body for diving underwater, a behaviour that is more relevant to marine mammals (and other diving species including birds) than to most humans.

The diving reflex is triggered by the contact of water with sensory receptors in the nasal mucosa, that are part of the anterior ethmoidal branch of the trigeminal nerve). This activates a control centre in the medulla that in turn triggers apnoea (cessation of breathing), bradycardia (slowing of the heart), and massive vasoconstriction of peripheral arterioles.

Although the diving reflex is a functional anachronism, it can be utilised to slow down the heart rate of a person who suffers from so-called idiopathic tachycardia. This is a condition in which the heart begins to race for no apparent reason. The rapidly-beating heart can often be markedly slowed in this situation simply by holding a wet towel on the face, thereby activating the diving reflex and slowing the heart rate.

Clinical considerations

There are a number of strategies that dentists should practise to minimise the risk of aspiration of foreign objects during treatment. Rubber dam will of course prevent objects outside of it from entering the pharynx. However, rubber dam clamps are themselves at some risk of aspiration, particularly if they accidentally spring off the tooth during placement. It is recommended that each clamp is secured by a length of dental floss with its free end outside of the mouth. Gauze packs are often used to prevent aspiration particularly during surgery and when intravenous sedation is being used. These should also be tethered by a length of floss to prevent aspiration. The dentist should be prepared at all times to remove foreign objects that enter the pharynx with high-velocity suction, or with an instrument or their finger.

Summary

A complex and interacting series of different defence mechanisms protect the lungs against the ingress of foreign particles and liquids, and deal with those that do get past them and enter the airways and alveoli. Despite the effectiveness of these mechanisms, dentists of course must do all in their power to prevent such incidents from occurring. This includes not only taking appropriate precautions during intra-oral manoeuvres, but ensuring where possible that patients are aware of the risks of having carious teeth or restorations that are susceptible to fracture. Perhaps it is wise for dentists to consider the consequences of such incidents in the context of the worst case scenario in which the patient is intoxicated by drugs or alcohol, or undergoing a general anaesthetic, when their defences will be substantially less effective.

Selected references

Cameron SM, Whitlock WL, Tabor MS. Foreign body aspiration in dentistry: a review. JADA 1996;127: 1224–1229.

Miller AJ. Oral and pharyngeal reflexes in the mammalian nervous system: their diverse range in complexity and the pivotal role of the tongue. Crit Rev Oral Biol and Med 2002;13:409–425

Nishino T. Physiological and pathophysiological implications of upper airway reflexes in humans. Japanese J Physiol 2000;50:3–14.

Shaker R, Lang IM. Reflex mediated airway protective mechanisms against retrograde aspiration. Am J Med 1997;103:64S–73S.

West JB. Respiratory Physiology: The Essentials. Lippincott, Williams & Wilkins, Philadelphia, 2000.

West, JB. Pulmonary Pathophysiology: The Essentials. Lippincott, Williams & Wilkins, Philadelphia, 2003.

Bone and calcium metabolism

Timothy S. Miles

Goals:
- To understand the aspects of bone and calcium metabolism that are particularly relevant to Dentistry.
- To describe the physiological mechanisms that regulate plasma calcium concentration and the effect of those mechanisms on bone.
- To understand the relationship between general bone health and periodontal health and disease, particularly osteoporosis.

Key words:
Vitamin D; parathyroid hormone; calcitonin; calcium balance; osteoporosis; bone grafts.

Introduction

The importance to dentists of understanding the biology of jaw and alveolar bone cannot be over-emphasised, as it is this tissue that ultimately supports the teeth as well as the various soft tissues that make the various functions of the orofacial system, including mastication, possible. This chapter reviews the physiology of human calcium homeostasis in the context of its relevance to contemporary clinical Dentistry. The primary focus will be the general physiological mechanisms that maintain the minerals in bone and the changes that result in states such as osteoporosis. The biology of the calcification of teeth is not dealt with here, as this specialised topic is dealt with extensively in other texts, including one referenced at the end of this chapter.

A brief description of the relevance of bone physiology to some specific procedures used in modern Dentistry is given at the end of the chapter. The detailed study of those topics is itself highly specialised, and also lies beyond the scope of this chapter.

Bone structure

Bone is a complex and dynamic tissue. It consists of an organic component which includes collagen glycoproteins, phosphoproteins, and mucopolysaccharides, and the inorganic component which is composed of hydroxyapatite: this gives bone its strength and hardness. Bones have an outer cortical layer which is densely calcified, and an inner cancellous structure. The cancellous bone includes a lace-like framework of *trabeculae*,

Miles

which are fine plates of bone that are arranged in a manner that gives added mechanical strength to resist specific patterns of forces applied to the bone. The cancellous bone also contains most of the cells that are responsible for the constant remodelling of the bone structure that occurs throughout life in response to hormonal and mechanical stimuli. The osteoblasts that deposit the calcified component of bone, and the osteoclasts that dissolve it are located in close relation to the trabeculae. The cells that are responsible for the formation of blood cells, and the osteoclasts and osteoblasts which differentiate from their progenitor cells, are also located within the trabecular bone.

The mandible and maxilla are generally similar in structure to the long bones, having a dense cortical shell overlying the inner trabecular layer. The alveolar bone in which the teeth are located is trabecular: however, the tooth sockets are lined with a thin layer of cortical bone into which the periodontal ligament is inserted. The trabecular bone and its capacity for rapid remodelling is what enables teeth to be moved by natural forces such as those that result from the extraction of an adjacent tooth, or by orthodontic intervention.

Calcium biology

While as dentists, we may think about calcium in terms of its role in the structure of teeth and bones, the mechanisms that control the deposition and removal of calcium from bones are really secondary to the mechanisms that maintain its concentration in plasma. That is, the bones are the first port-of-call for supplying calcium ions when they are needed to maintain the plasma $[Ca^{2+}]$: this variable must be tightly regulated because calcium is a critical factor in controlling the activity of all excitable cells. Changes in plasma $[Ca^{2+}]$ have a profound effect on the activity of these cells, with serious consequences for general homeostasis. Most excitable cells (i.e., those such as nerve and muscle cells whose membrane potentials control their activity) depend on the entry of Ca^{2+} from the extracellular fluid (where the $[Ca^{2+}]$ is relatively high, i.e. in the mM range) to the intracellular component (where the $[Ca^{2+}]$ is normally extremely low i.e. in the nM to μM range) to activate their internal machinery. As a consequence, excitable cells are highly sensitive to the level of plasma $[Ca^{2+}]$. The normal plasma concentration of the ionised free form is 1.07–1.27 mM. If this falls to critically low levels (hypocalcaemia), spontaneous contractions of skeletal muscle (tetany) may occur. If it increases (hypercalcaemia), neurological disturbances and cardiac arrhythmias are likely. To prevent these potentially devastating consequences, powerful feedback control mechanisms normally maintain the plasma $[Ca^{2+}]$ within narrow limits, and these mechanisms have important consequences for the integrity of bones, including those in the jaws.

Calcium is present in the plasma in two main forms. In this text, the expression $[Ca^{2+}]$ refers to *ionised* free calcium concentration which is the variable that is under hormonal control. However, of the total calcium concentration in the plasma (mean 2.55 mM), about 40% is bound to proteins (primarily albumin). Another 10% is bound to anions such as phosphate, carbonate, etc.

282

In addition to these important roles, Ca^{2+} are also involved in numerous other vital processes including the clotting of blood, formation of glandular secretions (including saliva) and regulation of the cardiac pacemaker. Most importantly for this chapter, calcium is of course the major component of bones: in fact, about 99% of body calcium is stored in the bones. Part of this store is available for exchange with extracellular fluid, and this fraction is the basis both for the maintenance of plasma $[Ca^{2+}]$ and the normal (and pathological) remodelling of bones that occurs throughout life. Note that under normal conditions dentine and cementum do not participate in this exchange process. Enamel is of course exposed to the extracellular fluid in saliva, and Ca^{2+} ions are exchanged freely between enamel and saliva (Chapter 1).

Calcium intake

Different authorities recommend somewhat different levels of minimal intakes: those shown below are fairly typical. It is important to note the variation in need at different ages and in different situations. While these recommendations are for minimal intakes for healthy subjects, the prevalence of both dietary deficiency of calcium and osteoporosis suggests that it is prudent to aim to exceed them.

Despite the many sources of calcium in western diets, the U.S. Department of Agriculture cites figures showing that only about 13 percent of girls and 36 percent of boys aged 12–19 in the United States consume at least the amount of calcium recommended in Table 1. This is a worrying statistic because nearly 90% of adult bone mass is established before the age of 20. If the skeletons of these people do not mineralise fully, their risk of developing clinical osteoporosis in later life is increased.

During growth, children and adolescents (in Western societies) are normally in positive Ca^{2+} balance with intake exceeding the loss in urine and faeces. Balance is usually then maintained until about 35–40 years, after which it tends to become negative with a net Ca^{2+} loss and the ensuing risk of osteoporosis. Both men and women lose Ca^{2+} at the rate of about 1% of the total body store per year after the age of 55; however, the loss accelerates following menopause in women. Following menopause, 3–5% bone is lost per year for about 5 years, before the rate of loss returns to the general age-related 1% loss per year. By age of 65, many women will have lost

Table 1. Recommended daily intakes of calcium for different ages and different conditions for healthy humans. Source: NIH Statement on Optimal Calcium Intake (2003).

Group	Recommended dailycalcium intake
Children 1–5 years	800 mg
Children 6–10 years	800–1,200 mg
Adolescents and young adults (11–24 years)	1,200–1,500 mg
Women 25–50 years	1,000 mg
Pregnant or lactating women	1,200–1,500 mg
Postmenopausal women with oestrogen replacement therapy	1,000 mg
Postmenopausal women without oestrogen therapy	1,500 mg
Men 25–65 years	1,000 mg
All women and men over 65 years	1,500 mg

as much as 25% of their total bony calcium. This clearly predisposes them to an increased risk of bone fractures including, for example, mandibular fracture during tooth extraction. It also reduces their suitability for a number of procedures used by periodontists and oral surgeons to supplement alveolar bone. Oestrogen replacement therapy (usually referred to as "hormone replacement therapy", or HRT) is effective in reducing the rate of this type of bone loss.

The major source of Ca^{2+} in the diet of European-derived societies is dairy products. However, this is not necessarily so for people of Asian and African descent, who may consume less dairy produce either for reasons of culture or availability, or because they are lactose intolerant; that is, their small intestine is deficient in the enzyme lactase which is important for digesting and absorbing lactose. Lactose intolerance does not interfere directly with Ca^{2+} uptake: rather, its consequences make the eating of dairy products less attractive. In the absence of lactase, the disaccharide lactose is not properly broken down in the small bowel and travels through the intestine unchanged. This stimulates the growth of bacteria that produce significant amounts of gas, causing abdominal cramping and diarrhoea. According to the National Institute of Diabetes and Digestive and Kidney Diseases, between 30 and 50 million Americans are lactose intolerant: the incidence is particularly high in adult African Americans (about 75%) and in Asian Americans (about 90%).

Although the gastrointestinal discomfort that arises from lactose intolerance leads to a decrease in the consumption of milk products by some ethnic groups, it is not yet clear whether or not it is associated with decreases in bone density even in post-menopausal women who are at highest risk. In many cases, the reduced intake of Ca^{2+} from milk is compensated by other sources of dietary Ca^{2+}, such as fish with bones that are eaten in some Asian diets, cereals, and some vegetables such as carrots, cauliflower and broccoli, in addition to the various calcium-fortified foods that are now available.

Note, however, that there is also the potential for inadequate Ca^{2+} absorption in vegetarian subjects whose diet is rich in phytates (found in whole wheat flour) and oxalates (which are abundant in leafy green vegetables). These anions bind to Ca^2 and form insoluble salts that cannot be absorbed.

■ Factors affecting calcium metabolism

The control of Ca^{2+} and bone metabolism is a good example of the complexity of operation of the endocrine system. These complex and interactive mechanisms give added layers of control to prevent potentially deadly changes in plasma $[Ca^{2+}]$.

Plasma $[Ca^{2+}]$ is primarily controlled by three hormones, namely, parathyroid hormone, 1,25 dihydroxyvitamin D_3 (1.25D) and calcitonin. The major target tissues for these hormones are the bones, the gastrointestinal tract and the kidney. These mechanisms are summarised in Fig. 1.

Parathyroid hormone (PTH)
PTH is the chief regulator of plasma $[Ca^{2+}]$. It is a polypeptide hormone that is secreted by the four parathyroid glands which are attached to the posterior surface of the thyroid gland or which are sometimes embedded within the gland.

PTH has important effects on the kidneys and the bones. PTH fine-tunes calcium balance by stimulating the kidney to increase the reabsorption of Ca^{2+} in the

Figure 1. Overview of the major hormonal mechanisms controlling calcium metabolism. These interactive processes maintain plasma $[Ca^{2+}]$ within a very narrow range. In this greater scheme of things, bone is, in effect, a reservoir for Ca^{2+} that may be required for replacing Ca^{2+} that is lost through the kidneys.

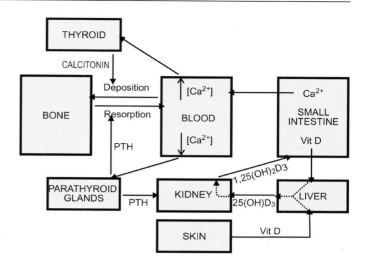

distal tubule and to inhibit the reabsorption of phosphate ions in the proximal tubule: both of these actions increase the plasma $[Ca^{2+}]$. It also exerts some control over the absorption of Ca^{2+} by the small intestine. This effect is achieved indirectly by stimulating the kidney to increase the rate of activation of vitamin D whose actions are described later.

The rate of PTH secretion by the parathyroid glands is controlled by a negative feedback mechanism *via* plasma $[Ca^{2+}]$. A decrease in plasma $[Ca^{2+}]$ is detected by the parathyroid glands which then secrete PTH.

The main direct action of PTH on bones occurs when plasma $[Ca^{2+}]$ falls significantly. The circulating PTH then activates osteoclasts (cells within all bones that can break them down) to produce acid and proteases which resorb the adjacent bone. It is believed that the Ca^{2+} ions are then removed by a cAMP-mediated pathway that results in the opening of Ca^{2+} channels in the cell membranes of osteoclasts, enabling Ca^{2+} to diffuse rapidly down their concentration gradient from the bony surface into the cell. The Ca^{2+} are then extruded from the cell into the extracellular fluid on the side of the cell that is not in contact with the bone, and enter the plasma. However, the loss of bone that would otherwise arise from the normal fluctuations that occur in $[Ca^{2+}]$ is prevented by intricate signalling mechanisms

The human calcium-sensitive receptor (CaR) is a membrane-spanning, G-protein coupled receptor that has been found in many tissues including parathyroid, bone, kidney and intestine. CaR is activated by extracellular Ca^{2+} and plays an important role in the synthesis and secretion of PTH. Mutations in this receptor cause disturbances in Ca^{2+} homeostasis and disease, e.g., increased sensitivity to Ca^{2+} (hypocalcemia) and decreased Ca^{2+} sensitivity (hypercalcemia). CaR is a new target for drug treatment of secondary hyperparathyroidism, the principle being that stimulation of CaR tends to normalise calcium homeostasis.

between the osteoclasts and the bone-forming osteoblasts.

Calcitonin

While PTH primarily regulates *plasma* Ca^{2+}, calcitonin is concerned with the balance of formation and resorption of *bone*. Not surprisingly, therefore, the action of calcitonin is particularly significant during growth, although it appears to be relatively unimportant in the mature skeleton.

Calcitonin is synthesised in the parafollicular cells of the thyroid gland. These cells are stimulated to secrete this hormone when the plasma $[Ca^{2+}]$ increases. Calcitonin is a highly-potent inhibitor of bone resorption, preventing osteoclasts from resorbing bone and inhibiting the differentiation of new osteoclasts. It is not thought to have a major role in maintaining plasma $[Ca^{2+}]$, and its importance may be more related to protection against excessive bone resorption particularly in growing children, and possibly during pregnancy. It seems logical that calcitonin could be used to replace bone in patients suffering from osteoporosis: however, such attempts have not been consistently successful.

1,25 diOH vitamin D (1,25(OH)₂D₃)

Despite its name, vitamin D is actually a steroid hormone rather than a vitamin. (Strictly speaking, a vitamin is an organic compound with a distinct biochemical role, which must be provided in the diet because it cannot be adequately synthesized by the body, and whose deficiency usually produces characteristic symptoms or a disease). Although a deficiency of vitamin D in the diet is associated with some diseases, it is not a true vitamin because it can be synthesised endogenously in the skin. Notwithstanding these objections, its name if not its status as a vitamin is firmly entrenched and its

chemical name of cholecalciferol is unlikely to be adopted in order to satisfy the needs of precise definition.

The provision of adequate amounts of the activated form of the steroid hormone 1,25D is essential to maintain appropriate plasma $[Ca^{2+}]$ and adequate mineralisation of bone matrix. The biosynthesis of this active form is regulated by a complex mechanism. Ultraviolet radiation of the skin converts circulating 7-dehydrocholesterol to vitamin D_3. Together with the D_3 ingested in the diet, this is converted to $25(OH)D_3$ in the liver. The final enzymatic reaction in which it is activated to the active form of the hormone, $1,25(OH)_2D_3$, occurs in the kidney.

The plasma concentration of $1,25(OH)_2D_3$ is regulated by the kidney, which senses the plasma $[Ca^{2+}]$ and $[PO_4^{3-}]$ and adjusts the output of the hormone accordingly by modifying the rate at which its precursor is hydroxylated.

Vitamin D_3 acts in concert with PTH and calcitonin to regulate Ca^{2+} and PO_4^{3-} metabolism at three principal target tissues.

It acts on the intestine to increase absorption of Ca^{2+} and PO_4^{3-}. The nature of this action is still not well-understood, but depends in part on the accelerated synthesis of *calbindins*, which are specific calcium-binding proteins in the small intestine: this process is regulated by Vitamin D_3. Calcium diffuses into mucosal cells in the duodenum and upper jejunum and is then bound to these proteins which promote its passage out of the cell by means of active Ca^{2+} pumps in the basal surface of the cell membrane. This has the effect of making more Ca^{2+} available for the formation of new bone by osteoblasts, thereby preventing a net loss of bone.

Vitamin D_3 acts on the bones by augmenting the action of PTH to resorb bone and release Ca^{2+} into the plasma.

Finally, it acts on the kidney by promoting Ca^{2+} retention. (Note that, even in vitamin D deficiency, 99% Ca^{2+} is reabsorbed in the proximal tubules).

Although the most obvious consequence of vitamin D deficiency is decreased mineralisation of bone, it is thought that the hormone does not directly induce bone formation.

The principal disorder of vitamin D deficiency is known as *osteomalacia:* in growing children, this disorder is known as *rickets.* Osteomalacia/rickets is really a group of diseases with a similar histological picture but diverse causes. The unifying feature is inadequate mineralisation of the bone matrix. Rickets does not occur in individuals with adequate exposure to sun and a diet sufficient in Ca^{2+} and PO_4^{3-}.

Vitamin D deficiency is also a risk factor for osteoporosis.

While vitamin D deficiency is not common in most industrialised nations, endogenous synthesis can be inadequate when there is limited exposure of the skin to ultraviolet light. This can occur as the result of the smog arising from industrial air pollution, and lifestyles that keep people indoors. Because only very small amounts of vitamin D are required in the diet to prevent deficiencies (Table 1), this potential problem is readily avoided by adding it to milk, for example.

It is clearly essential to maintain an adequate intake of vitamin D. However, the ready availability of oral supplements tempts some people to ingest "megadoses" of various vitamins. Prolonged intake of high doses of vitamin D (exceeding 2,000 IU or 50 μg/day) can result in toxic side effects that include the deposition of calcium in soft tissues, high blood pressure, kidney damage and other problems.

Other hormones affecting bone mineral metabolism

In addition to the major hormonal mechanisms that regulate Ca^{2+} that are described above, a number of other internal factors affect skeletal and bone homeostasis. These include a variety of other hormones (insulin, growth hormone, thyroid hormone, adrenal corticosteroids and the sex hormones), and vitamins A and C.

Insulin, growth hormone and the *androgens (testosterone)* are anabolic factors that promote bone growth and are especially important during fetal and childhood development. Testosterone contributes particularly

Table 2. Recommended Daily Allowances have not been established for vitamin D. However, the accepted daily intakes for adults recommended by the Mayo Clinic (Rochester, USA) are set out in this table. It should be noted that the requirement for vitamin D will vary depending on factors such as the total exposure of the skin to ultraviolet radiation (in sunshine). IU is the abbreviation for International Unit.

Age (years)	Accepted daily intake
19 to 50	200 IU (5 μg)
51 to 70	400 IU (10 μg)
>71	600 IU (15 μg)
Pregnant or breastfeeding	200 IU (5 μg)

Plasma glucocorticoid levels are often chronically elevated in psychological disorders such as depressive mental illness or the eating disorder *anorexia nervosa.* This is evidently sufficient to exert a measurable catabolic affect on bone, as there is a strong positive association between the presence of these psychological disorders and reduced bone density.

Table 3. Summary of major hormonal mechanisms controlling plasma calcium.

Hormone	Target Organ	Action
Parathyroid hormone	Bone	↑ Ca^{2+} resorption
	Kidney	↑ Ca^{2+} reabsorption
		↓ phosphate reabsorption → ↑ phosphate excretion
		↑synthesis of activated vitamin D
	Small intestine	Indirect effect from ↑ synthesis of 1,25D
Calcitonin	Bone	↓ osteoclastic activity → ↓ Ca^2 resorption
	Kidney	Minimal effect
	Small intestine	No known effect in humans
1,25(OH)$_2$vitamin D$_3$	Bone	Augments action of PTH to ↑ plasma [Ca^{2+}]
	Kidney	↑ Ca^{2+} reabsorption
	Small intestine	↑ uptake of Ca^{2+} (*via* calbindins)

to the pattern of bone growth that characterises the male skeleton.

Oestrogens are also important in the growth of bones during skeletal development. However, they are also important in relation to another critical aspect of bone metabolism that has direct implications in dentistry. When oestrogen secretion by the ovaries ceases at menopause, the rate of bone loss from the female skeleton accelerates dramatically. Women can lose up to 20% of their bone mass in the first five to seven years following menopause. There is now evidence that oestrogens and their receptors on osteoblasts are important for the osteogenic activity in bone that normally occurs in response to mechanical stresses.

Glucocorticoids such as cortisol are catabolic hormones that exert a negative effect on bone mineralisation. These adverse effects on bone include the inhibition of osteoblasts, the enhancement of bone resorption, the suppression of intestinal Ca^{2+} absorption and increased excretion of Ca^{2+} through the kidneys. These hormones exert their effects on bones through several pathways including a direct anti-vitamin D action, and by inhibiting osteoclast formation and activity. Demineralisation of bone is particularly prominent when these hormones are given in pharmacological doses for long periods for the treatment of chronic inflammatory disorders such as asthma, autoimmune disorders such as rheumatoid

Fluoride is of course an ion in which dentists are intensely interested because of its well-documented effect in reducing enamel solubility. Fluoride ions also substitute for hydroxyl ions in bone, and are incorporated particularly in bones that are growing or undergoing remodelling. As in enamel, fluorapatite is less soluble than hydroxyapatite. However, while fluoride treatment appears to increase bone density, it also alters bone structure. The current consensus is that high-dosage fluoride treatment is ineffective for reducing fractures resulting from osteoporosis, but that the ingestion of fluoride at levels recommended for reduction of tooth decay has no adverse effects on bone.

arthritis, disorders of the immune system such as Addison's disease, or to prevent the rejection of organ transplants.

Non-hormonal influences on bone mineral metabolism

External factors such as mechanical stress, pressure and gravity are also important for maintaining the mineralisation of bones. For example, confinement to bed causes dramatic loss of bone mass unless exercises are prescribed to reduce this. The importance of these factors was graphically illustrated during the first space flights. Because the importance of mechanical stress for bone health was not appreciated at that time, the first astronauts who were subject to weightlessness (and therefore absence of mechanical stresses) in space flights for as little as eight days lost up to 20% of their total bone mass. In addition to its intrinsic interest, this observation reminds us that virtually all bones are dynamic structures that are constantly being remodelled by a process of resorption followed by deposition of bone substance: at any given moment, 3–5% of bone mass (principally in the trabecular bone) is undergoing active remodelling, partly in response to the continually changing stresses to which they are being subjected.

◼ Pathological disturbances of calcium metabolism

A number of disease processes can interfere with normal calcium and bone metabolism. Primary amongst these are disorders of the parathyroid gland, the most common of which are briefly summarised below.

Hyperparathyroidism

Primary hyperparathyroidism is a dysfunction of the parathyroid glands in which they secrete uncontrolled amounts of PTH. This is frequently the result of either a benign or a malignant adenoma in the gland. The result of this hypersecretion is, predictably, an increase in plasma $[Ca^{2+}]$ which occurs as the result of resorption of bone, an increased tubular reabsorption of Ca^{2+}, and an increased production of vitamin D. Symptoms include kidney stones and depressed activity of the central nervous system. The treatment is usually surgical and, if all 4 glands are removed, the resulting hypoparathyroidism must be treated with appropriate administration of 1,25D and Ca^{2+}.

Hyperparathyroidism can also be secondary to other metabolic disorders such as renal failure in which the ability to retain Ca^{2+} is diminished: this results in hypocalcaemia which in turn triggers the increased PTH secretion.

Hypoparathyroidism

Depressed parathyroid function is usually the result of surgery of the parathyroid glands. However, because these glands are often buried within the thyroid, surgical removal of the thyroid gland can result in loss of parathyroid function as well. The loss of the parathyroid glands leads to hypocalcaemia, together with decreased bone resorption, decreased tubular reabsorption of Ca^{2+} and decreased synthesis of 1,25 vitamin D. The main signs and symptoms are the result of abnormal nerve and muscle activity.

Pseudohypoparathyroidism is less common, and results from a defect in the PTH receptor. It is treated in the same manner as primary hyperparathyroidism.

Radioactivity and bone health

Finally, it should be noted that the element *strontium* is a close chemical relation of Ca^{2+} and can replace it in many chemical reactions, including those that occur in bones. Strontium 90 is a β-emitting radio-isotope produced in nuclear reactors and by nuclear weapons. This isotope has a half-life of 29 years and, like calcium, is stored in bones. Children who are exposed to Sr^{90} have an increased probability of leukaemia and bone tumours as the result of long-term exposure of their bones and bone marrow to ionising radiation.

Osteoporosis and dental health

It is clear from the foregoing that there are numerous clinical conditions that result in bone loss. Of these, the most common is simply age-related osteoporosis. It should be emphasised again that age-related osteoporosis is not restricted to women. The component of bone loss that is strictly related to ageing is approximately equal in men and women. However, the decline in men occurs from a higher peak bone mass, and men do not suffer from the accelerated bone loss that is related to the menopause. As a consequence, men are likely to suffer osteoporotic bone fractures and related conditions much later in life than women.

While osteoporosis is an issue that has obvious major implications for general health, good evidence is also now emerging for a relationship between osteoporosis and periodontal disease. Dentists are familiar with looking for localised bone loss in dental X-ray images. However, it has now been demonstrated that the more bone general bone loss that occurs in osteoporosis is evident in dental radiographs, and indeed that these can be used to distinguish people with osteoporosis from those with normal bone density. In particular, mandibular bone density measurements have been shown to correlate with bone density measurements at other skeletal sites. It is possible, therefore, that dental X-rays may eventually come to play a useful role in the detection of individuals with generalised osteoporosis.

While every dentist knows that the periodontal disease that arises from an inflammatory process can result in tooth loss, there is now evidence that osteoporosis *per se* is also related to tooth loss. Several studies have shown that low skeletal bone mass is independently associated with loss of height of the alveolar crest. Furthermore, a recent study of post-menopausal women found that those who had osteoporosis of the hip also had fewer teeth and were more likely to have periodontal disease than the women without osteoporosis.

The relationship between osteoporosis and periodontal disease raises the more general question of whether interventions that reduce bone loss generally will also reduce damage to the hard tissues supporting the teeth. There is now associative evidence to suggest that this is so: this comes mostly from studies of ageing females (because of the higher incidence of osteoporosis in this group). For example, one study has shown that dentate women who were oestrogen-deficient have a greater loss in alveolar bone density than those who have pre-menopausal plasma oestrogen levels. At least two other studies have reported that older women using oestrogen replacement therapy have lower average rates of tooth loss than non-users and that the duration of oestrogen use is positively correlated with lower rates of tooth loss as well as with a more general reduction in bone density.

The issue of hormone replacement therapy to relieve the symptoms of menopause and to reduce bone loss is the subject of intense discussion at the present time: hence, it is not appropriate to recommend such therapies as a strategy to reduce alveolar bone loss until the present controversy about the side effects of oestrogen therapy is resolved. However, in general terms, it is reasonable to conclude that measures which reduce the severity of osteoporosis generally are likely to have a positive impact on the health of the tissues that support the teeth.

Dentists as applied bone biologists

Dentists and dental specialists are now employing highly sophisticated techniques to preserve and restore bone. Periodontists use methods such as grafting to encourage bone to regenerate in order to replace lost alveolar bone and improve the support of teeth. These grafts may be *autogenous* (often called autografts), which use bone from another site from the same patient: these are the "gold standard" for bone grafting. They may be *allografts* which use bone from other human subjects, or even *xenografts* (using bone from another species). A more radical source of bone graft material is coralline hydroxyapatite, a commercially-available material derived from sea corals.

There are many different techniques in use and more under development, but they all aim for one or more of the three following outcomes. **Osteogenesis** is the production of new bone directly from cells (osteoblasts and osteoprogenitor cells) contained in the graft that survive transplantation. Cancellous autografts (i.e., from the patient's own bone) are the only commonly used grafts that enable osteogenesis to occur. **Osteoinduction** is a passive process in which various active biological substances in the graft stimulate bone-producing (and cartilage-producing) cells in the host tissue. Finally, in **osteoconduction**, the grafted tissue

forms a scaffold into which capillaries and osteoprogenitor cells from the host tissue may grow. Cortical and corticocancellous grafts provide the most structured and stable scaffolds; however, cancellous grafts also have some osteoconductive properties.

While the foregoing techniques are used to replace bone, a different approach is used to replace teeth (or more accurately, tooth roots). The use of osseous implants is now accepted as a mainstream procedure in dentistry. In this process, titanium or ceramic prostheses are surgically implanted into the bone. Sometimes these prostheses are coated with an hydroxyapatite layer to encourage integration of the implant with alveolar bone. Alternatively, the prosthesis becomes secured to the bone by a fibrous connective tissue capsule. The bone is then allowed to repair, and the prosthetic post is eventually used as a platform on which to mount artificial crowns or perhaps to help support removable prostheses.

While these techniques are now routine, they were preceded by many years of unsuccessful attempts at implanting. It is worth noting that it was primarily the failure to understand the physiology of bones rather than breakthroughs in materials science that held back the development of this enormously valuable technology for many decades.

Finally, of course, orthodontists are also applied bone biologists who also manipulate bones, although usually by methods more subtle than surgery. For example, orthodontists encourage bone to grow in functionally desirable directions by manoeuvres such as gradual tooth movement and even by slowly separating unfused palatal bones (a procedure known in general terms as distraction osteogenesis). Orthodontists have also been at the forefront of determining the skeletal age of children from the study of X-ray images of bones such as those in the hand whose development patterns normally follow a clearly defined time course.

It is clear that, in addition to the well-established dental procedures for preventing bone loss, the rapidly expanding palette of options that is becoming available for repairing and reorganising bone is revolutionising the practice of dentistry. However, our understanding of bone physiology makes it very clear that interventions involving manipulation of bone by the dentist or dental specialist should be carried out only when the patient is in stable or positive Ca^{2+} balance. There is little point, for example, in undertaking complex and expensive surgical procedures to restore lost mandibular bone in a patient whose bones are in the process of slowly dissolving away because of progressive osteoporosis. In the future, it is certain that more emphasis will be placed on the use of systemic factors including hormones as well as local bone growth factors to support, supplement or even replace surgical transplants of bone.

■ Selected references

Nordin BEC, Need AG, Morris HA (eds). Metabolic Bone and Stone Disease 3rd ed. Churchill Livingstone London, UK, 1993.

Ferguson DB (ed). Oral Bioscience. Churchill Livingstone, ILondon, UK, 1999.

Favus MJ. (ed). Primer on the Metabolic Bone Diseases and Disorders of Mineral Metabolism. 4th ed. Lippincott, Williams & Wilkins, Philadelphia, 1999.

There is also a great deal of useful information on different aspects of osteoporosis on various National Institutes of Health (USA) websites.

INDEX

Tooth loads 178, 180, 181, 189, 197
Tooth sockets 178, 282
Tracheotomy 275
Transient pain 98
Trigeminal 22, 53, 63, 66, 67, 71, 72, 90, 97, 102, 103, 106, 107, 109, 114, 125, 129, 130, 131, 134–136, 143, 156, 158, 160, 162, 163, 165–167, 170, 174, 178, 180, 182, 200, 219, 220, 222, 224, 225, 231, 236, 242, 247, 248, 250, 257, 273, 278
Trigeminal motor nucleus 201, 223, 225, 231
Trigeminal nucleus 200
Trigeminal reflex responses 233

Umami 53, 58, 60, 61, 121
Urea 40, 62

Velopharyngeal sphincter 257, 258, 262, 264
Visco-elastic forces 227
Visual analogue scale 48, 120
Vocal cords 248, 249, 273, 275
Vomiting 132, 245, 252–254
Vowels 261

Wernicke's area 257

Xenografts 291
Xerostomia 17, 41–45, 47